T0329874

LEARNING TO SAVE THE WORLD

LEARNING TO SAVE THE WORLD

Global Health Pedagogies and Fantasies of Transformation in Botswana

Betsey Behr Brada

CORNELL UNIVERSITY PRESS   ITHACA AND LONDON

First published 2023 by Cornell University Press

Library of Congress Cataloging-in-Publication Data

Names: Brada, Betsey Behr, 1976– author.
Title: Learning to save the world : global health pedagogies and fantasies
    of transformation in Botswana / Betsey Behr Brada.
Description: Ithaca [New York]: Cornell University Press, 2023. | Includes
    bibliographical references and index.
Identifiers: LCCN 2022020480 (print) | LCCN 2022020481 (ebook) |
    ISBN 9781501762413 (hardcover) | ISBN 9781501762420 (paperback) |
    ISBN 9781501762444 (pdf) | ISBN 9781501762437 (epub)
Subjects: LCSH: AIDS (Disease)—Treatment—Social aspects—Botswana. |
    AIDS (Disease) in children—Social aspects—Botswana. | Medical
    anthropology—Botswana. | Public health—Anthropological aspects—
    Botswana. | Medical education—Social aspects—Botswana. | Health
    education—Social aspects—Botswana. | Transcultural medical care—
    Botswana. | World health—Social aspects.
Classification: LCC RA643.86.B55 B73 2023 (print) | LCC RA643.86.B55
    (ebook) | DDC 362.19697/920096883—dc23/eng/20220908
LC record available at https://lccn.loc.gov/2022020480
LC ebook record available at https://lccn.loc.gov/2022020481

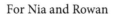
For Nia and Rowan

Contents

Preface

I have frequently considered titling this book *The Road to Hell* for two reasons. First, I wanted to underscore the sheer agonistic character that global health acquired in practice in southeastern Botswana's clinical spaces, a facet of my data that even other anthropologists of global health have struggled to accept as fact. Second, I wanted to emphasize the extent to which my analysis is not an indictment of my informants' intentions. Many earnest, well-meaning, and talented healthcare professionals appear in these pages, often locked in intense, even bitter conflict with one another. But it has never been my goal to convince the reader that any of my informants are bad people. If the problems that global health sets out to solve were amenable to good intentions, we would all be living in paradise. Instead, this book illustrates the tragic truth that profound conflict can arise even when everyone in the room wants to do the right thing.

Moreover, the global health that I write about in this book, with all its promises of transformation, has at times attracted me almost as deeply as it has perplexed me. Given the professional circuits I myself have traveled, but for a very slight change of fate I might easily have become too committed to that vision of global health to be able to write this book. My relationship to that vision, then, exists in a sort of no-man's-land between missed opportunity and happy accident. Susan Sontag once observed, "No one who wholeheartedly shares in a given sensibility can analyze it; he can only, whatever his intention, exhibit it. To name a sensibility, to draw its contours and to recount its history, requires a deep sympathy modified by revulsion" (1964). I offer this account, then, as global health's most ardent critic and its most ambivalent friend.

Acknowledgments

In early 2007 the physician I call Dr. Buyaga generously agreed to sit for an interview. Armed with my audio recorder, I began to recite the script that opened all my interviews. This script, which had been scrutinized by the University of Chicago's Institutional Review Board as well as Botswana's Ministry of Health, promised that, in conformance with standards of research involving human subjects, I would keep the contents of the interview private, confidential, and anonymous. Dr. Buyaga listened for a moment and then, to my great consternation, began to chuckle. I remained frozen in mid-sentence while his chuckle grew to a full-sized belly laugh. As he recovered, he swiftly identified between laughs the misalignment between my formal procedures and my circumstances: There is only one pediatric HIV clinic *in the entire country of Botswana*, he reminded me. How on earth could I possibly promise any kind of anonymity?

He was right. "Botswana is a small country," I was warned long before I set foot there or understood how small, tight, and overlapping social networks were, even across great distances. Part of my fieldwork involved becoming aware of how dimly I perceived these networks or their effects, let alone managed or usefully intervened in them. For that reason, I have employed pseudonyms beyond what other scholars of southeastern Botswana's clinical spaces have chosen. Doing so is less an attempt at impeachable anonymity—one that, as a chortling Dr. Buyaga pointed out, was impossible—than a veneer of dissimulation, a means of distraction that also, I hope, provides plausible deniability for my interlocutors.

As a consequence, there are a number of people I wish to acknowledge, but to do so would dissolve this thin veneer. I am grateful to all the Batswana, including patients and their families, who shared with me their time and their stories, and to all the healthcare and public health professionals in southeastern Botswana (Batswana and otherwise) who took time from their busy personal and professional lives to teach me what I know about HIV treatment and global health. I owe a large debt to the staff, patients, and families of the Superlative Clinic, the staff and students of EUMS in Botswana, and the staff and patients of Referral Hospital, particularly the adult and pediatric medical wards. Should you recognize yourself in these pages, please know that you have my deep gratitude. *Ke a leboga, bomme le borre, ka lo nthusitse le fa le ntse le tshwaregile ka go thusa ba bangwe. Kgetsi ya tsie e kgonwa ka go tshwaraganelwa; ke ithutile ka thuso ya lona. Ke lekile go kwala nnete ka bopelontle. Ke kopa maitshwarelo, bagaetsho, gore ke lo kgopisitse. Go tla mo Botswana go ne go solegela molemo.*

Andrew Horst shared with me both his childhood memories of Gaborone and his personal connections to BOTUSA. With the help of Greg Sawin, BOTUSA became a sort of base camp for this project, and I'm indebted to Marion Carter, Margarett Davis, William Jimbo, Poloko Kebaabetswe, Mary Kay Larson, and especially Todd Koppenhaver, Mpho Mogodi, Monica Smith, Fatma Soud, and Prisca Tembo for their interest in the project and their helpful advice. I was fortunate to also hold a position as a visiting scholar in the Department of Sociology at the University of Botswana. My thanks to Rogers Molefhi and Godi Mookodi for facilitating my appointment, and to Coryce Haavik, John Holm, and Isaac Mazonde for their help navigating UB's bureaucracy. Mabedi Kgositau, Oleosi Ntshebe, and especially Sethunya Mosime proved invaluable interlocutors. Neil Parsons generously invited me to sit in on his course on the historiography of southern Africa while my research approval was pending. Treasa Galvin took me under her wing and unstintingly offered excellent advice and encouragement. Weekly research meetings with her and Fanny Chabrol kept me buoyed up in moments of doubt.

Patrick Boikhutlo Monnaesi and Ntompe Jarchia provided vital services as interpreters, interviewers, and translators, for which I am immensely grateful. Both went far beyond merely collecting data, offering sensitive and intelligent insights into the social life of HIV treatment in southeastern Botswana. Members of Gaborone's medical and public health professional communities helped me glimpse the epidemic and its treatment programs beyond my field sites. My thanks to Ava Avalos, Ade Baba, Major Bradshaw, Diana Dickenson, the Rev. Rupert Hambira, Wemi Jayeoba, Stanley Mapiki, Brighid Malone, Tom Massaro, Howard Moffat, Charles Olenja, Ruth Pfau, Doreen Ramogola-Masire, Michelle Schaan, Debbie Stanford, Christine Stegling, Duncan Thela, Bill Wester, and Hélène Wong. I'm grateful to Rachel Xiaolu Han for sharing both her insights into global health pedagogies and an early version of the map of Referral Hospital. I owe much of my understanding of American biomedical training to Allison Arwady, Marcus Bachhuber, and Michelle Morse. Nandita Sugandhi invited me to shadow her for a week at Nyangabgwe Hospital and has been an enthusiastic critic ever since. Amanda Hillegas, John Holm, and Kirsten Weeks kindly offered me places to stay. No one can live by research alone; Verity Knight, Baz Semo, Carolyn Wilson, and the Gaborone Choral Society reminded me of life beyond work, as did Martin Dube and the members of Team Fred.

In Chicago, I had the great good fortune of Jean Comaroff's supervision. Discussing my research with Jean was a bit like stepping into a glass elevator and rapidly ascending several thousand feet. Whatever handle I had on the project's contours vanished, the shift in scale rendering it almost unrecognizable. Its significance and potential contributions were utterly transformed. I have never quite overcome the vertigo I feel after these conversations, but I truly appreciate the journey. In addition to Jean's breadth of vision, I am grateful for her good counsel and encouragement at every step and for the deep knowledge of southern Africa she has shared with me. Joe Masco, my first graduate adviser, improved this project beyond measure from its earlier iterations. My thanks for his sustained attention to the craft of writing and his patience with my early tendencies toward the polemic. I'm also indebted to Joe for gently but firmly pushing me out of the zone where medical anthropology's conversations tend to sit. If one is trying to get analytic purchase on the claims global health makes for itself, it is a very good thing to work with someone who critically engages the possibilities of nuclear apocalypse. Judy Farquhar's reputation for asking tough questions preceded her arrival in Chicago (or her return to it, depending on how you look at it). I was the fortunate beneficiary of her curiosity, her refusal to settle for easy answers, her careful reading (including marginalia in Chinese that sent me scrambling for a translation), and her enthusiasm for my successes. Sue Gal joined my committee after I returned from Botswana and, in addition to providing excellent practical advice on my writing, encouraged me to let my analyses be as (and only as) complicated as they needed to be, a lesson I still carry with me. Mark Nichter welcomed me into his network even before I got to Chicago. His outsider's perspective kept me grounded when, early in grad school, I feared I would float away on a sea of theory, and his career-long engagement with what has become global health helped me hone in on the specificities of the phenomena I analyze in this book.

The African Studies workshop at the University of Chicago was a site of intense intellectual formation. Ralph Austen, Jean and John Comaroff, Jennifer Cole, Rachel Jean-Baptiste, Emily Osborne, and François Richard fostered a lively and rigorous atmosphere. Beth Buggenhagen, Kelly Gillespie, Anne-Maria Makhulu, and Hylton White, all writing up when I arrived, set a high bar with the robustness of their analyses and their knowledge of the region. But I learned most alongside and from my age-mates: Rob Blunt, Bernard Dubbeld, Claudia Gastrow, Jeremy Jones, Kate McHarry, Erin Moore, Joshua Walker, and especially Bianca Dahl, a keen observer of southeastern Botswana in her own right. The Workshop on Medicine and the Body was similarly formative. I'm grateful to Summerson Carr, Judy Farquhar, and Eugene Raikhel for both the venue and their generous comments on my writing, and to Adam Baim, Lara Braff, Jen Karlin, Aaron Seamen, and Anwen Tormey for their enthusiasm for this project and their engagement with my work. Special thanks to Beth Brummel, Adam Sargent, China Scherz, and the late Michael Silverstein for encouraging my early forays into semiotics.

In its long journey from dissertation to book, this project has received aid from a wide range of sources. My field research was funded by the Wenner Gren Foundation and the Fulbright-Hays DDRA program. Write-up funding came from the University of Chicago in the form of a Social Sciences Collegiate Division Dissertation Teaching and Research Fellowship, and the Department of Anthropology's Watkins Dissertation Fellowship. A postdoctoral fellowship in Princeton's Program in Global Health and Health Policy provided invaluable time for thinking and writing in a truly interdisciplinary venue as well as funding for a follow-up trip to southern Africa. Thanks to João Biehl for inviting me to the Program, to Lauren Carruth, Peter Locke, Ramah McKay, Claire Nicholas, Yi-Ching Ong, and Bharat Venkat for camaraderie, and to Kristina Graff for her logistical acumen. Vincanne Adams and Claire Wendland both visited Princeton during my time there, and I'm grateful for the early career support they each offered me. A fellowship at Notre Dame's Kellogg Institute for International Studies provided time for a thorough reworking of my dissertation. My thanks to Denise Wright for ensuring my family and I landed softly in South Bend, to Terry McDonnell and Erin Metz McDonnell for making us welcome, to Maria Paula Bertran, Graeme Gill, Max Goedl, Victoria Paniagua, Ben Phillips, Diego Sanchez-Ancochea, and Veronica Zubillaga for making Kellogg a genial place to undertake the hard work of revisions, and to Paul Ocobock for his abundant good cheer.

I feel exceptionally lucky to have landed at Reed College. Charlene Makley and Paul Silverstein have created an environment that is lively and collegial while also minimizing demands on junior faculty. From the get-go, Char went out of her way to make my family feel welcome in Portland and has been generous time and again with encouragement, advice, and practical support. Paul has the kind of insider knowledge of Reed that I can only hope to acquire and is always ready to shed light on institutional workings within the college and beyond. I'm particularly obliged to him for lightening my administrative load during a challenging pandemic year. LaShandra Sullivan and Anand Vaidya are the kind of departmental colleagues one hopes for: congenial, fair-minded, and invested in making the department a better place for students and faculty alike. Troy Cross, Yaejoon Kwon, Mary Ashburn Miller, Radhika Natarajan, Tamara Metz, Suzy Renn, Sarah Schaack, Kristin Scheible, and Catherine Witt have all made Reed a place to thrive, not just work. Nora McLaughlin looked after me in difficult moments; I miss her care and wit in Wednesday afternoon meetings. Reed's generous junior leave policy, along with a sabbatical fellowship, made it possible for me to spend a much-needed year at Notre Dame. I'm indebted to Nigel Nicholson for helping me devise creative responses to administrative demands on more than one occasion, and to Emily Hebbron for her ongoing logistical support and for the care she took of me and my family in the most challenging moments of lockdown.

During my residency at Notre Dame, Beth Buggenhagen and Jennifer Cole invited me to present chapter drafts at Indiana University and the University of Chicago, respectively. I'm grateful for the opportunities to discuss my work and for the helpful feedback I received, particularly from Ilana Gershon and Eugene Raikhel. Lynnette Arnold and Teruko Mitsuhara provided critical feedback on chapter 3 via the Society for Linguistic Anthropology's junior scholars workshop in late 2020. Emily Yates-Doerr was a generous critic of the introduction and conclusion as the book neared completion. Thanks to Anna Eisenstein, Melissa Graboyes, Stacy Pigg, Noelle Sullivan, and Claire Wendland for their enduring enthusiasm for the project. A version of chapter 4 appeared in 2011 in a special issue of *Culture, Medicine & Psychiatry* on biomedical education, and a version of chapter 2 appeared in *American Ethologist* in 2013. I'm grateful to the editors and copyeditors of both journals, and to Seth Holmes, Angela Jenks, and Scott Stonington for inviting me to participate in the special issue.

Jim Lance at Cornell University Press has been a wonderful editor to work with. His enthusiasm for the project has endured in the face of challenges ranging from family emergencies to riots and global pandemics, and I appreciate his patience and encouragement. The close readings and excellent suggestions of two anonymous reviewers gave me the tools I needed to sharpen my points and hone my argument. Thanks also to Brian Balsley for preparing the maps and figures, to Paul Molamphy for his meticulous work on the bibliography, and to Ange Romeo-Hall and Michelle Witkowski for their assistance with production.

This project would have sunk beneath the waves long ago without the colleagues, many of them treasured friends, who breathed fresh wind into its sails. Since we met in Gaborone in 2007, Julie Livingston has been incredibly generous with her time, her advice, and her knowledge of southeastern Botswana. Julie has a knack for posing seemingly casual questions about my work that I grapple with for months or longer, and I'm particularly grateful for her thoroughgoing comments on the full manuscript. China Scherz was a member of my dissertation writing group and has never stopped cheering me on, treating me like a colleague with a contribution to make even when the book seemed a distant, even impossible goal. China softened my landing in both Portland and South Bend, and I'm grateful for her steady, practical advice in addition to our far-ranging conversations on Africanist anthropology. A fellow traveler just ahead on the steep path to a first book, Marissa Mika kept directing my eyes to the summit when it was all I could do to put one foot in front of the other. I cannot imagine how this book could have made it to press without her steady companionship and encouragement as well as her astute take on global health and its pedagogies. Lauren Carruth, Kate McGurn Centellas, Megan Crowley-Matoka, Rebecca Graff, Brady G'sell, Bea Jauregui, Jean Hunleth, Mary Leighton, Erin Moore, Krisjon Olsen, Michal Ran-Rubin, Jonah Rubin, Aaron Seaman, Anna West, and Emily Yates-Doerr kept a light burning for me in dark times. Special thanks to Naomi Caffee and Tamara Metz, who convinced me I was done and helped usher the book out the door.

I owe special thanks to my family and to friends who are like family. Robbie and Joe Brada raised me to be curious about the world and to consider the partiality of my perspective. I doubt they imagined that moving to Europe multiple times would result in one of their own children finding her way to sub-Saharan Africa, but I'm grateful that they regarded turnabout as fair play. Diana Steeble and Karin Johnson visited me in Botswana, and I'm grateful for their spirit of adventure, their confidence in me, and the love they show me and my family. Thanks to all the Bradas, Curtins, Dunies, Hornes, and Hurds who have supported me, my family, and this project along the way, especially Jenny Horne and the late Jonathan Kahana. Bryan Krol, Kate McKeon, and Rosalin Sakdisri keep reaching out, even when I'm too deep underwater to reach back. Robbie Brada, Susan Curtin, Gary Einhorn, Kelda Jameson, Marissa Mika, Libby Horne, and especially Jenny Horne cushioned us during bumpy times in Palo Alto. Finally, I'm grateful to Brian Horne for all the ways he made this book possible.

No anthropologist is truly outside their studies. Like many of us, my critical engagement with my object of study is intertwined with and complicated by my own unfolding biography. Due to circumstances surrounding the early childhood of my first-born daughter (into which my second daughter was thrust from the moment of her birth), this manuscript was repeatedly shelved, sometimes for years, as Brian Horne and I groped our way through highly specialized realms of biomedicine, including the heady mix of technoscientific wizardry and emotional turmoil that is pediatric organ transplantation in the contemporary United States.

My fieldwork in Botswana equipped me in strange and often unpredictable ways to move through the clinical spaces, roles, and languages that my family and I came to inhabit. If part of conducting ethnography is learning *how* to learn something, I had learned, among other things, something of how to learn biomedicine. I added new clinical terminology to my repertoire, using biomedicine's code like a crowbar to leverage information out of harried practitioners. I became the type of parent (if this truly is a type) whom a pediatric hepatologist would casually invite to palpate the edge of her own infant's spleen. I was also brought deep inside some of the phenomena I analyze in this book: American pediatricians' ambivalence towards children's families; the routine and often unacknowledged pedagogic practices entailed in biomedical treatment; the relentless affective disciplining of health professionals, patients, and families alike; the unacknowledged racialization of both expertise and suffering; the sheer violence of biomedical practice. Even as I write this book's final words, my own common-sense parenting practices, such as talking with my first-grader about her daily medications and routine blood tests using concepts drawn from biomedicine, overlap uncomfortably with some of the material I analyze in these pages, as does the pleasure I feel when she masters those words, ideas, and practices. It's not as simple as that—her budding proficiency with biomedicine's ways of seeing the world and my consequent pleasure. It is marked by the surpluses and excesses that locate medical anthropology's roots in the anthropology of religion, in existential puzzles classically framed in terms of termites and granaries, in questions my daughter has been forming since preschool: *Why me? Why now?* But I am teaching her to save herself the way I know.

Hypocrisy? That epithet falls far short of capturing the dynamics of cultural critique, the strangeness of being one's own field instrument, and the ephemeral boundaries of "the field" for anthropologists. Reflecting on his daughter's suicide in relation to his long-term fieldwork among indigenous communities in Venezuela's Orinoco delta through multiple deadly epidemics, Charles Briggs wrote, "Feliciana's death has changed my subject position in relationship to the death of children in the delta . . . I had thought that the people of the delta were informing me about their own lives. It turns out that they were preparing me for my own" (2004, 180). But the monumental force of biomedicine in my child's life and the gratitude I feel toward those who wield it on her behalf do not require that I temper my critique—any more so than the fact of having kin invalidates an anthropologist's analysis of kinship, or being a political anthropologist requires one to proselytize on behalf of democracy (Fassin 2012). Doing justice to what I have learned in the field sites I chose and the sites that chose me requires something both more refined and more robust than gratitude. Those of us who have felt the rough edge of biomedicine amid its soteriological mode know this.

This book, then, is dedicated to Nia and Rowan, who every day teach me to be brave whether I like it or not, and by whose side I have learned more than I ever wanted to know about biomedicine, and more than I ever could have imagined about love.

Acronyms

ACHAP	African Comprehensive HIV/AIDS Partnership
ARVs	antiretroviral medications
BDF	Botswana Defense Force
BHHRL	Botswana Harvard HIV Reference Laboratory
BHP	Botswana Harvard Partnership
BOTUSA	Botswana office of the US Centers for Disease Control and Prevention
CDC	US Centers for Disease Control and Prevention
CHAN	Children's HIV/AIDS Network
HAART	highly active antiretroviral therapy (i.e., ARVs taken in combination)
HIV/AIDS	human immunodeficiency virus / acquired immunodeficiency syndrome
HPRU	BOTUSA's HIV Prevention Research Unit (formerly the HPU)
HRU	Health Research Unit of Botswana's Ministry of Health
IDCC	infectious disease care clinic, i.e., HIV treatment clinic
IHSG	Institute of Health Sciences in Gaborone
MO	medical officer, i.e., nonspecialist physician
MOH	Ministry of Health
NACA	National AIDS Coordinating Agency
PEP	Postexposure prophylaxis to prevent HIV infection
PEPFAR	US President's Emergency Plan for AIDS Relief
PMTCT	prevention of mother-to-child transmission of HIV
PrEP	pre-exposure prophylaxis to prevent HIV infection
SAHIVCS	Southern African HIV Clinicians' Society

This guide is adapted from Klaits (2010), who adapted his from Suggs (2002). I use italics to denote syllabic stress; I also underline the sound being described in context.

Stress

In Setswana, stress tends to fall on the penultimate syllable. Modise is thus Moh-*dee* seh, Kenosi is Keh-*noh*-see, Kokeletso is Ko-keh-*leh*-tso. This generally applies to two-syllable words as well such that kitso is *kee*-tso. The major exceptions in this book are personal names that end in -*ng*, such as Tsile*ng*, where stress falls on the final syllable.

Vowels

a resembles the short *o* in English, as in *pot*, as in Mo*a*gi

e denotes both the low tone resembling the short *e* in the English *met* and the high tone resembling the long *a* in the English *late*. Both are present in this order in L*e*s*e*go.

i resembles the long *e* in English, as in *feel*, as in Mol*e*fi

o resembles the long *o* in English, as in *pole*, as in Karab*o*

u resembles the long *u* in English, as in *flute*, as in Chil*u*be

e at the end of the word is voiced, and vowels do not tend to form diphthongs. Moagi is Mo-*ah*-gi, Maikutlo is Mah-ee-*koo*-tlo, and Kgosietsile is Kgo-see-eh-*tsee*-lay

Consonants

g voiceless velar fricative; resembles the *ch* in the Scottish *loch* or the Yiddish *chutzpah*, as in L*e*s*e*go and Mo*a*gi; Gaborone is thus closer to cha-bo-*ro*-neh *kg*   resembles *g*, but has a rougher aspiration made by the preceding *k* sound, as in K̲gomotso

mm   resembles the *m* in English, but held for a longer duration, as in m̲m̲ele

ng   resembles the *ng* in the English word *thing*, as in bon̲gaka

nn   resembles the *n* in English, but held for a longer duration, as in n̲n̲a

rr   pronounced with a rolled *r*, as in r̲r̲a

tl   an explosive alveolar consonant made by bringing the tongue against the teeth at the sides of the mouth, as in Mai*ku*t̲l̲o

ts   resembles the *ts* in the English word *fits*, as in T̲sileng, or the *z* in German *Zeitung*

h   in consonant combinations (e.g., *ph*, *th*, *tlh*, *tsh*) denotes aspiration, as in T̲s̲hepo (*T̲s̲eh*-po) or Mp̲ho (*Mm*-poh); t̲hata is thus *tah*-ta, breathing hard on the first syllable; a similar principle applies to T̲s̲henolo (Tseh-*no*-lo) and Mot̲l̲habane (Mo-tlah-*ba*-nay)

Superlative Clinic

Dr. Buyaga, director

Dr. Amy, associate director

Dr. Grossman, founder and head of CHAN, the Superlative Clinic's parent organization

Squad Pediatricians

Dr. Alison	Dr. Natalie
Dr. James	Dr. Rachel
Dr. Mark	Dr. Wyatt

Medical Officers

Dr. Chibesa

Dr. Mokwele

Dr. Motlhabane

Nurses and Support Staff

Mma Kgosietsile, head nurse

Mma Modise, research coordinator

Mma Mokento, nurse

Mma Mokopakgosi, nurse

Mma Molefi, phlebotomist

Duduetsang, lab technician

Koketso, social worker

Malebogo, receptionist

Neo Baatlhodi, nurse

Tumelo, nurse

Patients

Karabo and his mother, Maikutlo
Kgomotso and her mother, Mma Kgomotso
Tshenolo and her parents

Eastern University Medical School (EUMS)

Dr. Baum, neurologist
Dr. Caffrey, faculty member, Division of Infectious Diseases
Dr. Goldberg, Chief of the Division of Infectious Diseases
Dr. Rosen, Director of EUMS's inpatient service on Referral Hospital's adult medical wards

EUMS Clinical Instructors

Dr. Frank   Dr. Matheson
Dr. Jackson   Dr. Tsileng

EUMS Trainees

Dr. Julie (resident)   Jessica
Adam   Molly
Amanda   Michael
Evan

Adult Medical Wards of Referral Hospital

Dr. Manisha, attending physician

Medical Officers and Interns

Dr. Lesego Balebetse   Dr. Tshepo Kokeletso
Dr. Chilube   Dr. Dineo Mogomotsi
Dr. Kgosiemang   Dr. Mpho Moseki

Patients

Kenosi

Miscellaneous

Dr. Mendoza, infectious disease specialist, Referral Hospital
Dr. Murewa, head of Referral Hospital's Intensive Care Unit (ICU)
Dr. Sibanda, biochemistry instructor, Institute of Health Sciences Gaborone
Dr. Sung, attending physician, Referral Hospital's pediatric medical ward
Rebecca, administrator, Botswana Harvard Partnership
Valerie, American public health professional

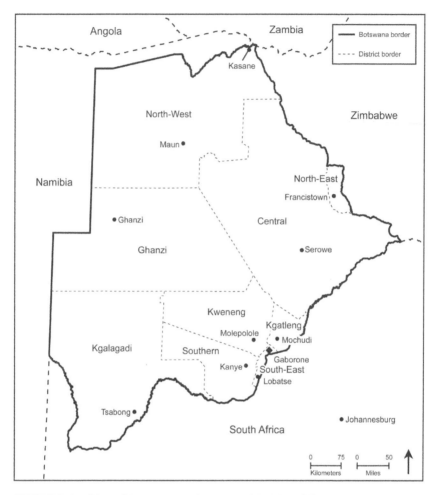

FIGURE 0.1. Map of Botswana (Brian Edward Balsley, GISP)

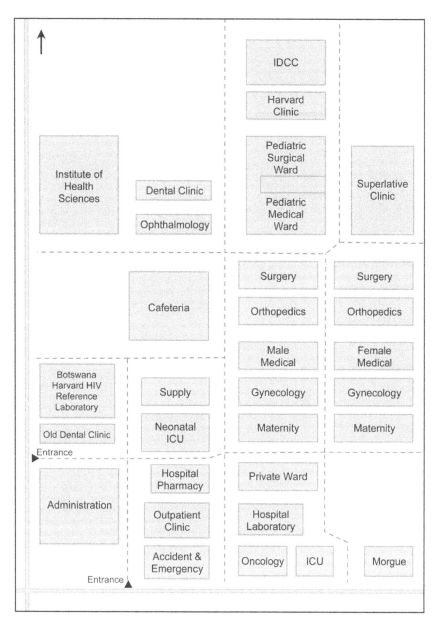

FIGURE 0.2. Map of Referral Hospital (Brian Edward Balsley, GISP)

LEARNING TO SAVE THE WORLD

In 2005, just before I returned to southeastern Botswana for long-term fieldwork, an argument broke out in *The Washington Post* over sub-Saharan Africa's most successful HIV/AIDS treatment program. According to a front-page article, US President George W. Bush's administration had circulated a press release in anticipation of the upcoming World Economic Forum claiming that the President's Emergency Plan for AIDS Relief (PEPFAR) had assisted more than thirty thousand people in Botswana in accessing antiretroviral therapies (ARVs), the medications that control HIV infection (Timberg 2005).[1] A landlocked southern African nation of approximately two million, Botswana had gained sudden international notoriety in the early 2000s for the world's highest HIV prevalence rate.[2] The operations manager of Botswana's treatment program told the *Post*'s reporter that the Bush administration's figures constituted "a gross misrepresentation of the facts": The number of Batswana whose treatment could be directly attributed to PEPFAR, he contended, was "zero."[3] Two weeks later, however, a letter signed by Botswana's Minister of Health and the White House's Global AIDS Coordinator appeared in the paper, emphasizing that PEPFAR dollars supported the program's logistical aspects and infrastructure, such as Botswana's national laboratory, in line with priorities set by Botswana's policymakers. The authors of the letter chastised supposed muckrakers for misdirecting attention to "alleged squabbles about who should take credit" for the program (Tlou and Tobias 2005).

This exchange hints at a profound anxiety that pervaded Botswana's HIV/AIDS treatment program and the American institutions that sought to support it: What exactly *was* the treatment program?[4] Was it a national public health program that happened to be animated by foreign health professionals, some of whom happened to be American? Was it an instantiation of a new global humanitarianism, the outcome of global treatment activism, and a response motivated by a conviction that "the idea that some lives matter less is the root of all that is wrong with the world"?[5] Or was it a sign of imperialism in a new and specifically American key, one that used African bodies to generate wealth through the expansion of pharmaceutical markets and clinical research under the guise of philanthropy and benevolence? When I visited Botswana for the first time the year before, fumbling across the complex institutional landscape of the treatment program, at once fractured and overlapping, the terms of this anxiety were *partnership* and its modifiers, *public* and *private*, and sometimes *African* and *American* and, muttered more softly and less confidently, *colonial, experiment, neoliberal, exploitation*. By the time I returned in 2006, however, the predominant term through which this anxiety was channeled was *global health*.

Over the past two decades, global health has become the watchword for a wide range of political entities ranging from states to international bodies to transnational nongovernmental organizations (NGOs). Its institutions and advocates, from the World Health Organization to Bono to Bill Gates, are numerous and powerful. Its stereotypes are well worn: the patient is dark skinned, poor, abject, and grateful; the heroic clinician has traveled great distances and voluntarily taken on hardships; the surroundings are described in terms of specific deficits (equipment, infrastructure, personnel, expertise, funds) and surpluses (pathogens, diseased and injured bodies, forms of violence). Its objects range from pandemics to famine to war. It has become a remarkably durable object in policy circles within and across national borders and in popular media. It is increasingly a standard component of biomedical education, and nearly as robust in the social sciences, not least of all in anthropology, and even offered as a field of study and set of credentials in its own right. Global health is all around us, albeit in some places more than others. Global health seems obvious, and it seems obviously good. Most importantly, it promises to *generate* goodness in those who participate in it.

This book begins from the premise that the "global" of global health is a "political accomplishment" (Biehl and Adams 2016, 124). Having attended to the complexities of global health programming in action, anthropologists are increasingly grappling with the slipperiness of the term itself, asking what it means to "do" global health or just how "global" it really is (Crane 2013, chap. 5; Dilger and Mattes 2018; Meyers and Hunt 2014; Pigg 2013; Yates-Doerr 2019).[6]

Yet disciplinary commitments make an analysis of the real-time production of global health, that is, the terms by which it is enacted and becomes recognizable as such, challenging despite—or as I suggest in the book's conclusion, due to—the discipline's own entanglement with global health. We rely on scare-quotes to signal our distrust of it, our disinclination to take it on its own terms. We reframe our own engagements as "*critical* global health studies" to distinguish our work from the interventions of overconfident positivists (Adams 2016c; J. Biehl 2016; Biruk 2018; Biruk and McKay 2019; T. Brown, Craddock, and Ingram 2012; cf. Herrick 2017; Neely and Nading 2017).[7] After all, we protest, we know it's not *really* global, and it might not even really be health, and anyone who claims to be *doing* "global health" is doing something with those words. We're just not sure what—or how.

This disquietude among anthropologists as well as our interlocutors drives my investigation. I proceed from the argument that global health itself is an argument or stance that provides the possibility for individuals to position themselves relative to other individuals and collectivities, to their own and others' institutions, materials, and ideas, and in terms of time and space. What follows draws on my own accounts of health professionals, patients, and their families engaged in the ongoing project of treating HIV in southeastern Botswana. I offer these accounts in order to undermine the seeming coherence of "global health" and highlight instead its contingencies and instabilities. My foremost concern is with the *pedagogies* of global health: how individuals learn to recognize themselves and others in terms of global health or, at times, learn to resist this and related categories altogether.

The central question of the book is this: How do people learn to use global health to stage the moral and affective transformation of themselves and those around them? These longed-for transformations of self and others are *affective* in the sense that, at their core, global health pedagogies are concerned about whether subjects "have the right feelings about what is wrong" (Berlant 2008b, 54; cf. Williams 1975). They are *moral* insofar as global health promises to both generate these "right feelings" and provide a means of determining whether subjects truly possess them.[8] They are *ideological* in the sense that the expression and recognition of these feelings presume and entail social identities. Most importantly, rather than adjudicate whether anyone was, in fact, transformed, I focus on the *fantasy* of transformation. In short, this book shows how the transformative potential that global health seems to hold—all the more potent for being so polymorphous—becomes affectively and politically powerful in itself. I track how my interlocutors wrestled with global health's inchoate nature and the labor they had to invest in learning to make places, activities, materials, and

people, including themselves, legible as global health so as to precipitate a transformation. This is what I mean by learning to save the world.

I focus specifically on the language of global health pedagogies. While the
pedagogies I examine entail a wide range of other material—from bodies to pills,
counting trays to spinal needles—it is predominantly through language that the
transformations at stake in global health are staged, that is, modeled, performed,
ratified, and contested. Taking its cues from semiotic anthropology, this book
views language as an embodied material practice through which historically specific subjectivities and institutions are constituted, become recognizable, and
undergo alteration (Irvine and Gal 2000; Schieffelin, Woolard, and Kroskrity
1998; Silverstein 1979; Woolard and Schieffelin 1994). The iterative dimension
of global health is discernable in ways of speaking that are demonstrated, mastered, critiqued, and refused by novices and patients as well as experts. My focus on the language of global health pedagogies demands a rapprochement
between medical anthropology and linguistic anthropology, subdisciplines
that often seem to discount the existence of one another's analytical tools even
when their objects of observation coincide.[9] One of my broader analytical aims,
then, is to persuade medical anthropologists that a semiotic approach to language in the analysis of global health is not merely useful but urgently necessary—
for analyzing global health, but also for understanding anthropology's own
relationship to global health as well. At the same time, for scholars of pragmatics, my study of global health pedagogies illuminates the real-time emergence of
a contingent spatial, temporal, and moral order. My focus on global health's iterative dimension is instructive insofar as it shows how the continuing coherence of
any scale-making project rests, at times precariously, on individuals aligning
themselves and the institutions they inhabit with one another across interactions.

Taking the language of global health pedagogies as a lens onto the real-time
production of global health also sheds light on how Batswana imagine the
state. Enactments of global health entail implicit assumptions regarding the
capacities of the state and its agents. As visiting Americans offered lessons to
one another regarding what one could expect from Botswana's national health
system and the ARV treatment program, Batswana, clinicians and patients alike,
offered their own commentaries on what the state could and should provide
and how visitors might offer help and commit harm. Global health pedagogies
illuminate not only how Americans imagine Botswana, but also how Batswana
themselves draw distinctions between public and private, and grapple with questions of what is local, national, African, or global. These subaltern accounts of the
political and institutional arrangements that undergird US-driven global health,
I show, contrast markedly from dominant narratives of global health with re-

gard to time, space, and moral action, drawing these narratives' basic assumptions into question.

What I know about learning to save the world comes from more than thirty months of fieldwork in and around Gaborone, Botswana's capital, in 2004, 2006 through 2008, and 2012, during which I observed and participated in the pedagogic practices immanent in everyday HIV-related clinical care at the intersection of Botswana's HIV treatment program and the private American institutions that supported it. I focus on two public-private partnerships based at a place I call Referral Hospital. Referral Hospital sits atop the country's tiered national public health system, a point of referral for the smaller district and primary hospitals throughout the southern half of the country. In the mid-2000s Referral Hospital served as a hub for most American institutions that sought to support the country's HIV treatment program. The first partnership, the Superlative Clinic, was the country's only outpatient pediatric HIV clinic. Located on the grounds of Referral Hospital, the Clinic was supported by an American NGO and a private American medical school.[10] During the bulk of my field work it was staffed primarily by American pediatricians assisted by Batswana nurses. The second partnership was directed by another private American medical school, Eastern University Medical School (EUMS). Focused on the inpatient adult medical wards, which handle the majority of HIV-related cases, the EUMS partnership had two goals. First, EUMS ran a six-week clinical rotation on Referral Hospital's adult medical wards that promised their students a pedagogic encounter with global health.[11] Second, because Botswana had no medical school at this time, EUMS promised clinical mentoring for the ward's medical officers (MOs), that is, junior physicians who held medical degrees but lacked specialized medical education, such as a residency.[12] This book offers an ethnographic account, based on this data, of the real-time interactive production of global health in southeastern Botswana, that is, how global health was made recognizable in one specific time and place, and the forms of transformation at stake in that production.[13]

In the remainder of this chapter, I illustrate the problem of stably locating global health in southeastern Botswana before situating Botswana's HIV/AIDS epidemic and ARV treatment program in the broader dynamics of British colonial rule and postcolonial governance. The portion of the chapter "Following Pedagogies" introduces my methodology and elucidates the significance of pedagogic language to my analysis. I then turn to two key analytical terms, scale and stance, to show how individuals strive to enact global health in an effort to transform themselves and others, offering a model of the mode of analysis the book as a whole employs.

Locating Global Health in Southeastern Botswana

Global health is a distinctly post-Cold War phenomenon. The discourses and institutions, not to mention the funds, that have coalesced around this term over the past two to three decades, have been shaped by shifts in US national security priorities, competition between the World Bank and the World Health Organization for control of health-related development programs in what used to be called the Third World, a reorganization and reinvigoration of philanthropic involvement in health programming, and the increased integration of both humanitarianism and military intervention in governance, at times in combination (Brown, Cueto, and Fee 2006; Crane 2013; Fassin 2007; Lakoff 2017; McGoey 2015; Nguyen 2009; Pandolfi 2003; Redfield 2012a).[14] It is also dominated in both definition and execution by institutions and individuals based in North America (Irvine and Gal 2000; Schieffelin, Woolard, and Kroskrity 1998; Silverstein 1979; Woolard and Schieffelin 1994). What exactly the term encompasses remains notoriously difficult to articulate, consisting of "more a bunch of problems than a discipline" (Kleinman 2010, 1518).[15] This is so in part because global health is not a unified field, as Andrew Lakoff argues, but is made up of multiple regimes framed by very different, if sometimes complementary, visions, problems, and solutions (2010).[16] But however anarchic global health might appear both conceptually and on the ground, it nevertheless assumes an ideal form, "a certain rhetorical universality" (Holmes, Greene, and Stonington 2014) that bears "the appearance of a shared moral and technical project" (Lakoff 2010, 59), even "a way of looking at the world" with which few would argue (Horton 2018, 720; cf. Metzl and Kirkland 2010). And while the rhetoric of global health tends to emphasize the porousness of geopolitical borders, whether in a register of humanistic interconnectedness or national biosecurity, global health is nevertheless "distinctly rooted in place; its primary symbolic register is not so much global, but African," and its dominant material focus HIV/AIDS and other infectious diseases (Biruk 2018, 213; Crane 2013, 152; West 2016).

But if global health is a post–Cold War phenomenon, its roots go much deeper. Global health in southern Africa builds institutionally and ideologically on the foundations of European Christian missionization from the early nineteenth century; colonial governance, including early twentieth century development projects; and the vicissitudes of postwar international health programming. In these encounters, biomedicine, far from a static set of universally applicable concepts and technologies, emerged dialectically at the intersection of missionary endeavors, capitalist labor regimes, colonial governmentality, and Africans' own efforts to safeguard their own welfare, preserve their sovereignty, and wield new instruments of power (J. L. Comaroff and J. Comaroff 1997a; Livingston 2005; Molefi 1996). This history is manifest in practices of clinical care in Botswana as well as its built landscape: Several of the district hospitals that refer cases to Referral Hospital began in the 1920s and 1930s as Christian missionary institutions.[17] Similarly, the country's postcolonial healthcare infrastructure reflects the emphasis on preventative public health over hospital-based care that briefly marked international health policy in the 1970s.[18] But what distinguishes global health is not merely the timing of its emergence but, as significantly, its objects: Rather than benighted souls (and the bodies housing them *pro tem*) to be saved for Christendom by means of a civilizing mission that compensated for the ravages of the slave trade, or citizens of postcolonial nation-states to be coaxed or bullied toward distant goals of self-determination and horizontality, the objects of global health are foremost "the poor," an abstraction defined less in terms of eschatology or development teleology than by sheer abjectness.[19] This depoliticized suffering productively intersects with categorical African-ness, a quality of those who belong, as President Bush put it in the dawn of the global health era, to "a nation that suffers from incredible disease."[20] "Africa" has provided a remarkably enduring imaginative field for European and American salvific projects from the early nineteenth century even as, despite these efforts, it remains the site of supposed "shithole countries."[21] Global health lies at the conjunction of these abstractions, new and old: abject suffering untethered from Christendom or nation-state and an enduring racism that denies Africans status as the subjects of history (Mbembe 2001, 2017; cf. Trouillot 1995).[22]

Emerging in tandem with global health, public-private partnerships are one of its defining features (Kenworthy, Thomas, and Crane 2018; Reich 2002). Through the late 1990s, as AIDS death tolls mounted worldwide, pharmaceutical manufacturers, under fire for allegedly contributing to thousands of deaths by pricing ARVs beyond the reach of those who most needed them, responded with high-profile initiatives, providing discounts to some countries through UN-sponsored programs, engaging in corporate philanthropy, and forming partnerships.[23] The institutional arrangements that emerged from this massive influx of funds and diversification of actors are part of a broader trend whereby "partnership has become a dominant modality for the bilateral engagements of international donors and aid agencies with governments of the global South" (Brown 2015, 345; Gerrets 2015). Like global health, however, the definition and execution of such partnerships tend to rest with individuals and institutions in the global North and, like global health, the content of the category is difficult to pin down.[24] Contrasted with top-down, donor-driven agendas, "partnership" can connote collaboration and reciprocity, a mutually beneficial endeavor, whether oriented toward treatment provision, scientific knowledge production, or some combination. In practice, however, partnerships are troubled by gaps between these ideals and their instantiation, including the role of the Global North in supporting the structural adjustment programs that dismantled African public health systems in the 1980s and 1990s, contributing to the very problems global health partnerships claim to address (Kenworthy, Thomas, and Crane 2018; Pfeiffer and Chapman 2010), and the fact that global health partnerships both require and reproduce the deep inequalities they seek to ameliorate (Crane 2013; Geissler 2013). Suspicions on all sides—of corruption and mismanagement, for example, or of neocolonial extraction—complicate the ideal of partnership that drives some (though not all) visions of global health, troubling those who attempt to act in accordance with it (Herrick and Brooks 2018).

I began my fieldwork in Gaborone by asking about public-private partnerships. Based on the extent to which they dominated the health policy literature at the time and have since come to dominate anthropological accounts of the expansion of HIV treatment and the rise of global health, they should have been easy to find. In fact, Botswana had been the site of an early, groundbreaking iteration of this trend: At the 2000 International AIDS Conference in Durban, South Africa, the President of Botswana at the time, Festus Mogae, had publicly declared his fear that Botswana faced "extinction," his determination to explore the feasibility of public treatment, and his appeals for international assistance (Farley 2001). That year, the Bill and Melinda Gates Foundation and the Merck Company Foundation, the philanthropic arm of the pharmaceutical giant Merck & Co., entered into an arrangement with the Government of Botswana to support the healthcare training and infrastructure the treatment program required. Each foundation initially donated $50 million, and Merck donated two antiretroviral medications (Ramiah and Reich 2005).[25] Ambitiously named the *African* Comprehensive HIV/AIDS Partnership (ACHAP) and thereby taking the entire continent as its object, the partnership began rapidly increasing the number of Batswana enrolled in treatment, flying in the face of international health policy, which emphasized prevention and palliative care outside North America and Western Europe.[26] The government began distributing ARVs in Gaborone in January 2002 and began slowly "rolling out" treatment via public health facilities, discarding a system of voluntary counseling and testing in favor of routine testing in order to streamline enrollment (Darkoh 2004; Heald 2006).[27] By 2005 the program had established thirty-two treatment sites across the country and enrolled more than twenty thousand patients, the highest ratio of HIV-positive citizens enrolled in treatment on the African continent at the time.[28] ACHAP was rapidly joined by other partnerships as new configurations of actors baptized themselves under this sign and other, older institutions retooled themselves in its image.

My search for partnerships, however, was met by Batswana public administrators with puzzled looks. *Do you mean Bee-Po-Moss?* they asked. I had no idea what that was. I explained again that I was interested in public-private partnerships for ARVs. *Yes, yes, that's Bee-Po-Moss,* they assured me. One civil servant sent to me another until someone finally explained that that the Ministry of Health had entered into an agreement with the Botswana Public Officers Medical Aid Scheme (BPOMAS), a health insurance carrier (in American terms) that was generally open only to public sector employees. The arrangement diverted some of the burden of the national treatment program away from the overburdened public health system and into the private sector. In short, private practitioners who held contracts with BPOMAS would treat HIV-positive patients, but the government would foot the bill.[29] I was confused: Was this a public-private partnership for global health? Partnerships were supposed to be transnational, multidimensional. BPOMAS felt homespun; indeed, few Americans I encountered in Botswana's public health sector had even heard of it, focused as they were on "the big ones" such as ACHAP and the Botswana Harvard Partnership. Even Americans familiar with the government rarely mentioned BPOMAS when discussing HIV partnerships in Botswana. On the other hand, some Batswana civil servants and health professionals swiftly corrected me when I described ACHAP as a partnership. "No," they insisted, "that's Government."

My emphasis on the pedagogies entailed in the production of global health stems in part from the sheer difficulty of discerning global health in Botswana. While Botswana may seem to epitomize a site of global health—a devastating epidemic, an overtaxed public health infrastructure, an African population in need of complex forms of medical care—demarcating institutions, forms of healthcare, or practitioners *as* global health or even as belonging to a global health partnership could actually be quite a precarious exercise, as the above example illustrates. On one hand, Botswana's public health infrastructure, oriented toward decentralized preventative public health, was unprepared for the burden of hospital-based care and ongoing debility to which the epidemic gave rise (Livingston 2004). Until the past decade, for example, the country lacked the capacity to train physicians within its borders, and the government has historically relied on a mixture of foreign health professionals and foreign-trained Batswana to fill positions in public hospitals.[30] On the other hand, even as the treatment program relied on American funds and institutions for the program's broader infrastructural requirements as well as for specialized medical expertise, Botswana's government has been heavily involved, both administratively and financially, from the very beginning. In contrast to South Africa, where political battles surrounding HIV treatment forced citizens to wrest life itself from a recalcitrant state, Botswana's ARV program has served as a means by which the state has shored up its legitimacy.[31] Accounts of the treatment program often emphasize the supposed weakness of civil society and, bemoaning a lack of popular mobilization, criticize the program as top-down, donor-driven, and unresponsive to popular understandings of the disease (Allen and Heald 2004; Kiley and Hovorka 2006; Swidler 2006). The Batswana I knew certainly had criticisms of their government, of the treatment program, and most emphatically of Referral Hospital, which was a site of intense fear and frequently subject to scathing public critique for mismanagement and dysfunction. That said, many regarded the treatment program as a manifestation of the state's obligations to its citizenry, a form of redistribution to which they were entitled (Livingston 2012). They readily recognized the state as the foremost provider of healthcare even when receiving those services from expatriates. Moreover, Batswana generally *expected* the state to work even when it did not, and they expected this work to entail an equitable distribution of healthcare resources regardless of who dispensed them.[32] As a consequence, and in light of the large proportion of expatriates in Botswana's national health system, Batswana did not always distinguish visiting Americans eager to "do" global health from other resources they attributed to the state.

As I moved through southeastern Botswana's clinical spaces, I quickly came to understand that the borders of these partnerships were sites of intense contestation. Tensions over what counted as the state, who counted as global, and what the epidemic signified made the ongoing production and maintenance of global health at once deeply necessary and incredibly fragile. Whether *anyone* was saving the world was often a painfully open question for some, even as it was also a presupposition for others. I came to see how global health took shape and meaning through pedagogic practices directed at individuals ranging from novice American clinicians to HIV-positive Batswana children, and the often-unequal struggles that resulted as individuals engaged in and opposed efforts to distinguish global from local, expert from inexpert, public from private, treatment from violence, and the present from the past. Global health, in short, proceeds from, rather than precedes, interaction. Pedagogic practices are key to capturing this phenomenon insofar as it is through these practices that individuals—local and visiting practitioners as well as patients and their families—staged global health from one interaction to the next as they learned to regard themselves and others in its terms, refuse those terms, or transform them altogether.

Gaborone in the HIV Treatment Era

Contrasting Gaborone with Johannesburg, a booming South African metropolis located some 350 km to the southeast, Tumelo, a nurse at the Superlative Clinic, once joked that, "Gaborone is just a town." Gaborone's population has rapidly increased in recent years, making it Botswana's most populous center and, increasingly, a hub for transnational medical and public health programming. In 2006 it was officially home to some 200,000 people, more than 10 percent of the national population. But as Tumelo's joke implies, Gaborone is far smaller than southern Africa's other major cities, which dwarf Botswana's entire national population.[33] But estimates of Gaborone's population do not reflect the extent to which Batswana circulate through the capital and its outskirts for work, schooling, and other opportunities. Indeed, many Batswana are quite mobile, moving among Gaborone and Francistown, smaller villages, and outlying farms and cattle posts. Population estimates also occlude the mobility of the urban population: many of Gaborone's residents, including Referral Hospital's Batswana staff, spent some part of the year in the villages of the surrounding districts, which ranged from small villages of a few thousand residents to "urban villages," capitals of Tswana chiefdoms whose populations ranged in the tens of thousands. The result was a surprising density of social networks despite the fact that Botswana is the size of Texas; when I traveled within the country, I frequently saw pairs of cars parked on the side of an otherwise empty stretch of road as the drivers, recognizing one another, had stopped to exchange greetings. "Botswana is a small country," I was warned and, hierarchies notwithstanding, the social distance between Batswana health professionals and the patients they encountered, even in the relatively large and heterogeneous spaces of Referral Hospital, could be very small indeed.

During the period of British colonization from the late nineteenth century to the mid-1960s, the Bechuanaland Protectorate, as it was called, remained largely undeveloped.[34] Shortly after independence in 1966, however, the government entered into an arrangement whereby the proceeds of mining extensive diamond deposits returned to the state (Gulbrandsen 2012). This arrangement generated one of the fastest-growing economies in the world and led to the rapid expansion of public services, including health and education. Botswana, like many other newly independent African states, focused on low-cost services related to childbirth and family planning, nutrition and water accessibility, child growth monitoring and immunizations, and the treatment of respiratory and diarrheal diseases (Høgh and Petersen 1984; Maganu 1997). Training for nurses has been available at missionary institutions since the 1920s, and at public institutions since around independence. These nurses staffed health posts and clinics in rural areas, referring serious cases to small hospitals from which patients might be transferred to one of two referral hospitals for more specialized treatment. The result was a large and powerful nursing profession and a much smaller cadre of physicians, with specialists concentrated at referral hospitals.

These infrastructural investments bore fruit: in the early 1990s UNICEF praised the near-universal access Batswana had to health services and primary education, and the World Bank reclassified Botswana as a middle-income country (1993). The country's burgeoning economy led to population expansions in urban centers: internal migration patterns joined established external ones as individuals and families moved among villages, farms, cattle posts, mines and other sites of industrial labor, and urban centers as schooling, farming, and other obligations demanded (Bryant, Stephens, and MacLiver 1978; Mookodi 2000; Townsend 1997). Lauded by observers as a "miracle" of democratic governance and steady economic growth, Botswana was frequently cited as an exception to the rules of poverty, corruption, and warfare associated with the region.[35] Botswana's government avoided debt to international financial institutions and the ensuing structural adjustment programs that dismantled public services in the region in the 1980s and 1990s even as the HIV/AIDS epidemic began to unfold (Pfeiffer and Chapman 2010; Poku 2006; Schoepf 2001). Yet these fruits were distributed unevenly: Despite the positive effects of public health campaigns in particular and better standards of living in general, poverty was pervasive, particularly in rural areas (Good 1993, 2008; Livingston 2005).

Botswana's HIV epidemic was thus shaped by contradictory dynamics of high levels of poverty and inequality despite rapid economic growth, expanded public services, and a burgeoning middle class as well as by the intersection of long-established patterns of regional migration with newly intensified internal ones (Hope 2001). Yet the epidemic bewildered outsider observers and Batswana alike: Foreigners did not expect an epidemic in a country hailed as a model of economic development and political stability, nor did Batswana recognize in themselves the deviant sexualities and general backwardness associated with the disease (Heald 2006; MacDonald 1996). The government launched awareness and prevention campaigns in 1987, eventually adopting the widely used ABC approach: Abstain, Be faithful, use a Condom. But in the years that morbidity and mortality rates remained low, Batswana regarded AIDS as a "radio disease" (Ingstad 1990) rather than one they directly experienced. ABC campaigns gained little traction locally, and popular enthusiasm around them quickly waned (Heald 2002). By 2000, however, Botswana had one of the highest prevalence rates in the world (UNAIDS 2014). The health system was quickly overwhelmed, unprepared for either the burden of hospital-based care that HIV, then the provenance of highly specialized physicians, demanded, or the chronic debility to which the epidemic gave rise (Livingston 2004, 2012). This was the context in which the treatment program and the partnerships supporting it emerged. Varying in purpose, with differing emphases on patient care, clinical research, and capacity building within Botswana's medical sector, they connected individual American clinicians, as well as their affiliated medical schools and NGOs, to new opportunities to treat patients, train students, mentor local practitioners, conduct research, and shape policy in an era of rapidly expanding American interest and investment in global health generally and in the AIDS epidemic in Africa in particular.

These partnerships, jostling one another as they reformulated their aims and increasingly overlapped in scope, were nearly all centered in one place: Referral Hospital. Built around the time of the country's independence and located in an older part of Gaborone, Referral Hospital housed inpatient wards, including adult medicine, pediatrics, surgery, orthopedics, and maternity, as well as the hospital laboratory, the accident and emergency ward, the outpatient clinics and dispensary, the laundry and cafeteria, and the towering administration block. Locally, the hospital was known for its cantankerous and neglectful nursing staff and its uneven if not downright dubious quality of care. The hospital often struggled to maintain basic supplies: the availability of beds and linens could vary greatly from one day to the next, one ward to the next. The medication supply was managed by the Central Medical Stores, and stock-outs were frequent. Overtaxed, under-resourced, and frequently the site of public moral panic, Referral Hospital served as a first point of care for Gaborone's growing population and the surrounding areas in addition to serving as the referral hospital for the southern half of the country.[36] Yet, in contrast to many other major African hospitals, admitted patients were provided with free linens and meals. They were charged two pula (about thirty cents in US dollars at the time) per night, but they were not charged for the individual medical services they received, nor were they required to purchase drugs and other medical supplies.[37]

Following Pedagogies

One afternoon in March 2007 I walked to the far edge of Referral Hospital's sprawling campus. The crowd at the Superlative Clinic had thinned since early morning, and the glassy cavernous waiting room, so different from the low one-story brick wards, rang with the sound of a cartoon playing on a television suspended from the ceiling. I walked behind the reception desk and down the hallway, where I found the head nurse, Mma Kgosietsile, sorting through papers in her office.[38] An older woman with ties to a chiefly lineage and a regal bearing, Mma Kgosietsile had been coaxed out of retirement from a senior management position, she told me, by the opportunity to work closely with patients. She had no illusions about the magnitude and severity of the HIV epidemic or the stakes of the treatment program. I was therefore surprised when she commented, "You know, this *thing*, this *terrible thing* was killing us." The Clinic's American pediatricians, concerned that the stigma of the disease negatively affected children's adherence (that is, the extent to which they consistently consumed their medications as prescribed), insisted on the term *HIV* and regarded substitutions, even Setswana translations, as insufficiently direct, too euphemistic. Yet here was Mma Kgosietsile, whose clinical expertise was unimpeachable, speaking in a manner that American pediatricians associated with frightened children and anxiously sought to censor and reform. I had to stop myself from glancing over my shoulder, aware that her words would be perceived by those pediatricians as a sign that even Mma Kgosietsile, unwilling or unable in that moment to name the "terrible thing," required their ongoing tutelage.

Pedagogy, scholars of southern Africa have shown, has long served as a site for the production, transformation, and contestation of social worlds and those who inhabit them (J. Comaroff 1996; J. Comaroff and Comaroff 1991; J. L. Comaroff and Comaroff 1997a; Ngwane 2001a, 2001b; Stambach 2010). From Tswana students' objections to toileting arrangements in early twentieth-century mission schools to the 1976 Soweto uprising to more recent efforts to "decolonize" South Africa's universities, contests over pedagogy reflect not only the legacy, however contested, of Protestant instruction, but also the Enlightenment project of marking out the terrain of the everyday as the site of individual transformation (J. Comaroff 1993; J. L. Comaroff and J. Comaroff 1997a; cf. Foucault 1977).[39] If colonialism was "an epic of the ordinary" (J. L. Comaroff and J. Comaroff 1997a, 35), wherein negotiations and transformations took place in and through pedagogies directed at how a house should take shape, how bodies should be cleansed and adorned, how and by whom fields should be tilled, then this scholarship directs our attention to the "unremarked ways of seeing and being" (J. Comaroff and J. L. Comaroff 1991, 246; cf. Bourdieu 1977; Gramsci 1971) at stake in how Mma Kgosietsile named the "terrible thing."

Methodologically, I had planned to "follow the drug," that is, let the movement of ARVs reveal the subjects and social relations they constituted and entailed, and the ideologies that structured their use and their relation to other forms of exchange (Bourgois 2000; Geest, Whyte, and Hardon 1996; Pfeiffer and Nichter 2008; Whyte, Geest, and Hardon 2002). Frédéric Le Marcis, for example, drew on the itineraries of HIV-positive residents of Johannesburg to create

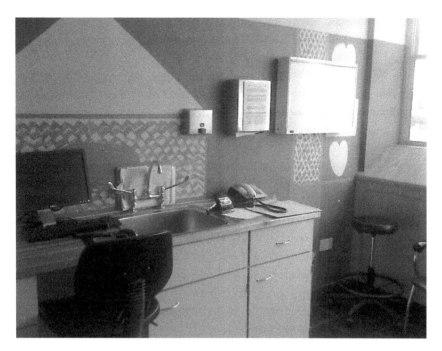

FIGURE 1.   Consultation room, Superlative Clinic (photo by the author)

a novel map of the city that illustrated how the movement of suffering bodies revealed and constituted boundaries between public and private (2004). I intended to combine an analysis of the global political economy of pharmaceuticals and its particular instantiations within Botswana with attention to the position of these medications within local social and semiotic orders. I began observing at the Superlative Clinic in early 2007, eventually participating in many of the Clinic's day-to-day activities, assisting where my help was wanted and my skills appropriate, such as counting pills, completing forms, running errands, and, because few American clinicians spoke even a few words of Setswana, serving as a makeshift translator in a pinch. I interviewed adults, mostly women, accompanying children to the Clinic. I also interviewed a wide range of public-sector health professionals, Batswana and expatriate, as well as American clinicians and administrators. I had thought my interlocutors would talk about drug security and informal pill sharing, revealing how ARVs transformed kinship and citizenship. Instead, they returned again and again to the topic of adherence: How patients could be made adherent; how clinicians could know their patients were, in fact, adherent. Indeed, American clinicians' claims as the arbiters of knowledge about Botswana's epidemic to its own national agencies as well as other, more distant institutions also hinged on adherence. The significance of adherence, I found, rested on a scalar logic, one that had to be painstakingly imparted to patients and clinicians alike.

Rather than following drugs, then, I found myself following pedagogies.[40] I paid close attention to how clinicians educated children about their infections and their medications, and to the deficits they saw in children's interactions with others, including children's families and the clinicians Americans called "local." At stake in these interactions was not simply a question of a clinician providing care for an individual child, but of clinicians *modeling* for one another (and for patients and their families as well as visiting anthropologists) the provision of care in a profession where the demonstration and observation of expert practice is a key pedagogical mode. I shifted to EUMS in late 2007, shadowing EUMS personnel and members of the Medical Department and serving in many of the capacities I had done at the Clinic. I was struck by the frustrations that emerged as hospital staff and visitors attempted to cooperate in the work of tending patients. Conflict simmered constantly, erupting at times and leaving many confused, disappointed, even resentful. In the clash of institutional norms and sites of authority, what stood out was the sheer difficulty, most acute among junior physicians and trainees, of framing the purpose and significance of their work as it pertained to their subjectivities. If this was global health, why did it feel so contentious, so antagonistic? Why wasn't it more gratifying? I spoke with a wide range of hospital staff and EUMS personnel, as well as patients and their families, with officials at the Ministry of Health, and staff at ACHAP, the Botswana Harvard Partnership, the University of Botswana, and BOTUSA, as the US Centers for Disease Control and Prevention field office in Gaborone was known at the time. I attended clinical conferences and meetings and followed up with both sites throughout 2008. To provide a contrast to the atmosphere of near-constant conflict at Referral Hospital, I spent short amounts of time at two other sites: a small mission-run district hospital that, by the choice of its chief medical officer, had little to do with any of the American partnerships, and Nyangabgwe Hospital, the country's other referral hospital in Francistown, which had fewer ties to American institutions than did Referral Hospital.

Recent scholarship has emphasized pedagogy's performative dimensions, focusing on how modes of being and orientations toward the world and the subjects and objects within it are modeled, rehearsed, and evaluated (Chumley 2016; Ho 2009; Wilf 2014). Language, these studies have shown, is a key site wherein trainees and educators work to constitute their objects of expertise and, in so doing, constitute themselves as proficient practitioners and experts (Carr 2010a; Goodwin 1994; Mertz 2007). Ethnographies of biomedical pedagogies, whether oriented toward patients or practitioners, have taken a different tact, focusing instead on the constitution of subjects and objects through embodied practices other than language, recapitulating an epistemological framework common to biomedicine wherein words and things are ontologically distinct and textual representations have no effect on the objects to which they refer (Kleinman 1995; cf. Daston and Galison 2010; Jakobson 1960; Silverstein 1998). A focus on the language of global health pedagogies illuminates the underexamined role language plays in the constitution of patient subjectivities, a process that, studies have emphasized, involves reforming the whole person into a therapeutic subject (Benton 2015; J. Biehl 2009a; Nguyen 2010; Rhine 2016; Robins 2006; Zigon 2011). Moreover, a focus on the language of global health pedagogies creates a bridge between studies of patient subjectivization in biomedical settings and ethnographies of biomedical training, two bodies of literature that rarely intersect.[41] Global health pedagogies, as the anecdote above illustrates, cut across diverse sites and encompass a wide range of actors, illuminating transformations anticipated, staged, and refused by experts, novices, and patients, dissolving and reconstituting distinctions between these groups. Following the language of global health pedagogies illuminates pedagogy's intersubjective dimensions and highlights how both expertise and the objects of that expertise, including patients, must be enacted across contexts and interactions. The next section offers a set of tools for analyzing that enactment.

The Pragmatics of Global Health Pedagogies

Global health is inherently an argument about scale. The massive expansion in ARV access that is entangled with the expansion of global health is commonly known in health policy as "scaling up" (Kenworthy 2017; Kenworthy and Parker 2014; Mangham and Hanson 2010); indeed, ACHAP's infrastructural support for Botswana's treatment program framed it as a model for the continent, asserting its scalability from the beginning. My more specific analytic project, however, is understanding first, how global health is enacted as a scalar argument, and second, how individuals use these enactments to transform themselves and those around them.[42] Drawing on insights from science and technology studies, anthropologists have emphasized the ways objects are enacted, that is, "brought into being, sustained, or allowed to wither away [through] common, day-to-day sociomaterial practices" (Mol 2002, 6), and rather than following objects up, down, or across scales, this scholarship highlights the labor entailed in making objects—hunger, "the offshore," even medicine itself—durable across space and time (Appel 2012; McKay 2018; Yates-Doerr 2015). As a consequence, analyses of scale have shifted towards the interrogation of "scale making" projects that interrogate "local" and "global" as effects, not stable locations, ontological givens, or preconditions (Hecht 2018; Helmreich 2009; Latour 2005; Strathern 1999; Tsing 2005, 2015).

Performative approaches in linguistic anthropology draw attention to the pragmatics of scale, that is, "the work required to bring scale into being and make it matter in social and cultural life" (Carr and Lempert 2016, 9). This approach allows us to back away from global health in order to examine it *as* a scale, a provisional argument that must be made and maintained and through which the people involved "orient their actions, organize their experience, and make determinations about who and what is valuable" (Carr and Lempert 2016, 9). The pragmatics of scale, in other words, offers us a methodology oriented toward investigating "the semiotic means by which social actors and analysts scale our worlds" (Carr and Lempert 2016, 8) and the conditions that make these scales durable and portable. Pragmatics of scale also reminds us that these semiotic processes are themselves ideological, that is, there are "frameworks of understanding" that "constrain which aspects of social life deserve attention, which merit comparison with what, and how they are to be measured" (Gal 2016, 91; Irvine 2016). Writing about the models that guide comparison across scale, Susan Gal reminds us that, "given political backing, they become models for ways of reorganizing relations, in order to match representations" (2016, 95). Scale, then, is a feature of how institutions create and maintain themselves and those within them, even as the scaling projects on which they rest tend to disappear from view. It is, after all, "the *institutionalization* of scalar perspectives that ensure that some scalar projects are relatively more effective and durable in the first place" (Carr and Lempert 2016, 16, emphasis in the original).

Pragmatics of scale is thus useful for a project that bridges medical anthropology, science studies, and linguistic anthropology insofar as "scaling projects typically rely on complex, heterogeneous, and sometimes far-flung assemblages that include extradiscursive forms" (Carr and Lempert 2016, 10). Attuning ourselves to the pragmatics of scale helps us see the ongoing labor—linguistic and otherwise—that is essential to making global health and its attendant categories make sense. Pragmatics of scale helps us see "how contextual boundaries are discursively drawn by social actors" (Carr and Lempert 2016, 10), drawing our attention to debates over who deserved credit for the success of Botswana's treatment program and to awkward comparisons between BPOMAS and ACHAP less in order to resolve them than to see how relations among individuals and institutions are maintained or dismantled, to chart the actions and positions made possible or foreclosed in these processes. "A scalar ideology" Irvine argues, "can pick out one degree of encompassment as counting the most" (2016,

227) such that BPOMAS seems merely national, hardly a partnership at all, or conversely, obviously national, a sign of the state's commitment to its citizens. Insisting that scales and scaling practices are ideological helps us orient ourselves to "how and why scales are made," whether among our informants or in the process of anthropological analysis (Carr and Lempert 2016; Gal 2016; Irvine 2016, 216).

Scale is a crucial element of the pedagogies at the heart of this book. Attention to spatial scales, for example, helps us see in chapters 4 and 5 the work entailed in making a heterogeneous group of clinicians born, raised, and trained in disparate settings across the globe into a group hailed by visiting Americans as *local* doctors. Spatial scales also draw our gaze to claims of encompassment, that is, moments when Referral Hospital stands in for all African hospitals, or one child's poor adherence to her ARVs becomes a threat to a manageable epidemic, or studies (anthropological or clinical) of Gaborone and Botswana's southeast stand in for a whole nation (Carr and Lempert 2016; Irvine 2009, 2016; Philips 2016). Attention to temporal scales highlights the crises clinicians undergo when their work fails to contribute to a future of progress, whether the horizon is the unfolding lifespan of an individual HIV-positive child or an entire "AIDS-free generation" (cf. Brodwin 2011; Irvine 2009).[43] A pragmatics of scale also attunes us to how the morality of global health emerges from its interscalability, "where qualities acted out in the here-and-now envelope of this interaction are meant to exemplify comparable qualities of something 'larger'" (Lempert 2016, 55; cf. Hecht 2018)—in this case, a moral project characterized by almost unquestionable urgency and necessity, a characterization that rests on and is reinforced by other scales.[44] Global health, after all, is about saving the world. Yet it is precisely this scalar narrative that holds global health's tantalizing promise of transformation, a framework for action that at times collapses into drudgery and frustration.

Medical students from EUMS arrived in Gaborone in groups of about eight or ten for six-week rotations. After a short orientation and tour of the hospital provided by EUMS personnel, their weekdays were fairly predictable: They arrived at Referral Hospital's medical wards in time for morning report at 7:30 a.m., when the MOs who had remained on call overnight or over the weekend discussed the status of the ward's patients and reported any new admissions. Students spent their mornings rounding on patients with their assigned firm, that is, a team led by a senior physician and composed of physicians at different levels of expertise. After lunch, students carried out the orders that had been placed during rounds: collecting blood, urine, and sputum samples, chasing down missing lab results, and familiarizing themselves with various diagnostic and therapeutic procedures. Around 4 p.m. students left for the apartments that

EUMS maintained for them. Upon returning to the apartments one evening, Evan, an EUMS student, complained to his roommates about Mma Gaoletswe, one of the older nurses assigned to the medical ward. Earlier that afternoon, he recounted, Mma Gaoletswe had flatly refused Evan's request that she translate between his English and a patient's Setswana, saying she was too tired. "I wanted to slap her face," Evan said, adding bitterly, "Don't they even *care* about their own people?"

If attention to scale-making practices helps us see the labor entailed in global health as an argument, then my second key term, stance, draws our attention to the kinds of subjects that are produced through this labor. Rather than linger over Evan's lack of empathy or the incongruity between the ideals of global health and his violent fantasy, I want to focus on what he did in this interaction and how. Because scale-making is necessarily positional, looking at how individuals "do" scale—that is, the stances they take in the process of assembling and using those scales—can shed light on the moral order they assume and how they position themselves and others in it. Most broadly, stance is a public act whereby one person positions herself vis-à-vis an object, whether epistemically or affectively, and, in the process, aligns herself with one or more other persons (Du Bois 2007; Englebretson 2007; A. M. Jaffe 2009b).[45] Stance entails a speaker's position, an evaluation of a stance object, and an alignment with at least one other person. This positioning may be verbal but may also entail bodily positions and movements (Matoesian 2005). Stance is intersubjective in the sense that the subjectivities of all participants are presumed, entailed in, and constituted through the interaction; it is indexical in the sense that it points to the broader cultural frameworks and contexts of interaction, including previous stances.[46] As public acts, stances have consequences, not least of all the consolidation of stances over time into identities and social relationships (Englebretson 2007; A. M. Jaffe 2009a). I focus in this book on the sociolinguistic aspects of stance, that is, how people construct, realize, and maintain social identities (Bucholtz and Hall 2005; Carr 2010b; Johnstone 2013; Ochs 1992; 1993; 1996; Silverstein 2004). But identities are not formed nor inhabited in a vacuum: stances point to and contribute toward a dynamically constituted shared framework while highlighting "point of view and action" (Du Bois 2007; Irvine 2009, 54).

Examining the stances individuals take through the scalar narratives that sustain global health helps us see the fantasies of transformation at stake. In the previous example, Evan shifted from Mma Gaoletswe to *they*, a term that in English, Joanne Scheibman observes, "is commonly used to evaluate groups that participants do not belong to, and often these assessments express disapproval or derision" (2007, 128). This unspecified *they*, a group or collectivity that encompasses Mma Gaoletswe but presumably not Evan or Evan's audience, "indexes a class of people with social and institutional relevance who are viewed derisively by the conversational participants" thereby "creating solidarity among [participants] themselves" (2007, 129). Evan's question evaluated two different kinds of subjects—people who care, people who do not—in relation to a stance object, "their own people." Evan's question positioned his audience, fellow EUMS students, as people who cared in contrast to a generalized *they*, illustrating how speakers use generalizations to "situate themselves in relationship to one another, to expectation, and to sociocultural beliefs" (2007, 113) and "to show alliance with other participants by confirming adherence to particular societal discourses" (2007, 115; Berman 2005).

These contrasting subject positions are also scaled: Mma Gaoletswe and her refusal to translate are encompassed within a broader category of failing to care, indicating the possibility that Mma Gaoletswe and people like her lack even a basic awareness of patients' needs. Moreover, Evan's use of *their* indicates a naturalization of a one-to-one correspondence between responsibility and an essentialized identity. In other words, Mma Gaoletswe and people like her are beholden by virtue of presumably shared qualities (nation, race, culpability for the epidemic, etc.) to care for the patients in question, while Evan, by offering care beyond this obligation, established himself and people like him, that is, his audience, as both capable of recognizing this obligation and passing judgment on its nonfulfillment. His unelaborated use of shifters *they* and *their*, with their potential to point far beyond Mma Gaoletswe to all Batswana nurses or even all Africans, was as much about positioning himself and his fellow students as arbiters of the content of that category as it was about its actual content at any given moment (cf. Silverstein 2003). Yet Evan's asserted scale and his confidence that his audience recognized and properly placed themselves within it only worked by virtue of their institutional "placement," that is, their "embeddedness within a highly distributed assemblage of practices that is designed to serve as a kind of scalar infrastructure" that "both makes plausible and narrows down what participants are likely to 'see'" in the interaction (Lempert 2016, 56).

The scales and stances that make up global health and that make it recognizable have institutional force behind them, but "global health" is a product of those interactions and the institutions that shape them, not a phenomenon that precedes them. Taken together, scale and stance illuminate not only how individuals imagine global health and how they imagine themselves vis-à-vis global health but also how they imagine others and the relationships they create with them in those terms (Carr 2009; Gal 2002, 2005, 2016; Irvine 2009, 2016). Denaturalizing scales and the stances they engender also draws our attention back to the language of global health pedagogies, that is, the interactions through which individuals make these scales make sense to one another, the stances they take in doing so, the social identities they solidify, and the moral orders that emerge. American pediatricians longed to transform HIV-positive children into adherent subjects and, in the process, affirm their own status as the humane practitioners they hoped they were. But their uncertainty as to whether these transformations had, in fact, qualitatively and stably transpired contributed to the tension that suffused their clinical interactions and made scaling those interactions an anxious endeavor. Moreover, individuals are not always compelled to take up the transformations to which they are recruited: One of Evan's listeners shared his violent fantasy with me, distanced herself from Evan's position, recruited me to recognize that distance, and invited me to align myself with her. Viewing scale-making projects as the consequence of stances taken over time and across institutions—stances that, in turn, shape subsequent stances—is key to approaching global health as an iterative project, the meaning of which is always emergent.

Looking Ahead

The first half of the book focuses on pedagogies directed at HIV-positive children and their families. Chapter 1 examines how the Superlative Clinic's pediatricians assessed whether children were taking their ARVs. When pediatricians concluded that a child's adherence was inconsistent, they had to decide whether to confiscate the child's ARVs in a bid to preserve their long-term efficacy. Focusing on the ways pediatricians scaled pediatric HIV treatment, I show how the uncertainties immanent in these assessments could cast doubt on the broader project of HIV treatment, while pediatricians' interest in preserving the efficacy of ARVs could, in the eyes of children's families and local clinicians, place the lives of individual children at risk. The problem of adherence in turn shaped how pediatricians taught children to talk about HIV, the focus of chapter 2. Concerned that children's families concealed their diagnoses from them, pediatricians stressed the need for transparency as a precondition for children's ongoing adherence and, thus, their very survival. But pediatricians' conviction that the word *AIDS* impaired children's ability to acknowledge their infections and adhere to treatment led them to silence representations of HIV as anything other than a manageable condition readily controlled by diligent children. Pediatricians' anxious efforts to shape children through speech were informed, I argue, by visions of catastrophe that could only be forestalled one child at a time. That the epidemic itself seemed to point to the inability of Batswana to acknowledge and intervene in it is the focus of chapter 3. I show how American health professionals used the metalanguage of HIV intervention—that is, talk about how people talk about HIV and its treatment—to insist on the inability of Batswana to confront the country's epidemic. American professionals, I show, used this metalanguage to project a scalar infrastructure across multiple sites—from individual interiorities to transnational funding arrangements—that positioned those "outside" Botswana as the arbiters of truthful claims about HIV within Botswana. The constitution of Botswana's epidemic as an object of American moral and technical expert intervention, I argue, was not a feature of the epidemic per se, but a project that relied on scalar claims asserted and maintained through the metalanguage of HIV intervention.

The second half turns to physician training on the hospital's adult medical wards. Chapter 4 examines how EUMS educators and trainees and Referral Hospital's own medical staff employed and contested terms such as *local* and *resource-limited* in their efforts to position themselves as experts and assert the value of their own and one another's labor. For EUMS personnel, global health emerged in contrast to a parochial, outdated, morally suspect biomedical practice ascribed to "local doctors," a position to which the wards' MOs responded in diverse ways, sometimes vigorously redrawing the terms of the encounter. Conceptualizing global health as a frontier, that is, as an imaginative project, rather than an arrangement of biological threats and expert practices, I show how American medical personnel's ability to "do global health" rested on their assertion of temporal and spatial contrasts between "global" and "local" and to enforce the boundaries of these categories. Chapter 5 looks more closely at the profound moral transformation Americans expected from global health as an embodied experience. Focusing on what I call the register of heroic American medicine, I show how EUMS personnel attempted to frame what might have been mere physical proximity or even violence into moments that both revealed and affirmed their moral rectitude. I contrast Americans' longings for these moments with the perspectives of the ward's young Batswana MOs, who regarded their own medical expertise as a means of aligning themselves with their patients in a project of national progress. In addition to capturing the terms of the ward's deep, ongoing tensions, this comparison helps us see the promised transformations of global health pedagogies as a fantasy grounded in institutional and national inequalities. Chapter 6 examines physician training at Referral Hospital as an instance of capacity building, highlighting African professionals' struggles to call attention to extractive aspects of American clinical pedagogies. I focus on clinical capacity building as a rhetorical strategy, illustrating how the rhetoric of clinical capacity building made it possible for clinical pedagogies themselves to function as a mechanism of extraction, inviting Batswana to consider themselves and those around them in terms of their contributions to American-driven projects of knowledge production and intervention. Clinical pedagogies, in short, promised to bring Botswana into "the global" even as they contributed to an enduring "local" site for American global health.

This book joins other critical accounts of "global" phenomena in highlighting the aspirational nature of claims to "the global" while tracking the possibilities these claims engender and foreclose (J. Comaroff and J. L. Comaroff 2000; Gupta and Ferguson 1992; Haraway 1991, 1997; Hindman 2013; Ho 2005; Ong and Collier 2005; Tsing 2000, 2005).[47] Indeed, this road is sufficiently well trodden that the argument that global health must be contingently produced in a historically and socially specific form might seem no more than a recapitulation of what we already know about postwar development and international health and, indeed, colonialism.[48] But while anthropologists may have heeded Arturo Escobar's call to liberate anthropology from the development encounter (1995), a critical account of global health will likewise "require a willingness to question the disciplinary identity" of anthropology (Cooper and Packard 1997; Ferguson 1997, 152). For if, as Didier Fassin argues, medical anthropologists resemble humanitarian workers—the "global apostles of health" (2012, 114)—we are also often apostles *of* global health itself. This obligatory moral orientation toward medical anthropologists' own object of study not only highlights the difficulty in getting at the analytic ground beneath our feet but indicates the risk one runs in doing so: Who among us dares appear so uncaring?[49] Yet a study of how individuals position themselves and others and the institutions they inhabit in terms of global health would be woefully incomplete if we did not include anthropologists ourselves in the analysis. The concluding chapter therefore offers a critique of the anthropology of global health that accounts for how medical anthropology as a subdiscipline has been participatory in constituting both the category of global health and the moral stances this category entails. I analyze my own recruitment to transformation through the recognition of suffering and call on anthropologists of global health to account for our own stakes in global health pedagogies in addition to illuminating what is at stake for our interlocutors.

Part 1

SCALING THE EPIDEMIC

SAVING MEDICATIONS VERSUS SAVING CHILDREN

One morning in January 2007 my research assistant, Patrick, and I were huddled in a small, windowless supply room behind the Superlative Clinic's reception area. "Caregivers," the Superlative Clinic's catchall term for the adults responsible for child-patients, often spent hours sitting on the plastic chairs that filled the reception area, waiting for the children in their care to be seen by one of the Clinic's pediatricians. Even when appointments went smoothly, they often went slowly, as nurses translated between English and Setswana.[1] The wait to be seen by a doctor was often followed by a second wait while one of the pharmacists filled a child's prescriptions. Even though some of these caregivers, most of them women, had arrived as early as 7 a.m., before the Clinic's doors even opened, a simple checkup could take the better part of a day, depending on the number of patients and on how far women and children had to travel. Malebogo, the Clinic's receptionist, knowing that a few of the women had particularly long waits, pointed them out to us so that we could ask if they would consent to be interviewed.

This was how we met Maikutlo. She arrived from the reception area looking harried, her young son in her arms. She shut the door behind her, muffling the din from the reception area, and maneuvered her way between file cabinets and an examination table to where a plastic stool stood waiting. Dressed in slacks and a large t-shirt, her long hair in braids, she did not look much older than thirty. Patrick, an affable university student in his mid-twenties, had trained as a prenatal HIV testing counselor and was adept at putting people at ease. After some discussion, Maikutlo agreed to speak with us. She set Karabo, who was snacking on toasted corn, down on the floor, and I offered him a small box of juice. His obvious enjoyment of these contrasted markedly with Maikutlo's visible agitation.

Karabo, about eighteen months old, was the youngest of Maikutlo's three children. About a year earlier Karabo, too sickly to try to crawl or to even move much, had been admitted to Referral Hospital's pediatric medical ward, where he had tested positive for HIV and been started on ARVs. Upon his release he had been referred to the Superlative Clinic. Maikutlo had brought Karabo faithfully to the Clinic every three months and had watched his health improve dramatically. The Superlative Clinic, she told us flatly, had saved her son. But this pattern of progress had been disrupted a month or so before our conversation when Maikutlo, pregnant at the time, had been admitted to Referral Hospital and ultimately suffered a late miscarriage. She had remained in the hospital for two weeks. While she was in the hospital, no one had been giving Karabo his medications. The staff of the Superlative Clinic, Maikutlo told us, had realized that Maikutlo had not been giving Karabo his ARVs and had taken the medications away. They had told Maikutlo that the medications would be stopped for two weeks. More than two weeks had passed, Maikutlo told us, and the staff had not yet given Karabo's ARVs back to her.

But how, Patrick asked, did Clinic staff know that Karabo had not been receiving his medications? Maikutlo explained that she and her children had been staying with her boyfriend, Thato, in Gaborone, though Maikutlo herself was from Mahalapye, a medium-sized town a few hours northeast of the capital. Thato was not the father of Karabo or of Maikutlo's two older daughters, aged thirteen and six years old. Maikutlo had told Thato nothing about Karabo's HIV-positive status, or her own. While still in the hospital, Maikutlo had arranged for Thato to meet her at the Clinic with Karabo so that she could accompany Karabo to his appointment. Just before Karabo was to be seen, however, a nurse had called Maikutlo back to the gynecology ward. Thato had taken Karabo into the consultation room, where an American pediatrician had begun questioning Thato about Karabo's medications. Quickly realizing that Thato did not know the reason Karabo attended the Clinic, the pediatrician had sent Thato away without explaining. Later, the pediatrician had told Maikutlo that it was important that she disclose Karabo's HIV-positive status to Thato.

Generally, Clinic staff maintained that a child's adherence to their medications depended upon the collaborative support of adults who were aware of a child's diagnosis and familiar with his or her medications. They stressed the importance of a "primary caregiver," that is, one adult who took ultimate responsibility for the task of giving a child his or her ARV. But they also emphasized the need for other adults in the household to know how to give the medications in the event the primary caregiver could not do so. They considered this support necessary because a child who received ARVs only intermittently risked developing resistance to a medication or even a whole class of medications, limiting their effectiveness in controlling HIV infection and forcing the child to switch from now-ineffective "first-line" medications to others that were often more difficult to take, were more difficult to store, had more severe side effects, and were more expensive.[2] Indeed, the Clinic considered adherence such a priority and adult caregivers such a vital part of a child's adherence that, before a child began treatment, at least one adult member of the child's family had to attend a morning-long training session. In this session Clinic staff explained to caregivers how ARVs worked and warned them that children must never miss even a single dose of their medications.[3]

Maikutlo had attended one of these sessions on Karabo's behalf. But her time in the hospital had convinced the Clinic staff that Thato's ignorance of Karabo's HIV infection and of his ARV regimen was detrimental to Karabo's adherence. They told Maikutlo that they would discontinue Karabo's ARV therapy until they felt assured that Karabo's adherence could be maintained, that is, until Maikutlo had disclosed Karabo's HIV-positive status to Thato. Clinic staff were bargaining that they could convince Maikutlo to adjust the circumstances of Karabo's care before he began to suffer the effects of interrupted ARV therapy and that doing so would better ensure Karabo's adherence, thus preserving the long-term efficacy of his medications or, in the Clinic's terms, "saving" them.

Unsurprisingly, Maikutlo felt trapped. Telling Thato about Karabo's HIV-positive status entailed disclosing her own. A young child's HIV infection is generally assumed to be a consequence of the mother's HIV infection, a matter of the virus having been transmitted during pregnancy, in the course of labor and delivery, or via breastfeeding. There was no good way around this. To suggest that Karabo contracted HIV outside perinatal infection—that is, to reveal Karabo's HIV-positive status but deny her own—would be to raise the disturbing possibility that Karabo had acquired the infection via sexual abuse or witchcraft.[4] Moreover, should Maikutlo disrupt her relationship with Thato, she and her children might find themselves with nowhere to stay. Maikutlo wanted to manage her relationship with Thato carefully. They had only begun the relationship a year ago, she told us, and while she felt Thato cared for her and wanted to have children with her, she feared that he did not care for the children she already had, adding that Thato sometimes "chased" the children (i.e., threatened them with punishment, possibly corporal punishment) and shouted at them.[5] The relationship was not yet secure enough for her to discuss these matters with Thato. One of the Clinic nurses, she told us, had tried to facilitate matters, offering to moderate a meeting between Thato and Maikutlo. Maikutlo had dismissed this suggestion out of hand.

Patrick gently suggested that the recent loss of Maikutlo's pregnancy had made her relationship with Thato rocky and wondered aloud if another pregnancy might help solidify it (cf. J. L. Comaroff and J. Comaroff 2001; Townsend 1997). The heart of Maikutlo's agitation, however, lay elsewhere: When Karabo had begun taking ARVs, Clinic staff had carefully counseled her that she must ensure that Karabo never missed a dose of his medications. Now the Clinic was making it impossible for her to do this because she would not disclose her status to Thato. "Is it OK that the medications have been stopped?" she asked us. Patrick and I glanced at each other, unsure how to reply. Patrick told her that if Karabo's *masole a mmele*—Setswana for "soldiers of the body" and a common gloss for CD4 cells, the white blood cells targeted by HIV—were strong, then he was not at risk, but the doctors would want to monitor the *masole*.[6] Wanting to reassure her, I added that if the *masole* were too few, the doctors would have to begin Karabo's medications again to prevent him from becoming ill. "Did they check the *masole*?" Patrick asked. Maikutlo replied that they had, but she had forgotten to ask whether they were strong or weak. Patrick and I were equivocating, and Maikutlo knew it. Karabo began to fuss, and as Maikutlo picked him up from the floor, she pressed us again: Was the Clinic harming her child by taking away his medications?

Saving Medicines versus Saving Children

Why would the Clinic save Karabo's life only to take away his medications, deliberately withholding the very objects that stood between Karabo's life and his death? This chapter focuses on adherence assessments, the processes by which Clinic staff determined whether children, with the help of others, were taking their medications as directed. I look beyond the practicality of adherence assessments as imagined by Clinic staff in order to examine their transformative effects on the people involved, that is, children, their families, and the Clinic staff, as well as their effects on ARVs and the Clinic itself. Through adherence assessments, I argue, the Clinic's pediatricians attempted to remake relations among individuals, establish authority, resacralize medications, and allocate blame through a careful pedagogical process. They did this, I show, by scaling adherence: positioning viruses, children, families, nations, medications, and the globe relative to one another and relative to time.

Tensions around the preservation of effective treatments and the looming threat of drug resistance, around physician authority and patient autonomy, and around individual lives and public welfare have shaped the epidemic from its very beginning. Indeed, as late as 2002, even after Botswana had begun to roll out public treatment, health researchers and policymakers alike argued forcefully that scarce funds were more wisely spent on prevention, claiming that ARVs in developing countries were not cost effective and that they held the potential to generate drug-resistant strains of HIV via "antiretroviral anarchy," an imagined "superbug" that crystallized and reinforced the security logics of global health (Crane 2013, chap. 1; cf. King 2002; Lakoff 2010). And while these arguments over clinical practice and health policy focused on patients' ability to adhere to treatment, Johanna Crane argues these disputes reflected broader debates over "inequality, citizenship, and Africa's relationship to globalization and modernity" (2013, 26). Adherence emerged as an index not only of the capacity of an individual patient to consume medications as directed but the capacity of African practitioners to administer these medications and monitor their use, and the capacity of African health systems to ensure drug supply and quality. It reflected the ability of Africans to engage a technology that Western policymakers framed as incompatible not only with poor infrastructure but with the position of the category of "Africa" in a linear developmental frame whereby paved roads, electricity, and more "basic" healthcare—themselves all indices of collective rational self-regulation—both preceded and justified the use of more "sophisticated" technologies like ARVs and cell phones (Crane 2013, 35–36; Ferguson 2006a). Adherence, in short, is profoundly scalar, expanding from viruses to individual patients to entire continents and, indeed, the whole world, and from viral mutation to moral subjectivity.[7]

Writing about the "deeper moral contours of clinical work," Paul Brodwin argues that clinicians experience a sense of futility not as a result of treating serious or even fatal conditions, but in the disjuncture between what they perceived as a necessary intervention and their capacity to intervene (2011, 189). I argue that pediatricians reframed the activity of seeing one HIV-positive child after another all day long by scaling it within understandings of a broader epidemic unfolding through time and of adherence as something with ramifications far beyond one child's body. By strictly policing adherence, pediatricians could regard themselves as intervening in a global epidemic one child at a time. "The argument against treating AIDS in Africa," argues Crane, "was remarkable in that it succeeded in framing the withholding of treatment from millions of people . . . as beneficial to public health" (2013, 34) because it preserved the efficacy of a small handful of medications. What is remarkable about adherence assessments, in contrast, is how they cast one child's adherence, and the efforts of an individual pediatrician to preserve that child's adherence, in terms of a capacity to save the world.

Yet, this optimistic project all too easily faltered. Even as the Clinic's pediatricians regarded the act of treating an individual child in terms of a broader epidemic, their efforts at scaling at times collapsed. While policing children's adherence might present a way of intervening in the broader epidemic, the obstacles American pediatricians perceived to children's adherence also pointed far beyond an individual child's body to include her family and more abstract and seemingly more insurmountable factors such as Tswana kinship norms. Faced with a child with poor adherence, pediatricians considered the harm that might ensue from withholding a child's ARVs against the harm that might ensue should the child develop resistance to those medications. But they also wrestled with scale, that is, balancing the harm caused to one child by withholding his ARVs against the good done by preventing that child from developing a drug-resistant strain of HIV that he might transmit to others in the future: saving medications versus saving children.

Maikutlo and Karabo's story draws our attention to the scale-making practices of pediatric HIV treatment: how Maikutlo's reluctance to disclose her HIV-positive status to Thato became part of Karabo's infection; how Karabo's missed doses became part of maintaining the efficacy of his medications; how the efficacy of Karabo's medications became part of broader anxieties about the feasibility of HIV treatment in Africa and the threats it posed. I sketch a brief history of the Superlative Clinic and its relationship to Referral Hospital. I then turn to the specifies of pediatric HIV treatment relative to adult models of adherence before turning to adherence assessments in action that illustrate how Clinic pediatricians projected poor adherence onto children's kin and, in some instances, onto Tswana sociality itself. Clinic pediatricians wielded adherence assessments, I argue, as a powerful and flexible tool to position viruses, children, families, nations, medications, the globe, and even their own actions, radically transforming their relationships one to another.

The Superlative Clinic

In what is now a common story of the epidemic at the turn of the century, pediatric HIV treatment in Botswana emerged from relationships among clinicians connecting the Global North and Global South. It was prefigured not by analogous treatment programs for other diseases in southern Africa but by the expansion of clinical research that accompanied both the HIV pandemic and post–Cold War geopolitical and economic rearrangements (Crane 2013; Nguyen 2005; Petryna 2009; Street 2014). In 1999, before Botswana's public treatment program had begun, a chance meeting between Dr. Buyaga, a Kenyan physician who was then head of the Pediatrics Department at Referral Hospital, and Dr. Grossman, an American pediatric infectious disease specialist who had become involved treating HIV-infected children in orphanages in Romania in the mid-1990s, laid the foundation for a clinical trial at Referral Hospital.[8] The trial was designed to evaluate the efficacy of a combination of two ARVs against the three-drug regimen that had become the standard of care in the US and elsewhere. The clinical trial, Dr. Buyaga explained to me in 2007, had seemed optimal at the time because ARVs were not yet publicly available in Botswana and the two physicians had hoped the two-drug combination would prove to be cheaper and perhaps even more easily tolerated by children.

The same year the trial began, UNICEF launched a pilot program investigating the feasibility and acceptability of programs to prevent mother-to-child transmission (PMTCT) of HIV in several African countries. These programs offered HIV testing to pregnant women and provided those who tested positive with a short course of ARVs that reduced the likelihood that the child they carried would contract the virus.[9] In 2001, as plans for a national public treatment program were underway, Botswana's government incorporated UNICEF's PMTCT program into its national health services. PMTCT was designed to interrupt HIV transmission and decrease the number of seropositive infants, but as screening pregnant women and their newborns for HIV became increasingly routinized and public awareness of the national treatment program grew, young children with chronic poor health were more frequently referred for an HIV test or, if they were admitted to a hospital, tested for HIV in the process, thereby creating a growing population of HIV-positive children enrolled in treatment.[10]

Buyaga and Grossman's first trial was halted in 2002 when the government of Botswana began rolling out treatment based on a three-drug regimen. By this time, however, the two physicians had turned their attention to establishing an outpatient clinic dedicated to pediatric HIV with the support of the American medical school that employed Grossman and the NGO he had founded, the Children's HIV/AIDS Network (CHAN), to promote his efforts to expand treatment for HIV-positive children. Modeled after the clinic Grossman had helped found in Romania, the Superlative Clinic in Gaborone opened in June 2003, with Dr. Buyaga as its director. It was located on the grounds of Referral Hospital, and Botswana's Ministry of Health, which governed the hospital, provided utilities, some medications, and laboratory support while sharing staffing and administrative costs with CHAN. During my fieldwork, the Superlative Clinic in Gaborone served as the "flagship" clinic in a network of clinics that CHAN developed across sub-Saharan Africa, each linked to Grossman's clinic in Romania, which retained its archetypal status, and his medical school and supported by the philanthropic arms of various pharmaceutical companies. At the time of my fieldwork, CHAN claimed that the Gaborone Clinic had the largest number of children enrolled in ARV therapy on the continent. As outpatient treatment for pediatric HIV rapidly expanded, Buyaga and Grossman began a second clinical trial that fit within the parameters of the national treatment program's guidelines.[11]

When I began observing at the Clinic in January 2007, tensions were running high between the Clinic and the rest of the hospital, as well as among factions of the Clinic staff themselves. In the first few years of the Clinic's operations, physicians in the hospital's Pediatrics Department had referred increasing numbers of HIV-positive children to the Superlative for follow-up care and outpatient treatment. The work of treating this rapidly growing population of children, however, had fallen largely to the Pediatrics Department's medical officers (MOs) who staffed the Clinic at the time, creating a bridge of sorts between the inpatient pediatric medical ward and the Clinic. The Clinic's reliance on these MOs, however, drew personnel away from the inpatient pediatric ward, generating friction between the new head of pediatrics and Dr. Buyaga. At the height of these tensions in 2005, half of the Pediatrics Department's physicians had resigned over working conditions, and the head of pediatrics withdrew most of the department's remaining MOs from the Clinic, insisting they were needed on the inpatient ward. Dr. Buyaga complained to CHAN, which responded to the Clinic's staffing crisis by sending the Squad, ten young American pediatricians, many of whom had only just completed their residencies and whom CHAN had recruited to serve one- or two-year contracts funded by the philanthropic arm of a major pharmaceutical manufacturer.

The arrival of the Squad pediatricians in August 2006 did nothing to ease tensions between the Clinic and the Pediatrics Department; instead, it reinforced the Clinic's isolation from the rest of the hospital. The Squad pediatricians had undergone a month-long training in the clinical management of pediatric HIV at Grossman's medical school, but they arrived in Botswana with no cultural orientation, no language instruction in Setswana, and no sense that these might be of any value. They also arrived bereft of leadership: Dr. Amy, the Clinic's American associate director who had been in Gaborone since 2003, was away on maternity leave, and Dr. Buyaga was out of the country. Dr. Motlhabane, a Motswana MO who had been treating HIV-positive children for years and who had worked hard to gain Dr. Amy's trust and fought to retain his position at the Clinic in the face of institutional turmoil, organized an orientation for the Squad. The

Squad refused to acknowledge his authority on the grounds that he lacked a pediatrician's credentials.

All this set the tone for relations between the Clinic and the hospital. The memorandum of understanding (MOU) between CHAN and the MOH stipulated that Squad pediatricians offered care under the auspices of Botswana's treatment program in accordance with MOH guidelines and that, like all other foreign practitioners, they were subject to Botswana's medical regulations. The Squad pediatricians, however, were determined to uphold the Clinic's mission to "elevate the standard of pediatric care in Botswana" and armed with what they considered universally applicable "best practices" backed by evidence-based medicine, asserted their authority to both dictate the terms of the Clinic's practice and to evaluate local practitioners' expertise, even barring some of the Pediatrics Department's MOs from the Clinic despite the MOs' long experience treating HIV-positive children.[12] Derisive toward what they regarded as these physicians' lack of training and lackadaisical, even negligent attitudes toward children's adherence, Squad pediatricians regarded physicians in Botswana's public sector as objects of mentorship at best, admitting very few as colleagues. Dr. Motlhabane, due in part to the close relationship he had formed with Dr. Amy prior to the Squad's arrival, retained his post at the Clinic, as did Dr. Chibesa, another MO in government service. But for most of my fieldwork, these two, along with Dr. Buyaga and an East African physician hired under the auspices of the Clinic's ongoing clinical trial, were the only African physicians in the Clinic. Unaddressed, these tensions grew ugly: More than four months after the Squad's arrival, Dr. Chibesa speculated to Dr. Rachel, a Squad pediatrician, that the reason most Squad pediatricians regularly failed to greet their Batswana colleagues upon arrival at the Clinic each day, a deeply antisocial practice suggestive of witchcraft (Alverson 1978; Livingston 2005, 2008), was that "they just don't like Black people." Relations between the Squad and the Clinic's nurses were less starkly negative. Squad pediatricians, reliant on nurses for clinical labor and translation, tended to regard them ambivalently, deriding them less systematically than they did the MOs. The nurses, supervised by Mma Kgosietsile rather than Dr. Amy, tended to keep to themselves, yet some complained to me that, rather than engaging in the practical work of nursing, they had been reduced to translating and the monotony of adherence assessments.

As the only specialized pediatric HIV clinic in the country, the Clinic endeavored to capture the population of HIV-positive children in southeastern Botswana and even as far as the Central District and the western edges of Kweneng and Southern districts, distances of more than three hundred kilometers from Gaborone. Many children had been referred from other public clinics and hospitals as infants or in early childhood, and Squad pediatricians encouraged this. Once Clinic staff had enrolled a child, they were loath to refer that child to another facility even if the child resided in a town where ARVs treatment was now available, arguing that children were not "little adults" and required specialized treatment that only pediatricians provided. In so doing, the Clinic also strove to establish the parameters of the pediatric subject. Across the public health system, children older than thirteen received treatment on adult wards, though children under eighteen could not make medical decisions on their own behalf and required a parent's or guardian's consent. Squad pediatricians balked at the fact that Batswana adolescents could not make their own medical decisions but also balked at sending those adolescents to the adult ARV clinics or the adult medical wards even as some children approached late adolescence.

These disagreements reflected a more fundamental disjuncture between Americans and Batswana regarding childhood and adolescence. Deborah Durham notes that for Tswana people, "social and behavioral factors"—not biological ones—"primarily distinguish various ages" (Durham 2004, 594; cf. Suggs 1987). One's status as a child, in other words, is assessed not in terms of age but in terms of one's capacity to be responsible for oneself and, perhaps more importantly, for others. The Tswana women I interviewed at the Clinic and in their homes frequently gauged a child's maturity in terms of her ability to undertake household tasks, such as cooking, cleaning, and minding younger children; they avoided naming an age at which a child could be held responsible for taking her medication without supervision. That said, most women expected children to take on a greater share of household labor than American pediatricians generally anticipated, and they expected a child to take ever more responsibility for the household as she grew. The idea of adolescence as a time of general rebelliousness did not have much traction, at least in the ideal (but cf. Dahl 2015, 2016). This view contrasted starkly with Americans' insistence that adolescents required more supervision than did little children. But even as Tswana adults expected children to contribute to household welfare in ways that mirrored their increasing capabilities, these adults remained suspect about even older children's ability to manage their own affairs, including healthcare decisions.[13]

Under these circumstances, the Squad might have retreated entirely into the Clinic, where their control was most readily, if not totally, maintained (see Brada 2016). Two factors prevented this: First, the MOU governing the Clinic required the Squad to rotate through Referral Hospital's inpatient pediatric medical ward.[14] Squad pediatricians had not anticipated this requirement; many deeply resented it. Beyond the more mundane aggravations of having to be on call at night and working in an unfamiliar setting without familiar resources, Squad pediatricians objected that they were being used as general pediatricians and regarded time spent on the ward as a misuse of their specialized knowledge. In other words, they refused to scale their knowledge and practice beyond pediatric HIV treatment within the Clinic. Second, two Squad pediatricians, Dr. Alison and Dr. James, organized "outreach" day trips to smaller hospitals in Botswana's southeast, intending to mentor MOs in general pediatrics as well as the clinical management of HIV by giving lectures, rounding in teams, and consulting on difficult cases. The two pediatricians argued fervently that their most significant contribution lay outside Referral Hospital as well as the Clinic but grew frustrated when the MOs they sought to mentor took their arrival as an opportunity for a break, or arranged for Squad pediatricians to treat patients alone rather than accompanied by an MO. "We're just seeing patients," Dr. Alison protested when her plans for outreach fell apart. "We're not building capacity." In sum, the site and scope of the Squad's activities oscillated unpredictably between the Clinic's tiny consulting rooms and Botswana's countryside and between one child and the national public health system as pediatricians attempted to scale the site of their intervention to their capacity to intervene.

The Specificities of Pediatric Adherence

These tensions over expertise, over ownership of the Clinic as an institution and over the terms of encounter between visiting Americans and Batswana crystallized in understandings of children as a vulnerable population and, in particular, over adherence as the key to their survival. Transnational HIV-related interventions frequently point to the defectiveness of local parenting practices (Wardlow 2012), and these criticisms have roots both in colonial projects and in the establishment through the twentieth century of children as a uniquely vulnerable population (Malkki 2010; Rosen 2007; Wark 1995; cf. Ticktin 2017). The idea of children's universal vulnerability, Didier Fassin (2013, 118) argues, has implied the culpability of their families and justified the intervention of public and private institutions in children's welfare. In the context of the African AIDS epidemic, he continues, "children become victims not just of disease but also of their parents . . . their parents appear incapable of assisting them, being either too ill or simply indifferent or irresponsible" (2013, 119). Squad pediatricians frequently articulated these attitudes: As I sat writing field notes in a corner of a consultation room, Dr. Wyatt, a self-styled sardonic Texan, joked drily to a visiting American resident: "Betsey's writing, 'These people [i.e., adult Batswana] are terrible. They don't take care of their kids.'"

Moreover, children's vulnerability vis-à-vis their families was heightened by their dependence on others for consistently administering their ARVs. While adult adherence models assume that the repercussions for poor adherence will ultimately manifest themselves on the body of the person held responsible for ensuring adherence, in pediatric HIV treatment responsibility for consumption and the act of consumption itself are distributed among two different subjects. For pediatricians, a child's body might reflect an adult's care and attention, or it might corporeally manifest an adult's failure to give the child her medications properly, a failure for which the child might suffer but could not be held responsible.[15] To compound problems, patients frequently could not give an account of themselves to their pediatricians, being too young to provide what pediatricians considered reliable recollections of their past actions, and perhaps too young to even speak at all. Pediatricians, in short, frequently grew frustrated as they relied on adult caregivers not only to administer children's medications but also to represent children's actions, experiences, thoughts, and emotions that were often further mediated through a nurse's interpretation from Setswana to English.[16]

Thus, while the adherence assessments that consumed so much time in the Clinic were ostensibly focused on a child's body, these activities made sense in terms of a scalar logic. In terms of temporality, pediatricians assumed HIV-positive children would require ARVs for all of their lives, selected from a finite (albeit slowly increasing) number of existing ARVs, only a subset of which were stocked in Botswana's national pharmacopeia. Pediatricians calibrated viral mutation, then, not only against a timeline of drug development but also a timeline of national development, that is, the medications that the government of Botswana could be expected to provide its citizenry. Pediatricians also calibrated viral mutation against children's unfolding sexual activity. As HIV-positive children have begun living into adolescence, the stakes in their survival have become more complex (Domek 2006; Gray 2010). Writing about Botswana, Beth Barr notes that, "The spread of drug-resistant HIV by youth in the future would have overwhelming implications for the cost and availability of ARV treatment in newly diagnosed patients" (2006, 26–27). A child's imperfect adherence to her regimen, then, threatened not only her health as an individual but also the epidemic's management more broadly in the sense that a child approaching adolescence who developed a drug-resistant strain of HIV might spread this strain to others directly through unprotected sex (Barr 2006). Even a child as young as Karabo was subject to these calculations. And while the pathological sign of drug resistance lay in an individual child's body, Squad pediatricians readily rescaled the source of the problem to include a child's immediate family members, Tswana norms regarding kinship and child socialization, a reified and demonized "Tswana culture," and the lurking stereotype of the dark heart of "African AIDS."[17]

Kgomotso: Adherence Assessments in Action

Mma Kgomotso arrived at the Clinic carrying tiny Kgomotso, aged four months, on her back, and a plastic bag full of all of Kgomotso's liquid medications in several 240-mL bottles. Kgomotso was taking the Clinic's standard regimen of three antiretroviral medications, a multivitamin, and a prophylactic antibiotic.[18] Mma Mokento, the nurse working with a Squad pediatrician named Dr. Alison, poured the contents of each of Kgomotso's medications into measuring cylinders one by one, rinsing the cylinders at the sink between each measurement, while Dr. Alison asked after Kgomotso's health and inquired about Mma Kgomotso's own CD4 count. The medications' consistencies made them challenging to measure: nevirapine was the consistency of hair conditioner, thick and semitranslucent; lamivudine, a clear syrup, was incredibly sticky. Some medication was unavoidably lost in the pouring back and forth between bottle and cylinder, and Mma Mokento lamented the inaccuracy of the measurements compared to counting tablets and capsules. Mma Mokento recorded the amounts of medication on Kgomotso's file, checked them against the pharmacist's record of the amounts given at Kgomotso's last appointment, and, pulling her cell phone from her pocket, calculated whether the correct amount had been consumed. While she did this, Dr. Alison examined the baby's body, looking for signs of illness before turning to the computer to retrieve the results of laboratory tests performed since Kgomotso's last appointment and to document Kgomotso's adherence, her physical condition, and Mma Kgomotso's responses.

Inside the Clinic's consultation rooms, the first order of business was not the state of a child's body but the state of the child's medications, that is, an assessment of the child's adherence. At the heart of the adherence assessment was the pill count. Nurses looked first for the drug sheet, a piece of paper on which a Clinic pharmacist should have recorded at the child's last appointment the amount of each medication that was dispensed and the date. Caregivers handed over their supply of unconsumed medications to the nurse. Using the dates and amounts listed on the drug sheet, the nurse calculated the amount of syrup or number of pills she expected to find in the bottles and packets the caregiver had handed her and compared them with what she actually found. Pharmacists normally dispensed a small amount of each medication beyond what was strictly necessary for a child between one appointment and the next to prevent the child missing doses in case circumstances should arise that prevented a child and her caregiver from attending the Clinic on the date indicated. The pill count was accompanied by a careful interrogation. Pediatricians and nurses questioned caregivers about the medicines, asking in a variety of ways whether there had been any

HOSPITAL PHARMACY ADHERENCE CHART FOR IDCC

NAME: _____ ACCOUNT NUMBER: _____

ITEM NO.	DATE →	A / B						
	DRUG ↓	A \ B	A = LEFT OVER		B = A+DISPENSED			
1.	CBV							
2.	NVP 200mg							
3.	NVP SYP							
4.	EFV 50mg							
5.	EFV 200mg							
6.	EFV 600mg							
7.	3TC							
8.	3TC SYP							
9.	D4T 15mg							
10.	D4T 20mg							
11.	D4T 30mg							
12.	D4T 40mg							
13.	D4T SUSP 10mg/ml							
14.	DDI 100mg							
15.	DDI 250mg							
16.	DDI 400mg							
17.	DDI SYP							
18.	DDI 25mg							
19.	DDI 50mg							
20.	AZT 100mg							
21.	AZT SYP							
22.	ABC							
23.	ABC SYP							
24.	RIT							
25.	SAQ							
26.	INV							
27.	KAL CAP							
28.	KAL SYP							
29.	ALUVIA TAB							

FIGURE 2. Drug sheet (Brian Edward Balsley, GISP)

problems with adherence. One American medical student explained to me that instead of asking, "Did you miss any pills?" one ought to ask, "How many pills did you miss?" and "Is there one you don't like?" thereby offering, the theory went, a less judgmental environment in which patients or caregivers could admit to missed doses.

Armed with plastic pill counter trays, graduated cylinders for liquids, and calculators or cell phones, nurses conducting pill counts sometimes found the amount of medication they expected, but many times they did not. Instances in which nurses found fewer pills than they expected presented several possibilities: Pharmacists might have recorded amounts incorrectly; medications, especially syrups, might have spilled; a child might have vomited after a dose and required an extra one. Caregivers, occupied with caring for a child or children, sometimes left heavy bottles of medication at home. Clinic staff, including pharmacists, chastised them for this because not knowing how much of each medication remained made it difficult to predict how much nurses ought to expect caregivers to bring to a subsequent visit. But while finding fewer pills than expected threatened to disrupt the record-keeping that ongoing adherence assessments entailed, finding more medication than expected, that is, pills or syrup that should have been consumed, was a cause for immediate alarm, a sign of "poor adherence" with all its ramifications. Faced with a child such as Karabo, who Clinic staff had identified as having "poor adherence" or, more importantly, a perceived pattern of poor adherence, the pediatricians might decide to halt a child's treatment. Ideally, clinicians imagined this temporary cessation of treatment as an opportunity to help the child's caregivers, with the assistance of key Batswana staff, identify and remove obstacles to adherence while still preserving the medications' efficacy by preventing intermittent exposure, that is, "stopping" them in order to "save" them.

Yet diagnoses of poor adherence, for all their disrupted consequences, were not nearly so straightforward as they might seem at first glance. In the instance that there were more pills or syrup than expected, pediatricians and nurses first questioned the caregiver. A caregiver sometimes admitted to having missed a dose or two or explained that she had left the child in the care of another person who had failed to give the child the medications. Some caregivers insisted that no doses had been missed or blamed a pharmacist's faulty record-keeping. Pediatricians compared caregivers' claims to other available points of data, including the amount of the discrepancy, the child's physical health, and the results of the child's most recent blood tests, as well as the child's triage measurements from that morning and any record of past adherence patterns in the child's medical records, a complex assemblage of paper and electronic documents. For example, an excess of pills and an increased viral load, that is, the number of copies

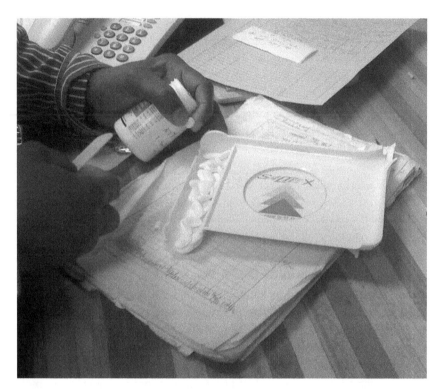

FIGURE 3. Counting pills in the Superlative Clinic pharmacy (photo by the author)

of the virus per milliliter of blood, might corroborate one another in indicating missed doses. No one method, however, was considered entirely reliable: Caregivers might not reveal their own or their family member's failure to monitor doses; pharmacists and nurses might miscount the pills; the child's medical records might be missing; the hospital's labs may have failed to perform, have improperly performed, or have lost a child's laboratory tests; a minor infection might cause an increase in the number of copies of the virus in the child's blood. Much to the deep and abiding frustration of the pediatricians of the Superlative Clinic, it could be difficult to determine whether a spike in a child's viral load was a sign of poor adherence, a common cold, or both.

Tshenolo

One morning in early April 2007 Tshenolo, aged twelve, arrived at the Clinic with her mother and her father for a checkup. She had just returned from Camp Lesego, the sleep-away camp run by the Clinic for ninety or so of their

HIV-positive patients aged nine to fourteen during the week-long school holidays that preceded Easter. Most of the children recruited to take part in Camp Lesego had been identified by Clinic staff as having poor adherence, a bad social situation, or often both. The camp had been held at a nearby private secondary school. Tshenolo and the other children had spent the nights in the school's dormitories, supervised by a cadre of volunteer counselors, including Peace Corps volunteers, visiting American medical students, and a few older students from the school. The campers spent the days rotating among sports, arts and crafts, and "life skills" sessions, such as a cooking class intended to encourage the children to consume nutritious foods. Counselors had collected all the children's medications upon their arrival at the school and then distributed each child's dose to them at mealtimes, where their consumption had been meticulously supervised by the Clinic's pediatricians (Brada 2019).

Because Tshenolo was known to Clinic staff to have a history of poor adherence, she was seen by Dr. Amy, the Superlative Clinic's Associate Director. Dr. Amy was so petite that she barely reached my shoulder, but she was not a woman to trifle with: her stature belied her forthright manner and sheer force of will. Unlike many of the Squad pediatricians, she had arrived in Botswana with previous experience treating HIV-positive children in clinical settings in the US. She was more familiar than many Squad pediatrician with ARV treatment and more accustomed to working with children and their families on adherence. Clinic staff referred particularly difficult cases to her, and some children with ongoing problems, such as Tshenolo, were scheduled specifically to see her rather than seeing the first pediatrician available as most children did. Looking Tshenolo over, Dr. Amy commented that she was looking well. As Dr. Amy began looking up the results of Tshenolo's most recent viral load test on the Clinic's computer system, she reminded the girl that her viral load test the previous month had been markedly high. "And that," she reminded the girl, "was how we *knew* there was a problem with you taking your meds." Giving Tshenolo, who was just about her own height, a level gaze, she said, "At Camp we could *see* you were taking your meds," adding with emphasis, "*That's* why you look better now."

Tshenolo's parents were both HIV positive, both on ARV treatment. Both had suppressed viral loads, and both insisted they watched Tshenolo take her medications. "I know from her blood tests she's not taking them," Dr. Amy maintained. Other pediatricians in the Clinic had suggested that Tshenolo could have developed a resistance to her ARVs, in which case even perfect adherence would fail to result in a suppressed viral load, but Dr. Amy had dismissed these suggestions. "I need to talk to Tshenolo alone," she told Tshenolo's parents firmly and marched the girl out of the examination room. Turning in the corridor to face Tshenolo more or less at eye level, Dr. Amy drilled her: "I *know* you're not taking them," she shot at the girl. "Why not?" Tshenolo traced a circle on the floor with her toe, played with the hem of her skirt and finally mumbled, "I just don't want to." When we re-entered the exam room, Tshenolo's parents were already trading accusations, each blaming the other for failing to realize Tshenolo had only been pretending to take her pills and had been throwing them away instead. "Parents always try," Dr. Amy told me later. "They just don't always succeed."

That adherence assessments posed an epistemological conundrum is only part of the story. Like the story of Maikutlo and Karabo, this set of interactions shows how Clinic staff, and pediatricians in particular, could use adherence assessments to powerfully remake relationships between Clinic staff and parents, between pediatricians and their patients, and even between parents and children. In the encounter mentioned previously Dr. Amy emerges as a figure capable of knowing things about children that even their parents do not and cannot know. Unlike Tshenolo's parents, Dr. Amy could extract Tshenolo's confession. But unlike Tshenolo's parents, Dr. Amy did not, in fact, need Tshenolo's confession to conclude her assessment of poor adherence. Instead, Dr. Amy positioned herself such that only through her could parents know what their children had done with their medications. Parents' knowledge of and representations of their children's actions, in short, required expert verification.

This was a profound assertion of the Clinic's authority. Dr. Amy maintained that even in the absence of definitive clues, she could discern poor adherence in her patients. "You just *know*," she insisted. "You can just tell." This ability to "just know" was, for Dr. Amy, a crucial component of professional expertise necessary to treat children with HIV, and she demanded the Squad pediatricians develop it. She grew frustrated with Squad pediatricians who, in her view, were overly hesitant to diagnose poor adherence and even more frustrated with doctors in the public health system, whom she criticized for their reliance on Botswana's national treatment guidelines. "You can't use them [the guidelines] like a cookbook!" she told me in exasperation. In these aspects, Dr. Amy resembled Bourdieu's "virtuoso," who "with a perfect mastery of his 'art of living' can play on all the resources inherent in the ambiguities and indeterminacies of behaviors and situations so as to produce the actions appropriate in each case, to do at the right moment that of which people will say 'There was nothing else to be done'" (1990, 107).

But in addition to framing the Clinic as a crucible for the radical transformation of social relations and the assertion of the Clinic's authoritative insights into children's behavior, Clinic staff used adherence assessments to insist on the exceptional nature of ARVs as objects. In Botswana's national health system many medications are dispensed free of charge or for nominal fees, and while

Batswana may fault the system for the quality of its services and even doubt bio-medicine's curative and diagnostic powers, this does not mean they do not value biomedical medications (Livingston 2004). Indeed, pills and tablets—particularly analgesics as encased in small plastic packets—are the ubiquitous sign of biomedical care in Botswana with all its limitations and disappointments (Livingston 2005, 2012) and a powerful manifestations of the state's commitment to its citizens. In contrast to the state public health bureaucracy, which had a vital stake in increasing the availability of ARVs, expanding their circulation and thereby positioning itself as the provider of abundance (Gulbrandsen 2012), Clinic staff sought to re-inscribe upon ARVs an aura of scarcity, to fetishize them, and to recruit caregivers and, especially, children themselves to recognize their power. Rather than regarding them as objects that merely improved an individual child's health or indexed the power of the postcolonial state, the Clinic's American pediatricians sought to frame ARVs as objects that held the capacity to save the world—and that they, as benevolent far-sighted experts, might need to withhold from children, families, even nations if the medications' scalar implications were not appreciated.[19] As chapter 2 illustrates, children beyond toddlerhood received careful instruction at each Clinic visit, learning to name each of the pills and recite the amounts they swallowed each morning and evening. Pediatricians frequently asked children to recall how sick they had been before they began ARV therapy or how sick poor adherence had made them, emphasizing the ongoing capacity of ARVs to transform children's bodies and lives. Through these assessments, Clinic staff insisted upon their power to verify adherence, to distribute or withhold ARVs, and to demand Batswana reconstitute their familial relationships in terms of the limits of ARVs reframed as children's needs.

The Bad Social Situation

It was with regard to adherence that Tswana kin relations were most pathologized within the Clinic. In the Clinic's terms, any adult responsible for a child's well-being was categorized as "caregiver," a term seemingly neutral with regard to the specific relationship to the child in question (e.g., mother, maternal aunt, paternal grandmother, adult sibling) and that on its face recognized the profound impact of Botswana's epidemic on how care among kin, and particularly care for children, was envisioned and carried out. But this seeming neutrality barely masked a deep ambivalence among American pediatricians toward Tswana social relations. On the one hand, pediatricians deployed the term "caregiver" to indicate that the specificities of the relationship between adult and child were immaterial as long as the child's ARVs were given consistently, the child's well-being was maintained, and the social relationship on which the child's adherence rested remained stable. On the other hand, Squad pediatricians, dependent on nurses to translate both what caregivers said and to situate caregivers' accounts against local kinship norms, were often quick to diagnose a "bad social situation" when faced with what they perceived to be disruptors to adherence, such as a child's moving among different households or among different sets of kin. While pediatricians avoided blaming children for their own nonadherence, in short, they did so by displacing blame not merely onto specific Tswana families, but frequently onto Tswana sociality more broadly.

A diagnosis of "a bad social situation" often emerged dialectically with a diagnosis of poor adherence; one frequently suggested the other, though it was possible, even heroic, for an individual caregiver or older child to maintain adherence in a bad social situation. For Clinic staff, the heart of the matter lay in determining whether a bad social situation posed an intractable barrier to adherence. "If we start a kid with a bad social situation on treatment," Dr. Amy commented once, "we might be hurting more than we're helping," that is, creating a situation wherein a child rapidly developed resistance and thereby reduced her treatment options. Many of the problems that characterized a bad social situation were, arguably, the purview of the social workers of Botswana's Department of Social Services tasked with providing services to orphans and vulnerable children (see Dahl 2009, 2014). Clinic staff did sometimes try to facilitate interactions between caregivers and social workers when it came to food baskets and other material services. More frequently, however, Clinic staff attempted to assess and intervene in the familial relationships that, in their eyes, disrupted the conditions for a child's adherence, "stopping" a child's ARVs until the adults who Clinic staff considered relevant to the situation agreed to a meeting at the Clinic, such as the meeting that Clinic staff had offered to convene on Maikutlo's behalf.

These meetings, conducted almost entirely in Setswana, were facilitated by Batswana staff, most frequently Koketso, the Clinic's trainee social worker, assisted by Mma Kgosietsile, whose age, professional rank, and personal background combined to make her the kind of *mosadi mogolo* (great or respected woman) who could both chide younger adults about their failure to take responsibility and speak to older adults without having to defer to them as seniors, as Koketso did. Batswana regard close kin relations as both somatic and sentimental, holding the potential to reciprocally "build up" bodies or induce physical illness through actions that constitute relationships over time (J. L. Comaroff and J. Comaroff 2001; Klaits 2010; Livingston 2008). Drawing on the idiom of family meetings that are often the locus of collective, if hierarchical, decision-making in Botswana, Mma Kgosietsile, Koketso, and other Batswana staff alternately scolded, exhorted, and cajoled adults to recognize and value their connections to children. "No, no," Dr. Motlhabane interjected, *Lo losika, lo tshwanetse go thusana* [You are family (lit. a vein), you must help one another], chiding one child's recalcitrant aunt, reminding the woman of her obligation to her niece just as the woman's elder brother might have done. Many children attending the Clinic had lost at least one parent, and while the vast majority of children remained with kin and Batswana continued to value such kin-based forms of care, the epidemic, as elsewhere in southern Africa, has transformed kinship, making it difficult for Batswana to care for their kin or demand care from them (Dahl 2009, 2014; cf. Block and McGrath 2019).[20] A young man in his early twenties, consumed with misery at the prospect of giving up his government scholarship to study graphic design in South Africa, stared at the floor as Mma Kgosietsile gently pointed out the skinny bodies, flaky skin, and swollen, bloodshot eyes of his younger siblings, aged eleven and thirteen, that bore witness to their elderly relatives' unwillingness or inability to supervise their treatment. Like other events, including births and weddings and, increasingly, funerals, that require Batswana to "reassess the terms of their familiarity with one another" (Klaits 2005, 48), meetings at the Clinic to assess a bad social situation forced Tswana to reckon kin ties and the obligations attendant upon them. Crammed into the small space of an examination room, these adults had to determine who would take responsibility for not only for a child but for her medications as well.

My argument is not that pediatricians diagnosed bad social situations in bad faith or that conflict within families did not negatively impact children's health. Instead, I draw attention to how these meetings revealed the fantasies and contradictions at the heart of the Clinic's attitude toward caregivers. The goal was deceptively clear: to arrange for the child's medications to be given consistently. But these negotiations emerged into the clinical gaze partially at best, and the relationships they revealed were often already pathologized in the eyes of Squad pediatricians unfamiliar with, and only ambivalently interested in, Tswana social norms. First, while pediatricians often maintained that it was most important that someone took responsibility as the "primary caregiver," they often grew suspicious of situations wherein that primary caregiver was not the child's mother. The fosterage of children within families, especially between adult sisters and between women and their own mothers, has long been a feature of Tswana kinship, but Squad pediatricians tended to view it with suspicion, particularly if the child's mother was still alive.[21] Second, pediatricians expected caregiving to be flexible in the sense that there should be other adults who could step in when the primary caregiver was unavailable, as in Maikutlo's case. But they regarded children's movement among family members' households, itself a consequence of high mobility among adults, as indicative of a too-flexible arrangement, a sign that a primary caregiver had not adequately assumed responsibility for the child and her ARVs. Third, while pediatricians relied on Batswana staff to translate, the pediatricians themselves often could not determine how much or what type of information they required in order to determine whether a social situation was, in fact, "bad." Dr. Wyatt groaned with exaggerated frustration, cutting off Mma Mokopakgosi, an older nurse, mid-sentence as she haltingly tried to explain that the "auntie" accompanying a child to the Clinic was the child's father's younger brother's wife and not, for example, a sister of either the child's father or mother, or wife of the child's mother's brother.[22] Yet, as often as Squad pediatricians complained about too much information, they complained about too little, reprimanding nurses for describing as a child's "mother" a maternal aunt who had assumed care of a child along with her own children, or using "parents" to encompass a child's elder kin rather than the two individuals of whom the child was the biological offspring.[23]

More than actually revealing or rearranging a child's social relations in a way that optimized adherence, however, the diagnosis of bad social situation and the meetings that produced it radically expanded the Clinic's domain of intervention, bringing an expanding circle of intimate relationships under clinical surveillance. For many Tswana, circumspection is a virtue that cuts across social and political domains (Alverson 1978; Bennett 1997; Gulbrandsen 2012; Klaits 1998; Z. Maundeni 2004; cf. J. L. Comaroff and J. Comaroff 1997b), and managing the concealment of elements of oneself from others, even—and sometimes especially—from close kin is a fundamental element of Tswana conceptualizations of personhood (J. L. Comaroff and J. Comaroff 2001; Durham and Klaits 2002; Lambek and Solway 2001; Livingston 2005, 2008). Yet regardless of how legibly a child's kin ties emerged in these meetings, Clinic staff asserted their demands for clarification, confession, and classification, justifying a drive for surveillance in terms of the needs of ARVs displaced onto and framed as the needs of the child. But pediatricians' ambivalence regarding how much they actually knew or even needed to know about a child's social situation revealed a deeper ambivalence regarding the scope of the Clinic's intervention. The sequential displacement of the object of intervention—from ARV to child, from child to caregiver, from caregiver to bad social situation—presented the possibility of diagnosing Tswana sociality *in toto* as pathogenic, as capable of nullifying children's futures in an apocalypse of national extinction and even global catastrophe. Nonetheless, the Clinic's pediatricians retained, even in the face of this ever-expanding scale of disaster, the power to retreat into the Clinic, into the temporal boundaries of their one- or two-year contracts, into clinical medicine's proper object, that is, the child—or more accurately, the medication—at hand.

"Like They Were Before HAART"

Even though only we two were chatting in her apartment in the quiet, high-walled gated apartment complex that CHAN had arranged as housing for the Squad, Dr. Natalie's voice took on a hushed tone as she told me about a letter sent to the Clinic by a high-ranking pharmacist in Botswana's national health system. In the letter the pharmacist had accused the Squad pediatricians of "killing the children of Botswana," claiming that by stopping medications, the pediatricians were "making things like they were before HAART," that is, before ARVs became publicly available. This was a horrifying accusation, but it was echoed in concerns I heard from MOs at the smaller hospitals around Gaborone, who were reluctant to stop a child's medications in the face of poor adherence not only out of concern for the child's physical well-being but also because withholding the medications, no matter how temporary or well intentioned, too easily resembled for both clinicians and a child's adult kin the nightmare they had only just escaped. Even the Clinic's nurses, drilled in the Clinic's strategies for the long-term preservation of ARVs, whispered or grumbled their misgivings in Setswana, rolling their eyes in impatience when pediatricians cut short their attempts to explain the dynamics of a family struggling in good faith to maintain a child's adherence. If for Squad pediatricians, the "global" in global health was both the site of clinical authority they claimed and the stakes of an uncontrollable drug-resistant epidemic that they felt responsible for forestalling one child at a time, MOs and nurses could still recall a global health that justified the sacrifice of the children in their care in its name.

Squad pediatricians could not solve the problem of adherence—that is, they could not directly supervise the adherence of all the Clinic's children—but quailed in the face of a seemingly pathogenic Tswana sociality. The next chapter turns to how these pediatricians sought to shape children's subjectivities, transforming their own self-understanding in terms of pediatricians' fetishized view of ARVs. The problem of poor adherence, in the eyes of the Squad, could most readily be solved by inculcating in Karabo, Kgomotso, Tshenolo, and others the dispositions necessary for continued adherence, recruiting them to the task of defending both their own bodies and the world itself against antiretroviral anarchy, obviating the need for the inadequate (in the pediatricians' eyes) supervision provided by children's families. Under Americans' careful tutelage, children could learn to save themselves, and indeed the world, by saving their own medications. We will see how, rather than remake children's families or argue with local clinicians over the management of medications, Squad pediatricians sought instead to do things to children with words.

HOW TO DO THINGS TO CHILDREN WITH WORDS

The Superlative Clinic's emphasis on children's speech was unique among the clinical spaces I observed in Botswana.[1] In other settings where children were present, both Batswana and the many foreigners in the national health system tended to direct words of instruction and advice to adults without much expectation of dialogue. "The etiquette of the clinical encounter in Botswana," Julie Livingston observes, "has long been based on a top-down model. Patients do not expect to ask many questions" (2012, 76). In those instances when they spoke to children, most clinicians, including medical officers and nurses, often spoke quickly in long strings of explanation and instruction punctuated by direct questions or requests for confirmation that the listener had understood. Children, prompted by the question, *A o utlwa* [Do you hear or understand], often merely nodded or said little more than *Ee* [yes] in response.[2] None of the parents I spoke with perceived this division of speaking labor as problematic, nor did the Clinic's nurses fear a lack of rapport with children. Across contexts, Tswana children are expected to receive advice in silence (Bagwasi 2012, 189).[3] Several nurses told me that children at the Clinic "should just feel free," that is, relaxed and comfortable, but the nurses' assessment of this sense of well-being did not rest primarily on whether children spoke or what they said. Instead, when nurses noted a child's comfort or happiness, or joked with a child or praised a child's maturity, they focused less on how much a child spoke or what they said, and more on the propriety of a child's actions and demeanor.[4]

Squad pediatricians, by contrast, put a great deal of time and energy into getting children to speak—particularly about themselves. In their exchanges with children, Squad pediatricians posed series of open-ended questions and strove to elicit personal preferences, such as a child's favorite school subject, favorite color, or plans for an upcoming holiday, and regarded a child's reticence as an excess of shyness or deference to be overcome.[5] Unfamiliar with Setswana and Tswana social norms, pediatricians often failed to grasp children's answers, and they often grew frustrated with children's one-word responses (and nurses' one-word translations). But the significance of the exchange lay in the fact that answers were elicited and recorded, creating a portrait of the child to which Clinic staff could refer and habituating children, however slowly and reluctantly, into speaking in the Clinic. In short, Squad pediatricians fostered what they saw as children's ability to "express themselves," that is, to reveal their presumed interior states through external self-representations, freed of the inhibitions of familial supervision and cultural constraints.

Even more exceptional than this emphasis on children's speech, however, was Squad pediatricians' commitment to systematically revealing children's diagnoses to them and their insistence that children learn to articulate those diagnoses themselves. The term *disclosure* in pediatric HIV treatment refers to the process by which children learn of their own infections. In the Superlative Clinic HIV-positive children learned about having HIV and taking ARVs by participating in a ritualized dialogue, a sequence of paired questions and answers that children rehearsed at each Clinic visit, often over the course of several years. "I take my medicines to keep me strong and healthy," each child learned to say, "and my medicines help my soldiers of the body [*masole a mmele*] fight bad guy." I gloss this ritualized dialogue as *disclosure catechism*. Some portion of this catechism took place in every consultation I observed in the Clinic, frequently taking up most of the time allotted for a consultation. "Talking about disclosure," as Clinic staff referred to it, occupied an enormous amount of time in a Clinic whose staff had little time to spare.

This insistence that patients articulate their diagnosis was in keeping with broader trends in HIV treatment. In Botswana, as elsewhere, how adults talked about having HIV was tied to their status as treatable patients and to continued access to medications. HIV-positive adults were required to declare their "readiness" to begin taking ARVs under a healthcare practitioner's scrutiny and to perform this readiness at each clinic visit by laying bare the practices by which they adhered to their prescribed regimen. Within southeastern Botswana's clinical spaces, any deviation from the "standardized formulas of self-declaration" (Jean Comaroff 2007, 204) accompanying ARV treatment became increasingly unavailable as anything but a sign of "moral cowardice" (Durham and Klaits 2002, 794). As forms of confession gained prominence within transnational HIV prevention and treatment efforts across Africa and Asia (Boellstorff 2009; He and Rofel 2010; Nguyen 2010; Robins 2006), the word *AIDS* and, to a certain extent, *HIV* came to index not only the speaker's knowledge of their medical condition, or solely their interpellation by clinical and public health institutions, but also their willingness to align a presumably objective biomedical truth with an external representation. In these contexts, *AIDS* possessed a singular purchase on truth and powerfully indexed the speaker's moral character and commitment to treatment.[6] Disclosure catechism revealed "an implicit assumption in the activist discourse about 'breaking the silence'" (Wood and Lambert 2008, 214–15) in southern Africa, namely, that the failure or refusal to name HIV/AIDS can only reflect secrecy, denial, the stigmatized nature of HIV, and stubborn reluctance to discuss sexuality.

In the context of pediatric HIV treatment, the ideological weight of naming the disease remained but was complicated by relationships among children, their adult caregivers, and healthcare providers. Since children tended to be accompanied to the Clinic by an adult, these appointments offered pediatricians an opportunity to reinforce the information adults received from the Clinic about ARVs and, more significantly, to model for adults how they should talk outside the Clinic with children in their care. This modeling had limited effects. Many of the women I spoke with told me they much preferred to leave these conversations to the Clinic staff. This was unsurprising; scholars of Botswana have emphasized the moral and existential stakes for Batswana in the management of negative sentiment, particularly among kin. For Tswana adults, the act of articulating a child's diagnosis held the possibility of causing children to "give up" and threatened the somatic and sentimental bonds within families. Writing about cancer treatment, Julie Livingston argues that many Batswana do not value the revelation of patients' terminal diagnoses to them in terms of patient autonomy or transparency, valuing instead "the social displacement of terminal prognostication onto relatives" (2012, 165).[7] Inside and outside the Clinic's walls Batswana were deeply concerned about how and with whom they should talk about HIV/AIDS. But they also faced the challenge of managing interpersonal relations wherein concealment plays an important, though not necessarily dominant, role in the ongoing constitution of moral subjectivities (John Comaroff and Jean Comaroff 2001; Durham and Klaits 2002; Klaits 2010; Livingston 2008; cf. Hunleth 2017, chap. 3).

The Clinic's forms of revelation gave little attention to these priorities. Squad pediatricians frequently grumbled that Batswana adults would encourage children to strengthen their *masole a mmele* by taking their medications but rarely moved from this to a conversation that, from the pediatricians' point of view, explained the significance of these actions in way that would motivate children's future actions. Thus, while the disclosure catechism, in its idealized form, provided a common ground for clinicians, child-patients, and their adult caregivers to discuss HIV and its treatments, this process was frequently disrupted by the reluctance of adult Batswana to name HIV in ways Squad pediatricians sanctioned. For their part, adults accompanying children to the Clinic were ambivalent: On one hand, many praised Clinic staff, as Maikutlo had done, for the love they showed children. On the other, while they could not entirely avoid conversations about *masole* if they wanted their children to receive care at the Clinic, they could displace onto Clinic staff the work of articulating a child's diagnosis, even if this meant being chastised by pediatricians for their reticence. Faced with this subtle resistance and often skeptical regarding the abilities of Tswana families to adequately care for children, Squad pediatricians sometimes dispensed with this modeling altogether, using the catechism instead to disarticulate children in early adolescence from their families by recruiting them to an exclusive set of interactions based on English language biomedical terminology and encouraging children to rely on the Clinic, rather than on their kin, for assistance and support. Tshenolo's invitation to participate in the Clinic's sleepaway camp and Dr. Amy's interactions with her were oriented toward such a realignment of loyalty, trust, and language.

This chapter grapples with how, in the midst of Botswana's epidemic, children's words became objects of ongoing scrutiny and instruction.[8] In chapter 1, I argued that Clinic staff viewed HIV-positive children as an ambivalent threat to the epidemic's manageability: If children refused to take their ARVs consistently, they might develop drug-resistant strains of HIV and transmit them via unruly sexual activity, giving rise to an epidemic and a generation beyond biomedical control. In this chapter I examine how these apocalyptic visions shaped treatment practices. Specifically, I analyze the pedagogies Squad pediatricians used in their efforts to shape HIV-positive children, specifically, the way they used language to teach children to about their infections. Fearing that children would understand the word *AIDS* to signal both their imminent deaths and their flawed moral states, pediatricians relied on the ritual speech of the disclosure catechism to reveal children's diagnoses to them in a highly circumscribed manner. By means of the disclosure catechism, pediatricians led children to what pediatricians perceived as the stable, objective fact of the virus in children's bodies and the need for medications to manage their infections. Pediatricians relied on euphemisms such as *soldier* and *bad guy* to cultivate children's positive affective orientation toward treatment, exploiting a provisional, if unplanned, correspondence between American biomedical conceptualizations of bodily integrity as national defense and a popular Tswana militarized nationalism. They gradually replaced these euphemisms with biomedically derived terms such as *CD4* and *HIV*, revealing the truth of children's infections to them with, from the pediatricians' point of view, the most truthful, accurate, and appropriate terms. By means of this militarized narrative, Clinic staff recruited children to inhabit a paradoxical affective stance vis-à-vis the epidemic, intimately acquainted with danger yet unafraid and capable of self-disciplined action. The result, in pediatricians' eyes, was children who could describe their infection and treatment with a clinical accuracy imbued with the catechism's affective values, a combination that would result in adherence.

Ideas regarding the effects of knowing and talking about one's serostatus have shifted dramatically over the course of the epidemic. Before HIV testing was available, prevention messages targeting US gay men encouraged them to approach all sexual partners as potentially infected yet unable to know or reveal their serostatus (Sheon and Lee 2009, 138). With the advent of HIV testing, "prevention interventions increasingly emphasized testing and disclosure, encouraging men to verbally discuss risks and negotiate condom use" (Sheon and Crosby 2004, 2106). These new prevention strategies rested on the idea that men who knew their HIV status would communicate it to their partners and would try to learn their partners' status before engaging in sex. The shift assumed that knowing one's HIV-positive diagnosis impels a person to seek treatment and actively avoid infecting others, an assumption that, Nicolas Sheon and G. Michael Crosby argue, "has never been supported by the data" (2004, 2106). Nonetheless, it underlies a position firmly articulated in the clinical literature: HIV-positive persons, and children in particular, benefit from knowing and talking about their infections. Clinicians point to increased adherence to ARVs as the most immediate benefit of knowing one's status, but they argue that the positive effects go beyond practical concerns to address the specific psychosocial needs of HIV-positive children, whose relation to HIV is gauged by what they say about it.[9]

The catechism rested on assumptions about children and about the relationships between speech and action. I call these assumptions, normally unarticulated in everyday activities, disclosure ideology. Disclosure ideology is a type of language ideology, or set of assumptions about what language is and can do (Schieffelin, Woolard, and Kroskrity 1998; Silverstein 1979; Woolard and Schieffelin 1994).[10] Attention to language ideologies illuminates how actors position themselves vis-à-vis present or imagined interlocutors and how subject positions constrain what may be said or by whom it may be heard (Bauman and Briggs 2003; Irvine and Gal 2000). Disclosure ideology shaped clinicians' presumptions that children infected with HIV must learn to articulate this fact in strict terms for the practical purpose of fostering the strict adherence Squad pediatricians considered necessary, as discussed in chapter 1. Prevention messages linking HIV/AIDS to immoral sexual behavior saturated southeastern Botswana, warning that, "AIDS kills." Squad pediatricians feared that children would understand the word *AIDS* to portend their imminent deaths. They feared these messages would shape children's understanding of their condition, negatively affecting their adherence to their ARVs. In short, these pediatricians assumed that children could not separate the word *AIDS* from a thing the word represented. That Tswana children could not encounter *HIV* as an affectively neutral reference to a biomedical object distinct from *AIDS*, in the pediatricians' eyes, was a function of popular public health campaigns and children's immaturity. But it also reflected what pediatricians perceived as the harmful obfuscating tendencies of Tswana social norms and the way stigma operated in Botswana (as described chapters 1 and 3). Against this, disclosure ideology framed disclosure as beneficial for a child's psychosocial well-being as a good unto itself (cf. Hardon and Posel 2012, S2). While pediatricians framed disclosure as a means of conveying the "facts" of HIV to children in a way that would ensure their adherence to their medications, disclosure ideology suggested a more thoroughgoing critique of Tswana sociality.

As a process of lexical reform, the catechism resembles what Summerson Carr calls "metalinguistic labor," that is, a dialogic process whereby experts ratify patients' utterances as expressions of a stable interior truth (2010b, 125). Claims regarding a subject's capacity to articulate these truths are necessarily intersubjective; they required an audience. Institutional arrangements matter deeply in these processes: "Institutions," Carr reminds us, "are not simply neutral contexts for talk but are instead organized to demonstrate and enforce the legitimacy of institutional authorities' linguistic strategies" (2006, 635; 2010b), thereby constraining "the truths that [a client] can felicitously propose" (2006 641; 646). But rather than ratify acts of inner reference (that is, children's claims about their own interior states), pediatricians sought to use the catechism to *prospectively* shape children into adherent subjects by positing an iconic relationship between an array of biomedical terms that should, in the ideal, be primarily referential and affectively neutral, and a set of affectively powerful if biomedically inaccurate euphemisms, and then substituting the former for the latter, a diagrammatic iconicity I examine in more detail later. Scaffolded by the catechism, a child's utterance of *HIV* should refer to a biomedical object while indexing the catechism's careful narrative of personal empowerment. In the framework of disclosure ideology, accuracy and persuasiveness, that is, the referential and performative functions of language, were linked, the former considered the precondition for the latter: only by learning to talk about HIV in a way pediatricians ratified could children become the kind of children pediatricians trusted to manage their infections.[11]

Disclosure poorly executed could hinder children's ability to regard themselves and their treatment positively light, negatively affecting a child's overall well-being as well as the child's adherence. But pediatricians imagined the consequences of improper disclosure to reach far beyond an individual child. Children who did not know and could not discuss their HIV-positive status might grow into adolescents who had no reason to take their medicines or who, betrayed by caregivers through faulty disclosure, refused to take their medicines. In both cases they would be at risk for developing drug-resistant strains of HIV. The ultimate fear was that they would transmit these drug-resistant strains to others either because they did not know their status or because the damage of subterfuge, lies, and betrayal led them to engage in "risky behavior" during adolescence. Standing on the brink of national extinction, HIV-positive children inhabited a fraught position vis-à-vis the future, at once the hope of the nation and the stuff of nightmares. In these apocalyptic visions, only children's relationship to their medications stood between them and a future too terrible to behold, a future characterized by a spiraling dynamic of "treatment failure" and "high-risk behavior," mutation and infection, ineffective medications and unprotected sex.

I argue that it was, in fact, the pediatricians who could not bear to hear children say the word *AIDS* with its implication of ineluctable destruction. The disclosure catechism highlighted pediatricians' profound ambivalence about the referential and performative powers of language. Pediatricians imagined that they knew the difference between words and things, that is, that calling something "HIV" or "bad guy" did not affect the virus itself or alter pediatricians' reaction to it. They imagined children differently, that is, they imagined that the word *AIDS* would cause children to fear for their lives. Pediatricians imagined that words like "bad guy" were persuasive enough to shape children's behavior because they invited children to take positive action but that these euphemisms had to be replaced by words like *HIV* that were (or should be) persuasive enough to shape children's behavior because, unlike "bad guy," they were true. Pediatricians imagined that lessons they taught children about HIV were accurate representations imbued with the positive affective that children needed to offset the indexical relationship popular discourse had established between "HIV/AIDS" and death. But pediatricians *also* needed to lead children to an understanding of HIV that fit within their vision of the ongoing management of the epidemic and that would be instrumental in bringing it to fruition. Pediatricians were more committed than were children to the power of the word *AIDS* to shape children's actions, to impair children's ability to manage their infections. And because these pediatricians believed—or believed that *children* believed—that the word *AIDS* holds such power, they barred it from the Clinic, excluding any consideration of the virus as something that might exceed biomedical management. In the disclosure catechism, treatment never failed.

This argument makes several broader contributions. First, an analysis of language ideologies in HIV treatment helps us rethink the role of language and affect in biomedical therapies and their place in medical anthropology. In keeping with contemporary medical anthropology's focus on the centrality of biological identities to contemporary forms of political belonging and access to care, analyses of testimonial practices in HIV care have focused on how speech, inhabitable identities, and material resources in HIV treatment become linked (Benton 2015; Biehl 2009a; Kalofonos 2008; Mattes 2011; Nguyen 2010; Rhine 2016; Robins 2006; cf. Biehl 2005; Petryna 2002; Rabinow 1992). These studies emphasize the role healthcare professionals and institutions play in producing intertwined forms of knowledge and subjectivity. While my analysis takes its cue from Foucault's analysis of the simultaneous production of knowledge and subjects in the clinic, Foucauldian theories of confession are inadequate to the task of analyzing the concrete processes through which subjects are constituted and recruited to role. Studying confession as mutually informed processes of subjectivization and knowledge production demands attention to how those processes became felicitous, that is, the circumstances that made them successful in the first place. Catechism's temporal orientation highlights this point: While both confession and testimony are retrospective, narrating that which has already transpired, catechism attempts to shape subjects as they unfold into the future, providing them with the means by which they might become confessional animals. Catechism, then, is better approached by an analytic that attends to ritual transformation, one that approaches catechism as an "exceptionally dense representation of spatiotemporally wider categories and principles" (Stasch 2011, 160; cf. Goffman 1967; Silverstein 2004).

Second, attention to what different actors imagined children could and should say also gives insight into the kinds of subjects different actors imagined children to be and the consequences they envisioned of children's speech in the context of pediatric HIV treatment. When a child was enrolled in the Clinic, at least one adult relative had to attend a one-morning training session that explained HIV's effect on the immune system and the importance of adherence before the child began receiving medications. Children were excluded from this session, and no effort was made in these sessions to engage these adults in building links between words and affective orientations over time. Catechism, then, assumed a particular affective plasticity in children, whose grief and fear toward their own infections could be preemptively mitigated by establishing a positive affective orientation toward treatment, emphasizing the increasing control of growing children over their daily medications as the pivot on which the treatment battle eventually turned. It also provided a metric by which Clinic staff measured their progress in shaping the affective orientations, and thereby the subjectivities, of the children in their care.

Examining the stakes imagined to lie in saying or not saying "HIV" or "AIDS" also draws attention to what count as illegitimate forms of secrecy and obfuscation within US-driven HIV-related programming.[12] As I discuss in chapter 3, disclosure catechism reflects an idea I found among many US health professionals in Botswana, namely, that the roots of Botswana's epidemic lay beyond Batswana's sexual behavior in their failure to properly reveal things to themselves and their intimates. Echoing the scalar logic that informed their deep ambivalence toward Tswana sociality, these professionals considered Batswana's apparent reticence regarding HIV as part of a larger pattern that included failures to specify kin relations, refusals to admit to extramarital affairs, reluctance to publicly queue for ARVs, and the use, even among health professionals, of euphemisms such as *this thing*, *this mogare*, even *this virus* to refer to HIV and the epidemic. Circumspection of any kind was suspect: Squad pediatricians tended to attribute all perceived failures at directness to stigma, and in the Clinic, disclosure was, in part, an attempt to mitigate stigma and its silencing effects. And while each individual child had to be catechized, disclosure catechism, like adherence offered a way for pediatricians to reform the social norms that, they imagined, drove Botswana's epidemic one child at a time.

Last, by drawing attention to the language ideologies underlying HIV treatment, this analysis questions a stance many anthropologists and others find attractive, namely, that the interests of those most vulnerable vis-à-vis the epidemic are best served by an insistence upon a certain form of speech that "breaks the silence," creating the conditions for HIV-positive individuals to "live positively." However laudable this stance may be, we should beware its ideological underpinnings. Michel Foucault (1978) cautions us against equating more speech with liberation. With this in mind, attending to what one can do with the words *HIV* and *AIDS* can illuminate subjugated understandings of the epidemic lost in the urgency of global AIDS programming. Only by bracketing the idea that language operates by more or less correctly referring to things can we attend to what actors imagine saying "HIV" or "AIDS" does, thereby shedding light on the ideologies governing the forms of transformation global health promises.

In what follows, I analyze disclosure catechism to illuminate disclosure ideology, that is, the ways pediatricians imagined their methods of soliciting speech constituted a well-adjusted and adherent pediatric subject. I examine the ways the pediatricians drew on and reinforced narratives of the militarized defense of bodies and national borders. I conclude with an example of a momentary disruption of disclosure catechism that reveals the apocalyptic visions that, in the catechism's terms, lay behind a child's utterances.

Modeling Disclosure in the Superlative Clinic: Lexical Reform in Action

Clinic guidelines stressed that children begin learning the names of their medications upon mastering the alphabet and, in its idealized form, catechism unfolded over the course of several years from approximately age four through age eleven or twelve. What follows are the questions and answers that composed disclosure catechism. In practice, lessons were taught and reinforced from one appointment to the next.

> Q: Why do you take your medicines?
> A: I take my medicines to keep me strong and healthy.

The first question, reiterated every time a child visited the Clinic, focused on instilling the "positive attitude" toward HIV treatment pediatricians regarded as a necessary facet of a subject who took proper responsibility for his or her healthcare, rather than on teaching the child the "facts" of his or her infection.

> Q: When do you take your medicines?
> A: I take my medicines at, e.g., seven in the morning and seven in the evening.
> Q: What are the names of your medicines?
> A: Ay-zed-tee, en-vee-pee, etc.
> Q: How do you take your medicines?
> A: I take, e.g., one in the morning, half in the evening.

These three questions aimed to cultivate adherence by normalizing the act of taking medicines and involving children in their routine consumption. Pediatricians emphasized the quotidian nature of taking medicines, comparing it to brushing teeth or bathing. They praised astute children who reminded adults to give them their pills on time or who mentioned reminders, such as cell phone alarms. Nearly all ARVs used in the Clinic had three-letter codes, and children learned to rattle off the combinations of letters corresponding to their medications. *Ay-zed-tee, three-tee-see, en-vee-pee*, a child might chant, indicating zidovudine (AZT), epivir (3TC), and nevirapine (NVP). Clinic staff also asked children to match the names of the medicines to their pills, distinguishing zidovudine's blue and white capsules from epivir's red diamonds and nevirapine's white ovals.

> Q: How do your medicines keep you strong and healthy?
> A: My medications keep my *masole a mmele* [soldiers of the body] strong. Strong *masole* keep me healthy.

Pediatricians sometimes began this lesson by asking a child about soldiers or about the Botswana Defense Force (BDF), hoping to elicit an idea of a positive, protective force comparable to the body's disease-fighting capacity (cf. Martin 1990). Staff then introduced the "soldiers of the body" that children assisted by taking medications each day. Having linked the regular consumption of their medicines to the continued protection of the body via *masole a mmele*, pediatricians expected children to explain that their medications (named, identified, and dosages indicated) helped their *masole* and that their *masole* protected their body, keeping it strong and healthy. These lessons in place, Clinic staff emphasized the causal relationship between children's health and the actions children took to help their *masole* by diligently taking medications. In many consultations, Clinic staff did no more than reinforce these links, praising children in good health by commenting on how strong the children's *masole* must be and how much they helped these *masole* by taking their medications as prescribed.

> Q: What do your soldiers do? Whom do they fight?
> A: My *masole* fight "bad guy."
> Q: What happens if you don't take your medicines?
> A: My medicines help my *masole* keep "bad guy" asleep. If I don't take my medicines, "bad guy" will wake up, and if I don't take my medicines, "bad guy" will be stronger than my *masole*.

These lessons introduced "bad guy," sworn enemy of *masole a mmele*. Clinic staff encouraged children to identify with and support their *masole* but tended to leave "bad guy" in relative obscurity. Instead, they emphasized the stakes for *masole*—and, by extension, for the child—in taking their medicines: medicines made *masole a mmele* stronger than "bad guy" and caused "bad guy" to sleep. Sleeping "bad guy" could not harm *masole a mmele*. Refusing to take one's medicines, however, weakened one's *masole*. "Bad guy" could wake and attack weakened *masole*. Weakened *masole* could not protect the body and keep "bad guy" asleep just as weakened soldiers cannot fight. The child who wished to protect his or her *masole* must take medications consistently. As clinic staff introduced the possibility that a wakened "bad guy" would fight *masole*, thereby reducing their numbers, they indicated that, left insufficiently defended, the child's body was vulnerable not only to "bad guy" but also to other illnesses. If "bad guy" woke, he might even become "tricky" by learning the children's medicines and reducing their power to make him sleep. Should this happen, the child would have to take new and more difficult medicines.

> Q: What's the name of "bad guy"?
> A: The name of bad guy is "HIV."

If the dramatic climax of catechism was the story of what happens to children who fail to take their medications, the revelation of the characters' "true" names was almost anticlimactic. Pediatricians encouraged a child to adjust the terms used to recount his or her ever-expanding answer to the question, why do you take your medicines? Children traded *bad guy* for *HIV* just as they traded *masole* for *CD4*. Knowing the name of "bad guy" concluded the catechism. At this point, a child should to be able to discuss HIV infection in the Clinic's terms. No longer dependent on the juvenile language of "the *masole* story," children could openly discuss their ARVs, CD4 count, and viral load with a clinician and talk about the implications of missed doses for their long-term health.

In its ideal form, then, catechism contained no moment at which the diagnosis was sprung on the child, the secret suddenly revealed. Upon being asked to name "bad guy," many children revealed what they already knew or suspected to be the case. Pediatricians emphasized that although the characters were unmasked, nothing about the relationship among them had changed. A child's medicines strengthened *masole* and kept "bad guy" asleep, just as ARVs increased CD4 counts and kept HIV in check. Nevertheless, Dr. Amy suggested making time to give children the opportunity to absorb the information and to ask questions. She urged her colleagues to "empower the child with knowledge" such that, in the final moment of disclosure, clinicians could help children view their HIV infection "in the context of what the child had already internalized," that is, "as long as you keep taking meds well and keep your soldiers strong, you can do everything that you want."

How to Do Things to Children with Words

Disclosure catechism was predicated on stepwise substitutions in which children gradually replaced terms pediatricians viewed as euphemistic with more accurate descriptions of HIV and the rationale behind ARV adherence. First, it relied poetically on diagrammatic iconicity, an analogy made between one thing and another on the basis of a similar arrangement of parts (Peirce 1932). Disclosure catechism linked words, affective orientations, and subject positions, comprising what Charles Briggs calls a "communicable cartography" (2007). Such cartographies "[project] a small set of shared and predictable circuits, [create] subject positions, [arrange] them in spatial, moral, and legal terms, and [make] only a very limited range of responses thinkable" (2007, 338). Children traversed the Clinic's cartography by progressively mastering a lexicon, and as they learned to deploy words Squad pediatricians considered capable of both generating and indicating corresponding interior states, children mapped themselves onto this cartography. Second, disclosure catechism projected a unidirectional temporality. From the pediatricians' point of view, children who learned to recite the disclosure catechism became children who took their medications, first, because they had positive associations with medications and, second, because they understood clearly why they should do so, and that set of accurate referents rested on a positive affective orientation. Most important, they would continue to take their medications even after learning they had HIV because their affective orientations toward treatment endured the substitution of biomedical terms for euphemisms.

Recruitment to and assessment of a positive affective orientation toward treatment pervaded every clinical encounter. Dr. Amy emphasized that ARV treatment required children to develop and retain "a positive attitude toward life." While HIV-positive children could become "productive adults," they required empowerment to learn to care for themselves. The timing of these subjectivization projects was critical. Koketso stressed that children attending the Clinic, many of whom had lost parents and relatives to the virus, knew more than their caregivers realized, linking words they heard at home or in the Clinic with radio or television ads about HIV/AIDS. "They may not realize the full meaning," Koketso continued, "but they'll get the connotation of 'H-I-V.'" Clinic staff regarded this inference as potentially harmful because children, responding emotionally to what staff regarded as misinformation, misunderstood their contagiousness, feared they were dying, or grieved over their flawed moral states.

Hoping to prevent these negative reactions, Clinic staff were anxious to cultivate a positive attitude toward treatment as early as possible because they regarded this affective orientation as fundamental for the child's future and because early efforts at disclosure exploited the adaptability of the younger child. "The earlier in life children are told about their HIV status," Barr insists, "the easier they find it to incorporate this information into their comprehension of the world and adapt accordingly" (2006, 93). Conversely, delaying disclosure "increases the likelihood that the information will cause significant psychological strain, as well as the need to place blame for their condition on someone" (2006, 94). Pediatricians documented children's moods, including their willingness to share elements of their personal lives with Clinic staff, as indicators of psychosocial well-being. While these exchanges sometimes formed the ground for an ongoing relationship between a child and a particular pediatrician, this documentation also ensured that a clinician unfamiliar with the child could extrapolate a kind of psychosocial profile from the child's clinical records.

For pediatricians, however, the most crucial aspect of disclosure was its relationship to adherence, the moment when verbal expressions and the ideas they presumably reflected shaped children's actions. Reflecting how disclosure ideology framed persuasiveness as something that must ultimately depend on accuracy, Barr observes that disclosure "has long been anecdotally reported at the clinic to have a beneficial effect on pediatric ARV adherence" (2006, 103). "Studies show," I was told repeatedly, "the sooner the child is fully disclosed, the better his adherence is." Disclosure, argues Barr, "provides the vital piece of the puzzle for a child to understand why they are taking daily medications even when they don't look or feel sick" (2006, 103). Children who understand their role in strengthening their *masole* regard their medicines in a positive light and feel empowered by their ability to contribute to their *masole*, doing their part to "fight AIDS" by taking their ARVs (Barr 2006, 103–104), joining pediatricians in a scalar imaginary of the epidemic whereby individual adherence can undermine or maintain control of the national, and even global, epidemic. Children lacking this understanding hide their pills, lie about taking them, or throw them down the latrine.

Catechism, then, was a matter of painstaking affective management as much as, if not more than, one of conveying information about HIV. The failure to disclose properly was potentially devastating. Squad pediatricians regarded talk that was too direct as harmful. Like many Batswana adults, pediatricians regarded telling children point-blank that they had "HIV" or, worse, "AIDS," as a deeply traumatizing event. Pediatricians thought that children would take the term *AIDS* to portend their imminent deaths and would become confused by the term's negative moral implications. At the same time, not everything a child might be told counted, from the pediatricians' perspective, as disclosure. For example, they disparaged Batswana adults who told children that their medications were for "tuberculosis." For the pediatricians, *tuberculosis* could not stand in for *HIV*; it was neither accurate nor correctly persuasive. They insisted this kind of substitution was harmful to children who, if told they must take medications because of ill health, resisted treatment once they no longer felt ill. Such obfuscation shaded into dangerous lies: Children who pieced together enough to realize, first, that they had been HIV-positive all along and, second, that their family had kept this fact secret, were "really angry, they feel betrayed," Dr. Amy told me. Pediatricians bemoaned children's "loss of confidence in caregivers" who relied on "secrets" and denied clinicians the opportunity to "dispel false beliefs" about HIV/AIDS. Both cases demonstrated a disruption in the alignment of persuasiveness and accuracy, verbal expressions and the actions to which they gave rise discussed earlier. In both cases, pediatricians' response was the same, a return to catechism's touchstone: "I take my medicines to keep me strong and healthy." "Never lie to children," cautioned Dr. Amy. "Do not say ARVs are for transient conditions, but rather are to make and keep them strong."

The idealized counterpoint to both traumatic directness and traumatic obliqueness is the catechized children who learn about their condition in developmentally appropriate ways, who maintain positive relationships with clinicians and adult family members, and who may struggle with the implications of the diagnosis but nevertheless take responsibility for their treatment as empowered, productive adults. Catechism's stepwise exchanges of words and subject positions were predicated on the idea that children who transform themselves into well-adjusted adherent subjects as they trade *masole* for *CD4* and *bad guy* for *HIV* come to a point at which they no longer need the catechism's lexical and affective scaffolding. But this idealized moment is deceptive: On the one hand, pediatricians were invested in making sure that children learned what physicians already knew: that one set of words possessed the capacity to accurately represent reality and thus persuade children toward adherence, and the other did not. Catechism provided a way for children to safely approach the word *HIV*. On the other hand, learning to talk about HIV in one way entailed learning not to talk about it in other ways. In the next section, I draw attention to these exclusions and the logics that give rise to them.

Learning a Productive Fear

The origins of the *masole* story, I was told, lay with a Ugandan NGO and had originally featured villagers responding to the threat of a lion. Analogies to agriculture or animal husbandry, activities with which many Batswana children are familiar, might have worked just as well.[13] But in the Superlative Clinic the story revolved almost universally around *masole* and "bad guy," and resonated in unanticipated ways with broader processes of militarization taking place in Botswana at that time (K. Good 2010; Makgala and Mmekwa 2009). To be enlisted in the BDF is an occupation considered available to those without extensive education or political connections, and because Botswana has never engaged in open military conflict, BDF soldiers run little risk of life and limb. Soldiers, then, generally connote a combination of patriotic pride and the benefits of a steady paycheck. Squad pediatricians frequently asked children what they would like to be when they grow up, and while a good many answered "doctor" or "nurse," not a few answered "soldier."

These broader processes of militarization were reflected in the slogan of Botswana's National AIDS Coordinating Agency (NACA), *Ntwa e bolotse* [the war is engaged/begun]. And while the only entity against which Botswana has ever declared "war" is HIV/AIDS, tensions between Botswana and Zimbabwe were high enough in early July 2008 that the government deployed a contingent of BDF soldiers along the border, prompting one of Botswana's nationally circulated weekly papers to ask, "Botswana prepares for war?" (Pitse 2008). Several scholars noted an increase in xenophobic attitudes in Botswana as the political and economic situation in Zimbabwe deteriorated and many Zimbabweans crossed into neighboring countries (Campbell 2003; Marr 2012; Nyamnjoh 2006). Zimbabweans figured prominently in the popular imagination as scapegoats, the ultimate cause of Botswana's ills. It should not be surprising, then, that the catechism could go awry in those instances when children answered that the BFD "chase Zimbabweans" or "beat" them rather than describing them primarily as a protective force. The figure of the "Zimbabwean" could easily stand in as "bad guy," a pathogenic entity who infiltrated Botswana in order to steal the nation's wealth and strength.

The power of the disclosure catechism's central metaphor, then, lay in the fact that it worked in two directions at once, framing the body as a nation in need of a militarized defense and casting the nation as a body in need of protection. Children learned to map onto their own bodies a topography of Botswana and its national threats. Yet, as children swallowed their medicines and aided the metaphorical "soldiers" who relied on them for assistance, they learned to extend this topographic model to the nation itself and locate themselves within it. Recall that President Mogae asserted that the epidemic threatened Botswana with national extinction. Just as "soldiers" within the body preserved it from a potentially lethal threat, so children who took their medications preserved Botswana from destruction. In this sense, HIV-positive children were simultaneously the front line of the battle for the nation's continued existence and the very stakes over which that battle was fought. And while Squad pediatricians may not have intended the catechism to index, let alone foster, ethnonational tensions, the key point is that they did not regard these military analogies as metaphoric. For the body to "fight" disease was, in their eyes, an accurate and thus persuasive description even if the names of the presumed combatants required adjustment.

But this symbolic condensation pointed to a profound contradiction: While the possibility of national extinction justified catechism, catechism itself framed the gestures with which HIV-positive children fought a "war on AIDS" as mundane practices of everyday hygiene, fostering what Joseph Masco calls an "emotional management campaign" (Masco 2008, 378; see 2014). In his analysis of the US government's deployment of images of nuclear disaster, Masco argues that defense theorists, hoping to avoid both mass panic and mass apathy, sought "an image of nuclear war that would be, above all, politically useful: the idea of an American community under total and unending threat" (2008, 363). The key to producing "this contradictory state of productive fear" lay in a familiarity carefully managed by the promulgation of a narrow set of representations and the exclusion of any others. The Cold War State, Masco argues, used specific representations of the bomb "as a mechanism for accessing and controlling the emotions of citizens" that, in turn, demanded "new forms of psychological discipline" (2008, 366) instilled through ritualized reenactments of nuclear war. This "productive fear" required those recruited to it to develop the "mental discipline" necessary "to live on the knife's edge of a psychotic contradiction—an everyday life founded simultaneously in total threat and absolute normality—with the stakes being nothing less than survival itself" (Masco 2008, 376; cf. Orr 2004).

Likewise, Abigail Kohn (2000) highlights the "ruptures in the emplotment process" that emerge as children with craniofacial abnormalities and their families attempt to navigate between visions of a "normal" future and one shaped by deformity and stigma. Clinicians, Kohn writes, "seemed to understand that one of the most difficult problems confronting parents of disfigured children . . . is how to help children define themselves as essentially normal while at the same time finding strategies for managing stigma" (2000, 217). The Superlative Clinic, with its tinted glass, air conditioning, imported cartoons, and American physicians, stood out dramatically among southeastern Botswana's clinical spaces. In this singular environment children learned they were "no different" from other children and could do "anything they wanted," re-inscribing their difference the moment Clinic staff attempted its erasure. And even as Clinic staff attempted to normalize children's relations to their own bodies, they could not but reinforce ambivalence: These children could do "anything they wanted" as long as "anything they wanted" included the reflexive articulation of their diagnoses, control of their sexual behavior, and the pharmaceutical domestication of the potential apocalypse they harbored.

These contradictions were best revealed in what went unsaid. When the treatment program began, its clinics were carefully named "infectious disease care clinics" and ubiquitously referred to as *IDCCs*. Similarly, neither the Superlative Clinic's name nor the name by which most Clinic and hospital staff called it referred to either "HIV" or "AIDS." While pediatricians insisted on "telling the truth" about children's infections, they were careful to correct speakers who used the word *AIDS* to refer to anything other than a clinical stage of HIV infection. Although the Clinic's raison d'être was an epidemic best known by its four-letter acronym, that acronym was effectively banned within the Clinic's walls. This policing allowed pediatricians to talk to children about HIV/AIDS and to require that children also talk about HIV/AIDS in a manner that pediatricians regarded as truthful and direct yet generative of proper subjectivities and positive social relations.

The recruitment of HIV-positive children to affectively orient themselves toward the threat of their own deaths and the threat of national extinction the HIV/AIDS epidemic posed echoes the recruitment of Americans to face nuclear terror. Recruited to a quotidian war they fought with gestures supposedly no more remarkable than a daily bath, children learned a productive fear by means of a carefully orchestrated oral recitation of the biomedical name of their own infections. This discipline dictated that the burden of responding appropriately to these threats—neither panicked nor consumed by grief nor apathetic—should rest squarely on their shoulders. The possibility that treatment could fail was, like the horror of a nuclear holocaust, simply inconceivable. Instead, disclosure catechism pointed children toward an endless temporal horizon of treatment, culminating in children and a nation under strict control, contributing to, if not inhabiting, an "AIDS-free generation."

Yet a representation of nuclear war, Masco argues, "'stands in' for the inevitable failure of the imagination to be able to conceive of the end" (2008, 382). The catechism could not entirely capture the proliferation of meanings to which a sublime horror is subject. This inadequacy gives rise to surplus signification, even within the narrow confines of disclosure catechism. The next section illustrates, first, disclosure catechism's failure to wholly define children's relationship to the epidemic's biomedical vocabulary and, second, the apocalyptic visions of the epidemic pediatricians attempted to constrain by means of the catechism.

Catechismal Failure

One morning, a little girl about five years old and her mother came into the room where Dr. Rachel and Mma Mokento were seeing patients. Perched on the exam table and swinging her ankles, the girl looked curiously about the room as Mma Mokento asked the mother about the girl's general health and adherence to her ARVs. Dr. Rachel performed a quick physical exam. Stepping back and slipping her stethoscope down her neck, Dr. Rachel addressed the girl, "So, do you know why you take your medicines?" Mma Mokento translated: *O nwa dipilisi tsa gago ka goreng?* The girl smiled up at Mma Mokento and answered brightly: *AIDS!*

All the adults in the room, including me, froze. There was a long silence. Tentatively, the girl tried again, mumbling: *Masole a mmele?* Recovering her voice, Mma Mokento attempted to regain control of the interaction: *Wena, o nwa dipilisi go nna thata, waitse?* [You take medicines to keep strong, right?]

If disclosure catechism consists of a series of stepwise exchanges of words and subject positions, this little girl had shot through the ceiling, rendering her unlocatable in the Clinic's communicable cartography. Inside the Clinic, *AIDS* slipped out only when the name of "bad guy" was revealed, and then only because in catechism's final step children still needed to learn that what infected them— what made the Clinic, the medicines, and the interaction in which they were engaged necessary—was "HIV," and emphatically not "AIDS." Silence or a mumbled *Ga ke itse* [I don't know] would have cued Dr. Rachel and Mma Mokento to return to first principles: "I take my medicines to keep me strong and healthy." Giving it all away in the first round—"AIDS!"—and in a bright, cheery tone, no less, utterly disrupted the alignment of affect, language, and action the Clinic strove to assemble and regulate. Dr. Rachel and Mma Mokento were faced not with a child who did not know but with a child who did not know how to know what she knew, a child who did dangerous things with language.

Rather than dismiss this outburst as an explosion of naïveté, I use the girl's answer to unpack disclosure ideology, the Clinic-eye view of what language can do and what is at stake in uttering "AIDS." But if the girl's statement cracked open the ground on which the epidemic and its interventions could be narrativized, we should be wary of slipping into the idea that she was "speaking truth to power," that her statement grasped a reality beyond language that catechism failed to reach except in its final moment. Such an argument would reflect, rather than critique, the language ideology I take as my object of analysis: that the words *HIV* and *AIDS* must be privileged beyond all others as the true representation of the condition in which this child and so many other Batswana find themselves, that these names are dangerous and uniquely powerful and must be revealed with care, and that one's moral character and perhaps one's life are at stake in one's willingness and ability to deploy those words.

The girl's outburst revealed what is at stake in the catechism in the relation of words to things, signs to what they represent. Michael Taussig uses Hans Christian Andersen's story of the emperor's new clothes to examine the ways adults displace their own inability to distinguish between a sign and its referent onto children, savages, and other incomplete subjects. Refusing both the logic of the "hidden truth," that is, the idea of the "real" behind the dissimulation, and Friedrich Nietzsche's proposition that "the whole of human life is sunk deeply in untruth" (1996, 30), Taussig complicates revelation by characterizing the adult's imagination of the child's imagination as a "stateless state" of "*nei-*

ther appearance *nor* depth" (Taussig 2003, 453–54; see Nietzsche 1969). Citing Georg Simmel's (1906) argument that the structure of modernity is that of a secret society, Taussig describes the modern state's secrecy as "public secrecy," or "a sort of active unknowing" (2003, 457). Like all secret societies, he argues, the modern state rests on the principle that "unmasking churns and thickens mystery instead of dissipating it" (Taussig 2003, 457). In the public secret, concealment and revelation become intertwined: "One can use revelation so as to conceal further, a trick writ firmly into the formula, 'knowing what not to know'" (Taussig 2003, 456). Such a distinction "provides the life energy of the society" (Taussig 2003, 457). Here transparency is inimical not only to the public secret but also to sociality itself.

Taussig offers two interpretations of Andersen's story. In the first, a child sees what everyone sees and no one will say and speaks "the truth"—here "truth" as "unsocialized being" (Taussig 2003, 458). In this interpretation, to "speak the truth" is to say that truth was there all along, waiting to be revealed by the righteous destruction of its concealment. Everyone knows the emperor is naked but knows not to know. The child is an "innocent" who lacks the capacity for dissimulation of the already socialized. The child of Taussig's second interpretation, by contrast, is not a speaker of truths revealed to the innocent eye but a player of games, capable of "taking advantage" of the adult's imagination of the child's imagination. This child, Taussig writes, "knows only too well what not to know, but for some reason . . . cannot but blurt it out" (2003, 459). Taussig introduces an economy of revelation based on secrets to be spent, sacrifices in Georges Bataille's (1990) sense, profitless losses that consecrate what they destroy. The structure of this secret resembles that of the gift insofar as the gift relies on a certain dissimulation or, more accurately, a suspension of disbelief. As instrumental as the gift might be, it must be treated by all concerned as altruistic. This contradiction illustrates what Taussig means by "neither surface nor depth": It takes as much social labor to reveal the gift as just an exchange as it requires to reveal the exchange as really a gift. For the well-behaved child, the key to these distinctions lies in knowing what not to know; for the player of games, it lies in "spending" the secret. In the second interpretation, smashing the rule—"AIDS!"—is an act suffused with pleasure, not a naïf's accidental, unconscious transgression.

For adults, Taussig argues, the child contains "a space of infinite possibility" spanning the distance between the player of games and the dupe who mistakes signs for what they signify, masks for what they mask. Adults distance themselves from the child's credulity, from a time before the distinction between appearance and depth was established. After all, what defines the child is "the inability to peel representations off from reality" (Taussig 2003, 462).

In the adult's imagination of the child's imagination, the child cannot distinguish the mask from what lies behind it. Yet, Taussig argues, it is adults who, despite any conviction they might have about the arbitrary nature of the linguistic sign, "cannot make sense without also believing the very opposite—namely, that there is a magical and mimetic link as strong as steel between words and things" (2003, 463). The adult's commitment to the magical nature of language, like the adult's commitment to the cloth draped around the emperor's body, is stronger than the child's. A childish child, so the adult imagines, might believe CD4 cells to be *masole*, but no pediatrician can allow "bad guy" to be called "tuberculosis." For Taussig, the child's supposed "literal-mindedness" allows adults to both engage and displace the unity of names and things without which adults cannot manage but to which they cannot wholly commit. The child, by contrast, exposes the arbitrariness of signification: So what if we call the condition "AIDS"? Isn't one name as good as another? And if children think all objects have unarbitrary names, this frees them to destroy and remake the signifying capacity of signs, "spending" meaning in "the exposure of the dadalike nonsense of the linguistic sign" (Taussig 2003, 464) with all its imaginative possibilities. In this scenario it is adults, not children, who tremble at the possibility of improper substitutions, who cannot separate the mask from what it conceals.

Where does this leave our little girl? My point is not just that her exclamation revealed the taboo in breaking it. Nor is it only that Clinic staff, in attempting one disenchantment of language, hoping to free it from its obscuring euphemistic and dangerous trappings, could not but engage in another set of magic words they hoped would affectively orient children as the kinds of subjects pediatricians imagined they need to be. By naming the reason she took her pills as "AIDS" and driving a wedge into the Clinic's communicable cartography, the little girl exposed a world in which what she has is, indeed, AIDS, a thing that kills, a sign of unassuageable grief and horror rather than a bad guy kept powerless by vigilant soldiers. In that world, one the Clinic tried by all means to deny and forestall, taking ARVs was a desperate act in the face of vast uncertainty. Treatment might not work—maybe for her, maybe for the entire country. In that world, the future is anything but a space in which she can do whatever she wants to do; to say so is to engage in a form of denial that borders on the grotesque.

The child who blurts out what she knows she ought not know, Taussig writes, "performs the basic split in belief that allows contradiction and conflict to persist, no less than multiple realities and interpretations" (2003, 459). The split in this instance, however, was fleeting. The silence answering the girl's exclamation and Mma Mokento's alarmed response indicated the Clinic's power to set the terms by which one could or, more pointedly, could not talk about "AIDS," and thereby the kinds of subject positions and futures of the epidemic one could legitimately inhabit. "What one can do with words in a particular time and place," E. Summerson Carr reminds us, "is largely determined by local ideologies of language, which establish the possibilities of verbal performance from the start" (2009, 321). Although subjects may attempt to refuse an assigned position within a communicable cartography, they may find it "impossible to construct an effective counternarrative" (Briggs 2007, 334). I do not want to suggest this little girl radically reshaped her own narrative constraints and subject position. But by momentarily shattering disclosure catechism and its painstakingly rationed economy of revelation, she helps us see disclosure catechism as a ritual of lexical reform with all its ideological underpinnings. Most importantly, she helps us glimpse ways of imagining the epidemic—such as the utter failure of treatment on interlinked individual and national scales, as sublimely catastrophic as a nuclear holocaust—that disclosure catechism forbids.

Of Futures, Fears, and Fantasies

This chapter focuses on pediatricians' efforts to shape HIV-positive children and the futures they inhabit through the language they used to teach these children about their infections. Eager to protect these children both from the horror they expected children to experience upon confronting the word "AIDS" and the decline in adherence this horror was assumed to provoke, pediatricians used the disclosure catechism to reveal children's diagnoses to them in an effort to ensure children took their ARVs, relying on euphemisms and replacing them with terms derived from biomedicine. Pediatricians dismissed Batswana adults' efforts to shield children from their diagnoses, insisting on catechism's purchase on the "truth" of HIV infection and its unique ability to contribute to children's survival. But these same pediatricians displaced onto children a conviction that the word *AIDS* impaired children's ability to effectively manage their own treatment, effectively silencing representations of the epidemic as anything other than a manageable condition so as to create a stable object of biomedical intervention.

My point is not that pediatricians were wrong in wanting to cultivate in HIV-positive Tswana children a sense of hopefulness. Who wouldn't want to console a sick, bereaved child in the midst of a devastating epidemic, to give her the tools her survival demanded? My objective has been to point out the tightly constrained contours of the moral and affective transformation pediatricians sought to bring about, and the extent to which it was oriented toward the fears and fantasies of American pediatricians, not the needs and experiences of Tswana children. This chapter and chapter 1 illustrate the moral tensions that suffuse adherence and the forms of knowledge organized around it both as a completed action that must be evaluated and as a future activity that must be coaxed into being. Both illuminate the precarious scales that link individual children, families, nurses, and pediatricians to the fantasies and nightmares of national and global proportions. But these anxieties were not confined to interpersonal interactions in consulting rooms. Chapter 3 follows Americans' efforts to scale their actions relative to the pandemic and their fantasies regarding the moral and affective transformation the pandemic demanded of Batswana out of the consultation rooms of the Clinic to Botswana's government agencies and distant international funding agencies, revealing another aspect of the scale-making entailed in the production of global health.

THE METALANGUAGE OF HIV INTERVENTION

In November 2007 Rebecca, an American administrator who had lived in Botswana for several years, showed me around the BHP building, formally known as the Botswana Harvard HIV Reference Laboratory, located on the campus of Referral Hospital. The BHP building, with its multistory facades of brick and mirrored glass, dominated the campus, which largely consisted of modest single-story red-brick wards connected by covered breezeways. As we stood at one of the upper-story windows and looked out over the campus, we could see just below us the hospital's old dental clinic. Rebecca told me that the dental clinic was being refurbished as the new IDCC dispensary. Once it opened, she explained, patients who needed refills of their ARVs would not have to wind their way through the hospital's many breezeways to the out-of-the-way corner where the IDCC stood. I was struck by how very public a site it was for this purpose. The hospital had two main entrances; the old dental clinic was immediately adjacent to one of them, in full view of all the staff, patients, and visitors entering or leaving the hospital or stopping to buy phone time, fruit, or cold drinks from the vendors whose tables and booths surrounded the gates and the adjacent parking lot. Mirroring the obliqueness of the IDCC's name, the virtue of its location was that it obscured the reason for one's presence at the hospital. Batswana in that part of the hospital might easily be assumed to be visiting ill family or friends, or seeking care at one of the hospital's specialty clinics; attending the IDCC was not a foregone conclusion. Surprised, I asked Rebecca, "Would people really want to queue for their medications with all their business on display?" Rebecca brushed away my concern: "It will help dispel stigma."

The Metalanguage of HIV Intervention

How had Rebecca come to see Batswana as so stigmatized that they had to be manipulated for their own good into the sort of public performance of disclosure the new dispensary's location would entail? What made the project of dispelling stigma by compelling Batswana into public performances make sense? As the previous chapters illustrated, American health professionals in Botswana regarded HIV-related stigma as a barrier to both adherence and disclosure, a threat not only to the health of individual patients but to the very manageability of the epidemic on national and even global scales. Rebecca's statement reflected anxieties that linked the intractability of the epidemic with the failure of Batswana to properly acknowledge it. My account of the Superlative Clinic has illustrated how these anxieties suffused interactions between Clinic staff and the HIV-positive children they treated. In this chapter, I follow these anxieties out of the Clinic and across multiple sites of Botswana's HIV treatment program. I show how American health professionals positioned themselves in contrast to Batswana who, Americans asserted, were unwilling or unable to fully acknowledge the epidemic and whom they sought to transform into the subjects that American-driven interventions demanded.

From the standpoint of American health professionals, acknowledging the epidemic was, I have argued, considered a necessary prerequisite to treatment. That the epidemic existed in the first place was taken by American professionals as a sign of broader social pathology. Previous chapters showed how Squad pediatricians' concerns about Batswana's inability to "face the truth" of the epidemic shaped their clinical practice in terms of how they assessed children's adherence and how they sought to shape children into adherent subjects. In this chapter, I illustrate how these concerns shaped HIV interventions in Botswana both within and far beyond the Superlative Clinic—from the Clinic's forms of documentation to interactions between Botswana's national agencies and distant funders. Americans' descriptions of these disparate practices converged around a specific set of words: honesty, transparency, accuracy, stigma, political, accountability. These terms are metalinguistic (Silverstein 1993, 2003), that is, they are talk about talk, and they highlight a sincerity problem, a presumed mismatch between external expressions and internal states, between appearance and depth (Keane 2007; Irvine 1982; Trilling 1972). This metalanguage, in short, constituted and reproduced a consistently skeptical stance, an assumption that one's interlocutor at best misrecognized the pandemic and was perhaps even disingenuous and dissimulating. By tracking this metalanguage across contexts, I shed light on how American professionals framed Botswana's epidemic as a site of expert American intervention by means of two related claims: The first claim was that (some) American professionals could accurately discern features of the epidemic and the elements that composed it—from individuals to institutions, intimate relationships to knowledge claims. The second claim was that Batswana, conversely, could *not* know the epidemic or its constituent elements, let alone intervene in them effectively, and that such knowledge could only be brought to their attention by actors who successfully positioned themselves "outside" Botswana. Moreover, these positions were relative rather than essential—that is, some Americans tried to make others seem insufficiently "outside" Botswana, thus unsettling their stances as experts.

Such claims draw our attention to the pragmatics of scale in global health—that is, how scales are made and are made to matter in context, the stances or processes of alignment entailed in scale-making, and the ideologies that shape and are shaped by these practices. Chapters 1 and 2 examined these phenomena from the vantage point of the Clinic's consulting rooms. In this chapter, I draw on data from across a broader range of social practices and institutions in order to track the dynamic relationship between the stances individual actors took by means of metalanguage and a "scalar infrastructure," that is, "a highly distributed assemblage of practices that . . . both makes plausible and narrows down what participants are likely to 'see'" (Lempert 2016, 55) in an interaction, shaping expectations and interpretations. The capacity of global health to offer the moral transformation of self and others, I argue, emerges from its interscalability. American health professionals used the metalanguage of HIV intervention to insist on the inability of Batswana to recognize the epidemic's true dynamics—from the national prevalence rates to their own interior states. These stances, whereby experts ratified the claims by individuals and institutions to know the epidemic, projected a scalar infrastructure that made such interpretations plausible, durable, and portable from one interaction to the next, one institution to another, blurring distinctions between technical expertise and moral judgment. The result was a pervasive scaling of moral accountability across contexts whereby to contest Americans professionals' authority was not only to refuse to acknowledge the epidemic but to actively perpetuate it. The constitution of Botswana's epidemic as an object amenable to American moral and technical expert intervention, then, was not a feature of the epidemic per se; it relied on sets of interlocking scalar claims, stances that had to be asserted and maintained through the metalanguage of HIV intervention. This chapter, then, is central to illustrating the book's larger point: that the scalar projects by which global health becomes recognizable as a particular spatial, temporal, and moral endeavor require institutional force behind them, but that global health emerges from those institutions and the stances taken by those within them; it does not self-evidently precede them.

Global health pedagogies, including claims regarding who and what was global to begin with, were thus confined to neither consultation rooms nor doctor-patient interactions. They traveled far more widely, constituting, challenging, and reshaping the scalar infrastructure of global health in the process. Because the effectiveness of such scalar infrastructures depends on their distribution (Lempert 2016, 64), this chapter follows the metalanguage of HIV intervention across three disparate sites, revealing the scale-making capacities of the power to authorize or delegitimize how people talked about HIV. In each case, authority was asserted through claims that only an "outsider" (a relative and contingent position) could see the truth of the matter. Were Batswana too stigmatized to recognize their own stigmatizing attitudes? Were national agencies too technologically unsophisticated to assess Botswana's epidemic and too invested in counteracting negative representations to concede this? This chapter is concerned, in short, with the *institutionalization* of scalar perspectives in global health (Carr and Lempert 2016, 16). This institutionalization, as this and subsequent chapters demonstrate, is a critical aspect of establishing who can be transformed by global health and how.

I begin by examining how American health professionals in Botswana talked about stigma. This "stigma talk," I argue, reveals their understanding of stigma as a pathogenic tendency to conceal—a tendency that, Americans contended, Batswana concealed even from themselves. Analyzing stigma talk reveals that, in the eyes of American health professionals, Batswana could not be relied upon to recognize, let alone intervene in, stigma in themselves or in others. American professionals thus constantly called on Batswana to reveal the truth of their stigmatized and stigmatizing interiors, but, as this and the previous two chapters illustrate, neither confession nor refusal could free Batswana from the need for outside surveillance insofar as the mere existence of the epidemic itself signaled to Americans that Batswana fundamentally could not confront its realities. I then turn to the documentary practices used by staff at the Superlative Clinic to produce epidemiological data. The Clinic claimed to represent not only the state of pediatric HIV in Botswana but the national epidemic as a whole; moreover, they attempted to set the terms by which the epidemic might be compared to other epidemics and the Clinic's own interventions evaluated. In the eyes of the Clinic's American staff, Botswana's national health system and those working within it could not be relied upon to gather the data necessary to accurately represent Botswana's pandemic, nor even recognize when their suspect clinical practices and political investments had biased their representations. I conclude by analyzing the failure of Botswana's National AIDS Coordinating Agency (NACA) to meet the Global Fund's reporting requirements, thereby putting further funding at risk. NACA was mandated by international donors to mediate between Botswana's government and the international funding agencies and institutions that claimed to be the state's "partners," but the agency's efforts to shape responses to the epidemic were undercut by the vested interests of "partner" institutions in *not* recognizing the state's authority. In the eyes of American health professionals, the state's efforts to place limits on "partner" institutions could only be the unacknowledged overinvolvement of a stereotypically pathological African state. Taken together, my three examples illustrate how American professionals established their expertise and constituted Botswana as a site of their expert intervention by means of a robust and portable scalar infrastructure that disavowed the moral and technical capacities of Batswana to know, let alone intervene in, Botswana's epidemic.

Two caveats: First, the danger in this analysis lies in the temptation to naturalize these scales ourselves, to assume their encompassment relative to one another: citizens by states, clinics by networks, national agencies by international ones (Hecht 2018; Irvine 2016). The stories in this chapter illustrate the fragility and contingency of claims to encompassment as well as their robustness. Likewise, these stories reveal the labor individuals and their institutions undertake to maintain these seemingly naturally nested scales and the eagerness, even desperation, of some actors to maintain these scales and the relationships to other individuals, other institutions, and other countries they authorize.

Second, often the anthropological impulse is to identify stigma as a form of suffering and cast revelation, even ethnographic revelation, as the alleviation of that suffering. Rather than searching for signs of liberation in my informants' performances of transparency, I take my cue from a long trajectory of scholarship that locates secrecy, rather than transparency, at the heart of society (Gluckman 1963; Goffman 1956; Piot 1993; Simmel 1906; cf. Jones 2014).[1] I focus on the intense demand for radical transparency ratified by foreign, predominantly American experts and their institutions that has suffused Botswana's epidemic, and the performances authorized and excluded in the process. Doing so shifts anthropology's own moral project from revealing the suffering concealed by stigma to asking how powerful individuals and institutions, including anthropologists, shape what counts as concealment, who is authorized to recognize obfuscation, and what is at stake in the ratification of these categories.

Dispelling Stigma through Brutal Honesty

On a bright Sunday morning in February 2008, I listened over breakfast as Valerie, an American public health professional, discussed HIV testing in Botswana. Valerie was employed by an American NGO that had seconded her to Tebelopele,

Botswana's state-run voluntary HIIV counseling and testing service. Tebelo-pele employed HIV-positive Batswana as "expert patients," that is, as educa-tors and counselors, hoping to counter stigma and promote voluntary testing by publicly deploying particular forms of HIV-positive subjectivity, known as "liv-ing positively," and to encourage prevention among those already infected, called "prevention for positives."[2] As we ate, Valerie griped about this policy, worried that it incentivized the acquisition of HIV infection. "We pay [expert patients] to be positive," she grumbled, "Why can't we pay people to stay negative?"[3] As breakfast continued, Valerie complained that many of her own HIV-positive Batswana staff claimed to have contracted the virus via "caregiver transmission," that is, in the process of caring for an infected relative or, for those who handled needles, through performing HIV tests. "I'm sorry, but that's *bull*shit," Valerie said, her voice rising with frustration. "I *know* the levels of sexual transmission in this country," she insisted. "They can't *all* be caregiver infections. They just won't admit they were fucking around."

Anxieties about stigma suffused Botswana's treatment program, spilling out into public spaces, highlighting a presumed failure among Batswana to talk about the epidemic. *Parents, let's talk to our children about HIV and AIDS*, exhorted billboards scattered around southeastern Botswana. To talk about HIV/AIDS, however, was not enough. Stigma was a matter of *how* people talked, as illus-trated by posters on clinic walls and combi stops depicting an intergenerational family meeting: *Le rona re bua ka mogare wa HIV/AIDS le ba malwapa a rona ka tshologa* [We speak about the HIV/AIDS virus with our families/households in an open/overflowing manner]. Such stigma talk in southeastern Botswana was largely the provenance of American health professionals and entailed evaluat-ing Batswana's actions, particularly (but not only) their verbal expressions, in terms of a capacity to reveal an interior state of stigma. In keeping with the lan-guage ideology that shaped the disclosure catechism in chapter 2, Batswana were encouraged to replace terms assumed to both reflect and perpetuate stig-matized states with a set of terms whose accuracy promised to preempt the con-cealment of stigmatization. Most broadly, stigma talk encouraged Batswana to foster an understanding of themselves as stigmatized, stigmatizing, or both, and to submit to experts' assessments of their stigmatized states. Stigma talk per-meated the Superlative Clinic, but it could also be found across public spaces and was promulgated through public media, reflecting international policymakers' hopes that the introduction of ARVs would normalize the disease, facilitating acceptance and increasing the efficacy of interventions (Castro and Farmer 2005; Roura et al. 2009; WHO, UNAIDS 2003).[4]

From the early days of the epidemic, anthropologists of Botswana have argued that HIV-related media campaigns have reflected the priorities of

Western, and particularly American, donors, featuring framings of the disease that map poorly onto local ones (Allen and Heald 2004; Heald 2002, 2005; Mac-Donald 1996). This section pushes this argument further, drawing attention to how American health professionals in Botswana's treatment program used stigma talk metalinguistically as a scale-making claim. Both stigma and sincerity are intersubjective: the former requires a second party to recognize the stigmatizing characteristic (Goffman 1963; cf. Hankins 2014); the latter requires a second party to assess the alignment of external expression and interior state. But this process of ratification may have far-reaching consequences, as any concealment or, more seriously, the inability or unwillingness to admit to concealment could be read by experts as a sign a subject was unable to align external expressions with internal states. In this section I argue American health professionals used stigma talk to diagnose individual Batswana with a pathogenic tendency to conceal. In the process, they scaled themselves vis-à-vis individual Batswana and, further, scaled their intervention from stigmatized individuals to a flawed nation, thereby establishing their professional credibility vis-à-vis global health.

A hallmark of the disease from its very beginning, stigma has been hailed by experts, policymakers, and activists as "a major barrier to effective responses to the HIV/AIDS epidemic" (A. P. Mahajan et al. 2008, S67; cf. Chesney and Smith 1999; Herek 1999). And while researchers across the social sciences, psychology, and public health cite Goffman's foundational text (1963), Goffman's emphasis on stigma as a feature of *relationships* rather than persons has given way in American public health and social psychology and, through them, biomedicine and health programming to an understanding of stigma in terms of a sociocognitive framework, that is, as "a relatively static characteristic or feature, albeit one that is at some level culturally constructed" (R. Parker and Aggleton 2003, 14). Across these fields, conceptualizations of stigma emphasize cognitive categories and processes over relationships or contextual factors (Link and Phelan 2001). In these "highly individualized analyses," Parker and Aggleton argue in their review of research on HIV/AIDS-related stigma, "words come to characterize people in relatively unmediated fashion . . . [and] stigma, understood as a negative attribute, is mapped onto people" (2003, 14) in a process framed as "essentially inimical to sociability" (Preston-Whyte 2003; cf. Hardon and Posel 2012).[5] In sum, from these research worlds to the interventions they inform, the problem of stigma has become a matter of revealing how people create negative stereotypes and apply these stereotypes to themselves or others and finding ways they can be made *not* to do so (Mahajan et al. 2008).

Valerie's outburst illustrates several assumptions American health professionals held regarding stigma and HIV in Botswana. The first was that Batswana did not, and perhaps could not, talk about having HIV or how they contracted the virus. Second, Batswana could not or would not recognize stigmatizing attitudes toward those with HIV, including, and perhaps most importantly, in themselves. Third, experts like Valerie were in a position to recognize this phenomenon—which ranged from deliberate concealment to unacknowledged avoidance to a kind of involuntary state of not-knowing—and to direct its remedy, that is, to convince her staff that an effective intervention into the epidemic required them to concede they were "fucking around." Anthropologists working in southern Africa have emphasized how stigma, in contrast to conceptualizations focused on static features or cognitive categories, operates instead as "a complicated, multilayered symbolic system . . . rooted in concerns about respect, maintenance of hope for the future, and a more general avoidance of illness" (Black 2013, 483; cf. Wood and Lambert 2008) that opens up the possibility for concealment as a gesture of compassion (Klerk 2012). But when Batswana used terms like *this mogare* or *this thing* or said, *O na le jwa radio* [he/she has the radio thing] and did not say *HIV*, American health professionals saw signs of deficient transparency embedded in Tswana culture that legitimized their expert intervention in the nation.[6] To whatever extent Valerie's staff, like other health professionals in sub-Saharan Africa, maintained among themselves "a secret sharing network" (Kyakuwa and Hardon 2012, S126), she regarded it as a misguided one that perpetuated the stigma that ultimately drove the epidemic.

Stigma purportedly hid inner truths from a stigmatized subject behind a barrier of denial born of shame and fear (cf. Carr 2010b, 92). Within the framework of stigma talk, American health professionals gauged the depth of a Motswana's stigma/stigmatization and her commitment to her own and her children's treatment, by the extent to which she used language Americans recognized as a sign that she had accepted her status and had confronted and overcome her feelings of shame and fear. While pediatricians nominally refused to disclose one person's HIV status to another, Maikutlo's story in chapter 1 illustrates that they would implicitly threaten to do so in the form of a family meeting in order "to identify and articulate the truth *on behalf of their clients*" (Carr 2010b, 101, emphasis in the original), that is, to bring the fact of Maikutlo's concealment of her serostatus and the harmful effects of this concealment to her consciousness. Conversely, Dr. Rachel had visibly brightened when Mma Mokento, translating for Mma Kgomotso, explained that Mma Kgomotso had found work as an HIV peer counselor and was "living positively." Yet these assessments were always precarious and subject to reevaluation. American health professionals like Valerie, Dr. Amy, and the Squad pediatricians, committed to assessing patients' and caregivers' stigma, faced the ever-present possibility that Batswana were "not be speaking inner truths precisely when they seemed to be" (Carr 2010b, 131). This is clear in Valerie's concern that expert patients leveraged disclosing their serostatus for material gain, instrumentalizing public disclosures of HIV infection rather than modeling how to "live positively" and, crucially, avoid infecting others.

A key aspect of stigma talk, then, was getting Batswana to recognize themselves as taking part in stigma, that is, perpetuating stigmatizing attitudes toward HIV/AIDS by harboring them, whether they directed those attitudes toward themselves, toward others, or both (cf. Pigg 2001). By means of such involuntary publicity as the relocation of the IDCC pharmacy would require of them, Batswana *for their own good* had to be forced to relinquish the dialectic of concealment and revelation that, as noted in previous chapters, is foundational to Tswana conceptualization of personhood, a particular manifestation of a more general phenomenon Goffman called the "ritual game of having a self" (Goffman 1956, 497; 1967). Chapter 2 illustrated how American physicians recruited children to a stepwise pedagogy by means of the disclosure catechism; American health professionals' approach to adults was quite different. American physicians reprimanded adult Batswana for even minor evasions, like keeping out of sight until an acquaintance had departed the clinic, or seeking treatment in Gaborone, which might afford more anonymity than a village clinic, or facilitating treatment through trusted kin. These health professionals equated denial, however unconscious, psychologically protective, or culturally mediated it might be, with death; this equation was further complicated by the transmissibility of HIV and American physicians' imaginations of adults' sexuality, a marked contrast to the emphasis in the Clinic on children's *future* sexual encounters. In this view, Batswana who, like Valerie's staff members, admitted to HIV infection but could not or would not admit they were "fucking around" not only engaged in dissimulation but exacerbated the epidemic by refusing to link their HIV transmission to their sexual behavior. This gave them an "out" from the moral position, which, in Valerie's eyes, they were obliged to occupy and, by occupying it, normalize it.

The metalanguage of HIV intervention pervaded these interactions, grounding survival in a project of surveillance that Batswana could participate in only by transforming seeming concealment into public display. Dr. Natalie, discussing with me a ten-year-old patient who had been raised by his aunt after his mother's death some years ago, explained that she needed to find out how the boy's mother died. "If it was AIDS, we need to tell him," she explained. "We have to dispel stigma through brutal honesty." This project, however, was confounded by Barr's own finding that children whose adult caregivers feared stigma on the part of family members actually had *better* adherence than children whose caregivers found their own families to be more accepting. One woman, Barr observes, attributed her careful monitoring of her daughter's adherence to her desire to keep her kin from deducing the child's condition (Barr 2006; cf. Thupayagale-Tshweneagae 2010, 262). Maintaining a child's adherence, Barr observed, also reduced the likelihood that Clinic staff would pressure a caregiver to disclose the child's infection to other family members, as they did when a child became resistant to first-line ARVs (2006, 121). Rather than telling clinicians what they knew clinicians wanted to hear, caregivers did what they knew clinicians wanted them to do—that is, they maintained their children's adherence—in order to avoid having to say what they, caregivers, wished to avoid saying.[7]

But instead of reading in such avoidance a simple desire to maintain a measure of privacy, some experts worried that it indicated Africans' stigmatizing attitudes toward *being recognized* as harboring stigmatizing attitudes toward HIV to begin with. In other words, experts worried that any seeming absence of stigma was, in truth, a barrier of shame and fear toward *admitting* stigma that concealed beneath it feelings of shame and fear about HIV that had become unacceptable to admit and that motivated a second layer of concealment. In neighboring South Africa, researcher Jo Stein worried that reports indicating lower levels of stigma with regard to HIV/AIDS "could merely indicate that most people in South Africa . . . are now aware that discrimination is 'wrong' and want to appear to social science researchers as more accepting of HIV positive people than they actually are" (2003, 96). By contrast, no such worry of dissimulation accompanies southern Africans' admissions of stigma: individuals' confessions of stigmatizing attitudes were generally taken at face value, the African epidemic's axiomatic truth. But Stein suggests that South Africans who claim to have overcome their stigmatizing attitudes may in fact feel so stigmatized by the stigmatizing attitudes they hold that they will not admit them to researchers, thus generating yet another "dirty secret" that conceals a "hidden truth" (2003, 96). Using the metalanguage of HIV intervention, experts such as Valerie could assert that the truth is only visible to those "outside" the epidemic, authorizing expert scrutiny even when experts fail to uncover stigma. This is a scalar claim that serves to uphold the importance of external expertise. The result is an ever-receding horizon in which the ability of southern Africans to recognize, let alone articulate, their own interiorities is constantly in doubt.

The Networked Clinic

Across the landscape of Botswana's HIV/AIDS-related programming myriad nurses, doctors, students, and outreach staff roamed hospital wards and clinic corridors in the capital and the countryside. Armed with paper forms and ballpoint pens, they meticulously recorded people (patients, trainees, recipients), activities (testing, mentoring, touching, traveling, examining), and materials (needles, blood, the number of lines on an HIV test, pills). The seemingly endless activity of documentation also provided an endless source for discussion as Batswana and expatriates alike debated its minute and particular demands, expressed concerns about its incompleteness, and harbored suspicions about its accuracy and relevance. Where did all these numbers go? What did they do when they arrived at their destinations? What, if any, were their effects?

Anthropologists of global health have analyzed how numbers have come to dominate global health, shaping how those who "do" global health imagine their sites of intervention, how they design interventions, and how they assess the efficacy of these interventions. Rather than merely reflecting objective truths, they argue, numbers "constitute and reflect the particular social worlds and infrastructures necessary to birth them" (Biruk 2018, 168; Erikson 2012; Tichenor 2017).[8] In this section I focus on how numbers are deployed in scalar claims, that is, how some numbers acquired a capacity to point to or encompass contexts beyond themselves while others pointed only to the condition of their production. While scholarship on global health has emphasized how transnational interventions contribute to the disorganization of clinical data (McKay 2018, chap. 6), I highlight instead how the Superlative Clinic's administrators used the metalanguage of HIV intervention to frame the Clinic as a transnational intervention in the first instance through the disaggregation and even disorganization of clinical data.

Like stigma talk, debates over numerical representations of Botswana's epidemic were metalinguistic in the sense that the heart of the disagreement was about what the numbers pointed to and what they encompassed (Gal 2016; Irvine 2016). These debates posed a sincerity problem insofar as they called into question the willingness and ability of institutions to represent the epidemic. In this section, I show how the Superlative Clinic's administrators, while participating in processes of patient data collection authorized by Botswana's Ministry of Health, mobilized a parallel system in an attempt to "upscale" (Bauman 2016; Irvine 2016) their numbers as the only reliable *national* representations of HIV in Botswana. Employing the metalanguage of HIV intervention, administrators argued that by limiting their analysis to the data they themselves produced, they more accurately assessed the state of pediatric HIV in Botswana. More strikingly, they claimed that although their data were limited to children, the Clinic nonetheless captured a more accurate representation of Botswana's epidemic as a whole than the state could extrapolate from its own much larger collection of data. The capacity of the Clinic's data to capture Botswana's epidemic, in turn, legitimized the Clinic's reliance on CHAN's network of pediatric HIV clinics in Eastern Europe and across sub-Saharan Africa, rather than Botswana's national institutions, to set standards of practice and to assess the credibility of epidemiological claims. Within this network, each clinic took its cues from CHAN's US-based headquarters, and each claimed to know what the nation-state in which that particular clinic was located could not. These assertions drew on and reinforced a broader scalar infrastructure that positioned the epidemic in each of these places as visible only to outside experts.

Documentation formed an integral part of consultations at the Superlative Clinic. Fundamental to both the production of adherence assessments and processes of disclosure, documentation took up a significant portion of clinicians' and patients' time. Each child attending the Clinic had an archive composed in multiple modalities and stored in multiple locations. The process often began before a child even set foot in the Clinic for a checkup. Before the end of the workday, a few nurses went upstairs to the file room on the second floor to pull the binders that corresponded to the children scheduled to be seen the next day. These binders, the first component of the archive, were then piled behind the reception desk. The next morning, adults and children arriving at the Superlative Clinic began by registering at the desk with Malebogo, who handed them a pink numbered card indicating their place in the queue and began arranging the binders to correspond to that order. One by one a nurse called the children to a small room off the reception area to be triaged: their height, weight, and temperature were measured and recorded and any signs of severe illnesses examined or referred to the hospital's inpatient pediatric medical ward. Each child then returned to the reception area until a pediatrician or nurse called the child's name a second time, at which point the measurements gathered from triage and the child's binder accompanied them to a consultation room.

The second component was the child's outpatient card, a pink or blue card upon which every clinic visit was meant to be recorded, along with the stamp that accompanied all encounters with the public health system.[9] The card also ideally recorded the child's weight and height, childhood vaccinations, prescriptions, and treatments. If a child's card became full, another would be attached, and many adults who brought children to the Clinic had crafted some kind of folder to protect a child's growing collection of outpatient cards. Information was meant to be chronologically arranged (Bussmann et al. 2006); in practice, this was not always the case. Clinicians struggled to decipher other health professionals' handwritten notations; annotations, admonitions, and corrections abounded as a child's outpatient card moved through different points in Botswana's public health system.

Each consultation room was equipped with a networked computer and a printer. During the consultation clinicians intermittently turned to the screen to refer to documentation from prior visits or turned to the keyboard to enter the results of their assessments and document the counseling they performed. The second component of the archive consisted of Meditech, an electronic health record system used throughout Botswana's referral and district hospital system. Developed by an American company in consultation with its South Africa branch (Snyman et al. 2007), Meditech allowed Clinic staff to look up the results of CD4 counts and viral loads as well as less complicated tests such as complete blood counts that were conducted outside the Clinic at the Botswana Harvard HIV Reference Laboratory and the Referral Hospital laboratory, respectively. Meditech promised a centralized location for patient data, making it possible for clinicians to track patients and their test results from one clinic to another. American clinicians throughout the hospital, however, complained bitterly about Meditech frequently "going down," and Squad pediatricians frequently held their breath or gritted their teeth as they attempted to look up the results of a child's most recent tests.

The third component of the child's clinical archive was the Clinic's in-house documentation system, a cumulative set of one-page Microsoft Word documents stored on the Clinic's server in an electronic file labeled with a child's first and last name. This system predated Meditech, and, in effect, served as a backup electronic health record system when Meditech was unavailable. Indeed, Squad pediatricians often sighed with relief as they turned to the in-house documentation system. A new Word document was created for each visit, and clinicians copied patient information from the record of a prior visit—usually, but not always, the most recent visit—and pasted it into the new Word document. As she copied and pasted information from one Word document to another, a pediatrician obtained a brief account of the child in front of her with whom she might be unfamiliar. Unlike Meditech, furthermore, these Word documents frequently provided Squad pediatricians with another Squad pediatrician's account of a child's adherence and her social situation, which they used to frame their assessments. Pediatricians recorded a child's current state of health, the results of her adherence assessment, her progress with regard to the disclosure catechism discussed in chapter 2, any laboratory results available in Meditech, and any changes to her social situation. Despite its comfort and familiarity, however, the in-house system could prove cumbersome as pediatricians, who had varying degrees of familiarity with Setswana names and were often unaware of Setswana lexicographic rules, such as use of the letter *H* to indicate aspirated consonants in names such as *Tshenolo* or the voiceless velar fricative of *G* in *Kgomotso*, found themselves sorting through multiple files belonging to one child whose name had been spelled three different ways by three different American pediatricians at previous appointments.

Pediatricians saved the new Word document on the server and printed two copies. Nurses punched holes in this first copy and placed it in the child's binder, which contained a chronologically ordered set of all the Word documents from prior visits to the Clinic. The binder served as an offline backup system for the Clinic's in-house electronic health record system and the repository for the pen-and-paper notes that were the final fallback resource when both Meditech and the Clinic's server were down. The second copy was stapled to the child's most recent outpatient card, where it joined an ever-expanding collection of such documents, a medicalized life course in paper form. On the reverse side of this collection of papers was the Clinic's drug sheet, with a new one stapled on top of the previous one as needed (see figure 2 in chapter 1). As the child left the Clinic, a nurse or pediatrician returned the binder to a shelf just behind the reception desk so that it could be returned to the file room that evening, where it would wait to be retrieved when the child was scheduled to return to the Clinic.

This duplication of data could be extremely time consuming. On days when Meditech was down, the pediatricians spent their afternoons synchronizing patient data by hand in either Meditech or the Clinic's in-house system, as Dr. Rachel often did over a makeshift lunch of French fries and Fanta. But the possibility of isolating the Clinic's data from other clinical data in Botswana provided the Clinic's administrators, primarily Dr. Amy, opportunities to scale the Clinic and Botswana's epidemic in particular ways. First, it allowed her to discount Meditech. For one thing, she distrusted the ability of public-sector clinicians to accurately account for their patients. But even if she had considered the data an accurate representation of public-sector clinicians' practices, American pediatricians tended to assume pediatric HIV treatment in Botswana outside the Clinic was substandard: in their eyes, local clinicians ignored children's poor adherence and thus failed to capture drug resistance. This distrust could extend within the Clinic itself, complicating distinctions between inside and outside (Brada 2016; cf. Gal 2002). Dr. Chibesa told me that Dr. Amy, examining a patient's records, would sometimes ask a caregiver, "Who wrote this? Was it a *Black* doctor?" He had heard about this from the nurses, to whom the caregivers would recount the exchange in Setswana, sheltering the conversation from American ears. "Look what this *lekgoa* [white person, i.e., Dr. Amy] is asking me," caregivers demanded of nurses, affronted by Dr. Amy's invitation to participate in her disparagement of African physicians.[10] In short, for Dr. Amy, comparing outcomes of pediatric HIV treatment across clinical spaces in Botswana could be significant only insofar as it illustrated both the superiority of the Americans' treatment practices and the relative accuracy of the Clinic's self-assessment. The data from inside and outside the Clinic could not, from this point of the view, be aggregated. Americans might uncover irregularities in the spelling of children's names as they compiled numerical data from patients' files, but they considered these inconsequential mistakes in contrast to other clinicians' faulty clinical assessments.

Further, if, from Dr. Amy's points of view, Meditech provided an account of faulty pediatric treatment practices at best and inaccurate data about those practices at worst, then the Superlative Clinic could most accurately represent the state of pediatric HIV in Botswana on a national scale. As discussed in chapter 1, the Superlative Clinic attempted to enroll HIV-positive children from far beyond Gaborone and its surrounds, arguing that HIV-positive children required specialized treatment that only the Clinic could provide. Rather than one inaccurate piece of an inaccurate national puzzle, as another clinic's Meditech data might have provided, Clinic administrators positioned the Superlative Clinic's in-house data as the most accurate *national* perspective available on Botswana's pediatric HIV epidemic. This claim, in turn, provided the Clinic with the grounds to compare its data on pediatric HIV in Botswana with analogous representations of other countries. Rather than comparing what they saw as incommensurable treatment practices across Botswana's clinical spaces, Dr. Amy and her colleagues were much more invested in producing data commensurable with the network of pediatric clinics that CHAN supported, reinforcing a scalar infrastructure that linked the existence of national epidemics to the untrustworthiness of national epidemiological data. Across this network, treatment protocols and assessment methods could be standardized with the aim of comparatively evaluating ARV regimens and failure rates enacted and assessed by pediatricians whose relationships of trust were mediated by CHAN and reinforced at its annual meetings. "We want to be able to see if we're improving," Dr. Amy explained once, but the scale of comparison was in terms of CHAN-sponsored clinics, which Superlative Clinic's American staff considered commensurable both in terms of the practices used to treat pediatric HIV and in terms of the data collected to reflect those practices, not other clinical spaces in Botswana.

Participating in a global conversation about pediatric HIV thus meant using the metalanguage of HIV intervention to scale data from Clinic to nation, and scaling both treatment practices and data collection methods from local idiosyncrasies to authorized standards, reflecting ideological claims whereby some forms of encompassment count more than others (Irvine 2016; cf. Bowker and Star 1999; Timmermans and Epstein 2010). It entailed reading Dr. Chibesa's documentation as a reflection of his presumably inferior clinical practices rather than of his patients' adherence; it also entailed rejecting other institutions' claims to capture anything beyond themselves, even when those claims were articulated by Americans.[11] Dr. Mendoza was an American physician who had relocated to

Botswana in the early 2000s to work for ACHAP on the treatment program's guidelines. She had stayed on in Gaborone, working in Referral Hospital's Failure Clinic, where she treated adults enrolled at the hospital's IDCC who had developed resistance to first-line ARVs. She was so busy that she could only make time to speak with me while she was running errands in her car. As we drove around Gaborone, she told me that the national failure rate for adults on first-line ARVs was around 4 percent. When I repeated this statistic to Dr. Amy, she snorted derisively, estimating that the failure rate for children attending the Superlative Clinic was around 33 percent and dismissing the possibility that the IDCC's failure rate could be one-eighth the Clinic's. Confident in both the stringency of the Clinic's adherence assessments and the quality of its data, Dr. Amy asserted the Clinic's capacity to capture the epidemic's dynamics at a national scale while refusing the Failure Clinic's data to reflect anything other than the idiosyncrasies of the Failure Clinic at best and at worst, as Dr. Amy hinted, Dr. Mendoza's professional investment in the treatment program's success.[12]

Dr. Amy's claims reflected and reinforced a scalar infrastructure wherein health professionals positioned within Botswana's public sector simply could not accurately account for their own patient population or generate data that reflected anything more than the image of itself the state desired. Even the national prevalence rate, which might seem like a basic fact concerning the epidemic, was a source of constant tension. UN-sponsored surveys in the early 2000s had estimated Botswana's HIV prevalence rate to be about 37 percent, but this rate was extrapolated from women attending antenatal clinics (UNAIDS 2004).[13] In 2005 the Central Statistics Office issued the second Botswana AIDS Impact Survey (BAIS II), a national population-based household sexual behavioral survey that concluded with an average national prevalence rate of just over 17 percent, with a slightly higher rate for females than males (Government of Botswana 2004). Although the government continued to refer to the results of BAIS II as official representations of the epidemic, some American health experts, Valerie among them, flat out refused to believe the results, faulting the government survey's methodology. The low rate, she and other American professionals argued, was "political," that is, an index of the government's desire to manage its image that had corrupted its methodology and blinded it to the magnitude of the epidemic, thereby necessitating the intervention of outside experts who could assess the epidemic dispassionately. The claim that the prevalence rate was "political," like the suspicion of a stigmatized attitude submerged in denial, reinforced a spatial, temporal, and moral scalar infrastructure whereby "outsiders" could see the epidemic's true contours while "insiders" remained indefinitely mired in denial and vested interests. For American health professionals to claim that a lower prevalence rate might merely reflect a state agenda ignores the fact that the higher number was itself useful to American organizations (and indeed, to anthropologists) appealing to funders. As the next section illustrates, while statistics might be the "science of the state," the state sometimes appeared *least* equipped to know and represent its own epidemic (Foucault 1991, 96; cf. B. Anderson 1983; Appadurai 1996; Scott 1998).

Being Seen Like a State

In 2006 The Global Fund for AIDS, Tuberculosis and Malaria formally withdrew its commitment to provide Botswana with P54 million (US $9.5 million), the second installment of a US$18 million grant, on the grounds that Botswana's National AIDS Coordinating Agency (NACA) had failed to meet the conditions of the first term of the grant, including failing to submit a country report detailing how the first installment of the grant had been disbursed.[14] The scandal had, to an extent, been forewarned: In 2005 an auditor general's report had raised concerns about NACA's lack of control over the funds from the first installment of the grant that it had channeled to local nongovernmental organizations (Muzinda 2007). As the debacle unfolded, NACA insisted the blame lay with its own grantees who, NACA claimed, had failed to submit their own reports, thus depriving NACA of data it required to report to the Global Fund (Muzinda 2007; Serite 2006; Sharma and Seleke 2008). In response, four of Botswana's largest NGOs published statements in local papers and through their own public relations mechanisms expressing dismay at having been publicly and unfairly blamed by NACA and insisting that they had regularly reported to both NACA and the Ministry of Finance and Development Planning. Turning the tables, they had accused NACA of lacking a "proper funds management system" (Sharma and Seleke 2008, 331; *Mmegi* 2007).

In early 2007 NACA sought to reassure the public of its good relations with the Global Fund. While the National AIDS Coordinator at the time, Batho Molomo, admitted that Botswana had been unprepared to manage the grant's first installment, he also pointed to the situation's silver lining, namely, that, "unlike in other countries, the withdrawal [of the commitment to provide the grant's second installment] has nothing to do with corruption in the utilization of the funds by any of the players."[15]

Thus far, I have argued that both stigma talk and epidemiological representations of HIV in Botswana offer examples of the metalanguage of HIV intervention. American professionals used this metalanguage to determine who could be knowledgeable about Botswana's epidemic and who, by contrast, could only be the subject of knowledge and intervention from "outside." In so doing, American health professionals anticipated and reproduced a scalar infrastructure across clinical interactions between American health professionals and HIV-positive patients, and in American health professionals' claims regarding the epidemiology of Botswana's epidemic. This section extends this argument by examining the relationship between Botswana's National AIDS Coordinating Agency and the Global Fund as a site of this scalar infrastructure. Rather than stigma or accurate epidemiology, however, what was at stake was "transparency" as a principle of "good governance."[16] Like my previous two examples, transparency reveals itself as metalinguistic: the model it offers "presumes a surface to power that can be seen through and an interior that can, as a result, be seen" (Sanders and West 2003, 16), thus requiring their calibration. I argue that NACA's failure to represent its activities to the satisfaction of the Global Fund and other international funding agencies was an inevitable outcome of the scalar infrastructure of global health. In other words, these international institutions were structurally predisposed *not* to recognize the country as capable of adequate self-knowledge and self-representation. Furthermore, activities that might have been construed as good governance, such as the state's efforts to account for health-related activities within its borders and to uphold its own regulations, were received not as signs of state capacity but as the opposite.

NACA was established in 1999; its head reported directly to the National AIDS Council, which was chaired by the President of the Republic. It was a foundational element of what James Putzel calls an "organizational template" for HIV/AIDS programming worked out in the World Bank's funding requirements and perpetuated by the Global Fund through its funding mechanisms and by UNAIDS' conceptualization of the epidemic (2004). This template framed the epidemic as a crisis of development as much as of health, thereby widening the scope of interveners and legitimizing the involvement of the Bank and other development agencies. In addition, it requires the creation of independent National AIDS Commissions, bypassing state agencies, including national Ministries of Health, in order to emphasize "civil society" and private sector "stakeholders" (Putzel 2004, 1311). As an institution NACA represented "an implicit assessment of the inability of organizations within the state, or public authority, to implement HIV/AIDS programs" (2004, 1138), a position that itself reflects the legacy of structural adjustment policies and "an implicit, virtually ideological belief, that NGOs, religious organizations and private sector organizations will be able to do better" (J. L. Comaroff and J. Comaroff 1999, 18; cf. Pfeiffer and Chapman 2010).

Furthermore, the funding requirements and programmatic strategies laid out by the World Bank, Global Fund, and other funding agencies reflect an approach to that epidemic that privileged international expertise over forms of knowledge produced at the national level, let alone district or municipal, one, and emphasized the horizontality of comparisons among nation-states over local histories.[17] In her analysis of HIV-related policy planning in India and South Africa, Manjari Mahajan argues that international experts drew on "foreknowledge," that is, "an already existing, generic template of an AIDS epidemic," that shaped the way they perceived any national epidemic, emphasizing tools, categories, and interventions that could be made commensurable from one country to another, including an emphasis on "civil society" and nongovernmental organizations (2008, 585–86; cf. Escobar 1995; Ferguson 1990; Pigg 1997; 2001). Remarking on the "profoundly generic" and thus portable character of models of the epidemic, Mahajan observes that this "template" renders an epidemic measurable, albeit limited to national terms, thereby making the planning of a national response possible, but also carries the potential to shape the epidemic itself through this response (cf. Briggs and Nichter 2009). Furthermore, as with both stigma talk and national epidemiologies, the standardization of models, tools, categories, components, and interventions itself "carries a moral valence" (Mahajan 2008, 588; cf. Bowker and Star 1999; Lampland and Star 2009; Riles 2001; Scherz 2014, chap. 5). Chief among NACA's responsibilities, then, was to demonstrate Botswana's capability to meet the requirements of the template itself. Not only did the report and its adherence to expectations carry a moral weight but the government's willingness and ability to represent its own activities reflected a bid toward the modernity of Botswana's national government and, by extension, the entire country.

Mahajan argues that in India the structure of "foreknowledge" lent itself to a dynamic in which national actors found themselves responding to the dictates of already established international expertise rather than setting the terms by which the epidemic should be understood and addressed (2008, 90). In Botswana, NACA and other agencies, particularly the MOH, had to contend with an emerging consensus among American health and development professionals that the state was unwilling or unable to temper its inappropriate involvement in HIV/AIDS programming. Some scholars have argued that, accolades regarding its political and economic stability aside, Botswana is more an authoritarian state than a democratic republic, a *de facto* one-party system in which political and economic domination and bureaucratic ineptitude masquerade as good governance and pretensions to modernity (Botlhomilwe, Sebudubudu, and Maripe 2011; K. Good 1992, 1996, 1999; Holm and Molutsi 1992; Molutsi and Holm 1990). Anthropologists and others have challenged this view, arguing that its formalism misses the heart of how politics "works" in Botswana, that is, as a durable orientation toward constituting and reworking social and political relationships through absorption, incorporation, and evasion rather than confrontation (Botlhomilwe and Sebudubudu 2011; J. L. Comaroff and J. Comaroff 1997b; Durham 1999; Gulbrandsen 2012; Z. Maundeni 2004; Tsie 1996; cf. J. Comaroff and J. L. Comaroff 1991, chap. 4).[18] During my fieldwork, however, the former view held sway among American health and development professionals who bemoaned the state's interest in their operations, its demands for reports, and its sway over local NGOs, and who longed for more distance, even antagonism, between "civil society" and the state. "Botswana *has* no civil society," the director of the Botswana office of one large American NGO unequivocally declared to me, while the director of PACT, another American organization that was tasked with administering PEPFAR funds to small NGOs in Botswana, described Botswana's civil society as "the weakest on the continent" (Strain 2008, 32).[19] Civil society may be, as Jean and John Comaroff note, a "modernist conceit" that is "impossibly difficult to pin down" (1999, 6, 5); nevertheless, the Global Fund demanded that NACA demonstrate that a civil society existed in Botswana that met the Global Fund's expectations and requirements.[20]

As the number of stakeholders, including NGOs, partnerships, and government ministries, increased in response to ongoing pressure from international agencies to decentralize the country's HIV/AIDS programming, NACA's role as a coordinating mechanism grew both more necessary and less possible. In the wake of the 2006 scandal, NACA was reported "to be struggling in enforcing its authority for command, coordination, and control over several organizations operating at the central as well as local government levels" (Sharma and Seleke 2008, 330). But as the point of mediation between the national government and the international institutions that insisted upon a civil society on their terms, NACA could not *but* fail. While international funding agencies required it to exist to disburse funds, and American institutions and NGOs, including global health partnerships, needed it in order to continue to receive a portion of those funds, American institutions and organizations in Botswana *also* had a vested interest in NACA's institutional weakness insofar as this weakness provided the conditions for them to continue to claim the state was generically "African" and incapable of asserting itself as a modern institution and could thus be disregarded. For Americans professionals and institutions to disregard the state and its directives, like the public placement of the new IDCC clinic, could even seem beneficent, an action taken on behalf of Batswana for their own good.

The metalanguage of HIV intervention, including generic templates of the epidemic and of the individuals and institutions participating in the response, thus anticipated and solidified American health professionals' approach to Botswana's government as an institution that fundamentally could not coordinate the response to its own epidemic or even represent the interests of the nation and could only reflect Africa's failed bid to modernity. Americans read NACA's supposed failures not as the logical consequences of inequitable transnational institutional arrangements, but as evidence of a scalar distinction between what Batswana could know and do about the epidemic and Americans' own perspectives and actions. In a sad irony, the government's efforts to shape policy, enforce regulations, and even determine which organizations operated in the country were seen not as governance but as the state overstepping its authority. American pediatricians complained bitterly that the government insisted on keeping the age of consent for HIV testing at eighteen years while public hospitals admitted children older than twelve years to adult wards, not pediatric ones; expatriate development professionals were shocked when PACT, headed by a notoriously uncivil individual, was asked by Botswana's government to cease its operations in the country.[21] A number of civil servants, however, complained to me of a double standard: Botswana's agencies were required to strictly observe the funding, operational, and reporting requirements of the Global Fund and the US government, not least the byzantine requirements of PEPFAR funding (cf. Reynolds 2014a, 2014b). Americans, by contrast, regularly disregarded Botswana's regulations, dismissing any "local" objections as the pedantic overinvolvement of an inept state. Some members of the Pediatric Squad, I was told more than once, received permission to practice medicine in Botswana as specialists before they received Board certification as pediatricians in the US. but without undergoing any equivalent examination in Botswana. In Dr. Jonathan Frank's words, this had entailed the Clinic' leadership "muscling them [i.e., Squad pediatricians] through" the Botswana Health Professions Council's registration process. Some "local" physicians, including expatriate (but not American) members of the BHPC, complained that American physicians seemed to assume that American training obviated any need for Botswana's own regulatory processes. Yet "local" doctors' complaints that Americans were violating Botswana's policies by treating noncitizens under the auspices of the national treatment programs or by letting American medical students perform duties beyond their level of training were received by Americans not as signs of their own overreach or as manifestations of transnational and institutional inequalities, but as claims whose illegitimacy was grounded in the fact that the state and its agents were articulating them in the first place.

Scaling the Epidemic

This chapter has argued that the constitution of expertise in Botswana's epidemic rested on an observer's claim that she knew something about the observed that the observed themselves could not know—something, indeed, that the observed may not even know they did not know. I focused specifically on the metalanguage of HIV intervention, that is, a skeptical stance toward one's interlocutor's ability and willingness to match inner states and external representations. Following this metalanguage out of the Superlative Clinic's consultation rooms and into contests over epidemiological data and accounting practices, I showed how American health professionals positioned themselves in contrast to Batswana who, Americans asserted, were unwilling or unable to fully acknowledge the epidemic, and who they sought to transform into the subjects that American-driven interventions demanded. Tracking the metalanguage of HIV intervention helps us look beyond individual actors' stances to the scalar infrastructure that both assumed and reinforced these stances, a scalar infrastructure that disavowed the moral and technical capacities of Batswana to know, let alone intervene in, Botswana's epidemic.

Attending to the pragmatics of scale reminds us that the scalar infrastructures that made Botswana's epidemic seem to self-evidently fit within the project of "global health," while remarkably durable, are also incredibly fragile: their portability across interactions and institutions cannot be assumed; their continuing coherence requires ongoing labor. While this chapter has emphasized the durability and portability of a scalar infrastructure of global health in southeastern Botswana, the subjects and stances that constituted it were not foregone conclusions and, as aspects of global health pedagogies, could be open to contest. Chapter 4 turns to the question of how Referral Hospital's staff and American visitors grappled with the positions assigned to them in global health's scalar infrastructure while engaged in the everyday business of treatment and training on the hospital's adult medical wards.

Part 2

FANTASIES OF TRANSFORMATION

THE GLOBAL HEALTH FRONTIER

The first half of this book examined the constitution and inhabitance of the social categories of global health through language by focusing on pedagogies directed at patients and the scalar infrastructure that they presumed and entailed. The book's second half examines these processes at play in pedagogical practices oriented toward clinicians. In this chapter I offer a close examination of how EUMS physicians and students and Referral Hospital staff used instances of clinical instruction to constitute and contest the terms of global health. I argue that "global health" and the "resource-limited settings" in which it takes place are not born, to borrow Simone de Beauvoir's terms (1989); they must be made. For if, as scholars of science and medicine have argued, experts must constitute the objects of their expertise and, by so doing, constitute themselves as experts (Carr 2010a), this should be as much the case with "global health" as with any other realm of professionalized practice. What makes global health "global," I argue, has much more to do with how practitioners discursively configure space and time and the claims to expertise and moral stances these configurations make possible than it does with the geographical distribution of medical experts and expert practices, or with the universal and interdependent, if also uneven, distribution of threats to health and well-being.

In what follows I bring together anthropological arguments about place-making, the world-making capacities of language, and pedagogy and expertise to show how professionalized spaces and regimes of transnational expertise are made, inhabited, and sometimes dismantled. I examine how physicians and medical students affiliated with EUMS and the Superlative Clinic and the medical personnel they call "local" constituted, recognized, reinforced, and contested "global health" and its attendant terms in pedagogical moments on the wards of Referral Hospital. Using concepts drawn from linguistic anthropology, namely, indexical orders and chronotopes, I examine what some actors could accomplish by using or contesting the terms of global health. I focus more on how actors deployed and contested the terms of global health, such as "local" or "resource-limited," rather than on the words "global health" themselves.[1] Attending to the circumstances under which something can be called "local" or "resource-limited" helps us see what is at stake for different actors in naming places, subjects, and activities in terms of, or in contrast to, global health. More generally, attending to these terms also helps us observe how medical trainees and educators constitute their objects of expertise and, in so doing, constitute themselves as experts and as moral actors (Carr 2010a; Goodwin 1994; Mertz 2007).

After introducing the concepts grounding my argument, I situate EUMS's presence at Referral Hospital in terms of the rise of global health in biomedical education. I then offer a close reading of an orientation speech given to a group of newly arrived EUMS students that lays out the terms of what I call the global health chronotope, followed by examples of how so-called local doctors responded to the terms of the chronotope and how some of them contested and reconfigured these terms. I end with an anecdote that emphasizes the flexibility of the chronotope in delineating the spatiotemporal frames within which global health can be located. The remarkable flexibility of the terms of global health, I argue, highlights the potential for global health to operate as a frontier, that is, as an ideological project the spatiotemporal parameters of which practitioners may attempt to delineate and redraw (Tsing 2000, 2005). This imaginative project of the global health frontier, I will show, not only makes possible a variety of stances but also legitimates an endless horizon of intervention.

Constituting Spaces and Subjects through Language

"From at least the time of Durkheim," Gupta and Ferguson remind us, "anthropologists have known that the experience of space is always socially constructed" (1992, 12). For any seemingly self-evident unit of space, "the globe" included, the task remains to analyze "the processes . . . that go into the construction of space as place or locality in the first instance" (1992, 8; cf. Haraway 1991, 1997; Tsing 2000). And as places are made, so are subjects. Stacy Pigg shows how development experts in Nepal craft their object of expertise in the form of an abstract, generic place inhabited by an abstracted, generic type of subject, while Nepalis circulate, contest, and transform these generic types and the relations between them (1992). She demonstrates first how *bikas* ("development") and "village" are constituted in relation to one another, and second, how ideas about "the village" formed in opposition to *bikas* congeal in an idea of a generic village. In the institutional context of "development work" in Nepal, "the village" "encapsulates" a wide range of sociocultural phenomena and, once this has taken place, subjects can be similarly fixed (1992, 504). With regard to "the villager," Pigg notes, one's position vis-à-vis "development" and "village" lies in one's ability to authoritatively point to the distinction: "One cannot be one to see one" (1992, 507). These now-generic subjects and the generic places they inhabit seem readily amenable to interventions, including biomedicine, that are construed by the experts who deploy them as universal.

Interventions must also be calibrated to these spaces and subjects. Drawing on feminist critiques of science and technology as well as actor-network theory, scholars of science and biomedicine have long questioned the ontological status of universals, demonstrating instead "the multiplicity that characterizes the products of technoscientific network" both in terms of the political stakes congealed in the objects of technoscience and in terms of science's "disunity" (Berg and Mol 1998; Berg and Timmermans 2000; Hacking 1996). Taking up the problem of the constitution and maintenance of universals, Marc Berg and Stefan Timmermans argue, first, that any universality—whether idea or practice—is only ever a "local universality" that "always rests on real-time work, and emerges from localized processes of negotiations and pre-existing institutional, infrastructural, and material relations" (Timmermans and Berg 1997, 275). Second, they argue that rather than replacing disorder with order, universals require a certain amount of flexibility in order to be maintained by the network that supports them and that scholars need to account for how orders give rise to and encompass their own disorders (Berg and Timmermans 2000). The universality of biomedicine is subject to the same contests as other objects of technoscience: it must be maintained; it must be flexible enough for agents to deploy it across contexts; and efforts to order it generate and shape its disorder.

These arguments help us approach claims of biomedicine's "universal" applicability or a "local" doctor's provinciality with a degree of skepticism. Nevertheless, we require a mechanism for explaining how spaces and subjects come to acquire the meanings they do. In his work on indexical orders (1993, 1995, 2003), Michael Silverstein draws on Peirce's notion of an index as a sign "where the occurrence of the sign vehicle token bears a connection of understood spatiotemporal contiguity to the occurrence of the entity signaled" (Silverstein 1995, 199; see Peirce 1932). Indexes are of two kinds: referential indexes, or shifters, take their meaning from the context of their utterance (such as the personal pronouns *you* and *we* and the spatial and temporal deictics *here* and *now*); nonreferential indexes presuppose and entail social meaning (Benveniste 1971; Jakobson 1971). Indexical orders refer to the relationships between linguistic forms and their social meanings, or to what an index can be understood to "point" in a stabilized manner, and are subject to recalibration. In this way, social meanings are "laminated" (Silverstein 2003, 222) onto linguistic forms as subjects take stances by deploying particular linguistic forms. The stances made available by any indexical order depend upon the connection between indexicals of different yet proximate orders.

The lamination of social meaning onto shifters facilitates the constitution of chronotopes, a feature of narrative characterized by an "intrinsic connectedness of temporal and spatial relationships" that is "always colored by emotions and values" (Bakhtin 1981, 84, 243). The spaces, objects, and practices defined by or in contrast to "global health" mark less a particular institutional arrangement of biological threats and expert practices in the world than they index arguments about the world and the actors and actions within it. We may more fruitfully regard the terms of global health as chronotopic, that is, as indicative of spatial and temporal positions and their attendant moral claims. Taking the terms of global health as a set of arguments obviates the need to delineate the contours of "global health" as a thing-in-the-world. Rather than argue over what it *is*, we can look instead at how it is made. Thinking about global health and its terms as chronotopic also helps us attend to its temporal dimensions as well as its spatial ones, for as much as global health imagines another country as the past, it also imagines it as the potential future (Munn 1990). The authors of an article justifying the expansion of international medical education in a "globalized world" warn that "the emergence of a new public health threat in one part of the world becomes a concern throughout the world" (Drain et al. 2007, 226). The "global" that joins global health to "globalization" imagines not only that "their" present is "our" past, but also that "their" present could well become "our" future.[2] For American medical students, going somewhere that seems to recall America's past is concomitant with preparing for, and possibly shaping, that future (cf. Hanrieder 2019).

The Rise of Global Health in Biomedical Training

EUMS's involvement in Botswana had its origins in the early days of the treatment program. In 2001 a nurse who had worked at EUMS before taking a position at Merck & Co. reached out to Dr. Byron Goldberg, Chief of the Division of

Infectious Diseases of EUMS Medical School, asking if he would send two physicians to Botswana for six months to a year to help the Ministry of Health devise the initial treatment guidelines for the ARV rollout. Thus began a process of EUMS physicians, particularly infectious disease specialists, rotating through Gaborone on a short-term basis, staying anywhere from a few weeks to a few months at a time. Once the initial treatment guidelines were in place, the EUMS physicians in Gaborone turned their attention to the clinical treatment of HIV infection at Referral Hospital, initially in the hospital's Infectious Disease Care Clinic (IDCC), the outpatient clinic in which HIV-positive patients were treated, and later on the medical wards. They also began working within a program based at the Botswana Harvard Partnership that trained members of Botswana's national health service in the management of HIV infection.

In these early years a few EUMS students found their way to Referral Hospital for short periods of time. This process gained considerable traction in early 2004 when Dr. Jackson, a young internist who just finished his own residency and the first physician to be appointed by EUMS as full-time staff at Referral Hospital, began an EUMS inpatient service on the medical wards of the Hospital. Fourth-year medical students began arriving from EUMS for six-week rotations under Dr. Jackson's supervision.[3] Students had to have completed a subinternship, that is, a rotation wherein they assumed the role of an intern (i.e., first-year resident) under close supervision. They received credit for the elective at Referral Hospital and were supervised and graded by EUMS's clinical instructors, not "local" staff. The launch of the inpatient service coincided with the launch of EUMS's new Global Health Program; by 2007 the inpatient service at the Hospital had become the GHP's flagship project. As Eastern University formalized its presence at the hospital as a partnership with the Botswana Ministry of Health and increased its staff, EUMS also received a PEPFAR grant to "elevate" the level of clinical teaching on the ward for "local" MOs and interns. Residency trainings were only just beginning to be developed in Botswana, and both MOs and their supervisors complained that MOs had insufficient mentoring and opportunities for further clinical education. EUMS personnel regarded their two goals, that is, providing EUMS students with a "global health experience" and mentoring "local" interns and MOs, as compatible. Moreover, since Botswana did not yet have a medical school, EUMS students could "fill a niche," to use the words of Dr. Rosen, director of the inpatient service, in the hospital hierarchy that was unoccupied by any "local" medical students.

EUMS's inpatient service on Referral Hospital's medical wards was part of the explosion of interest in global health in American academia, particularly in biomedical education (Kerry et al. 2013; Macfarlane, Jacobs, and Kaaya 2008; Merson 2014; Merson and Page 2009).[4] Such short-term global health rotations became enormously popular in American medical education over the past decade in conjunction with a rapid expansion of international clinical volunteering and clinical tourism in "resource-poor settings" (Berry 2014; Prince and Brown 2016; Sullivan 2018; Wendland 2012b).[5] These programs are shaped by tensions in American biomedicine with regard to the relationship between technology and care, the bureaucratization of healthcare, and the allocation of blame, topics I explore further in chapter 5; more concretely, they are highly valued for offering contemporary medical students a pedagogical experience at once technical and moral. On one hand, the rationale for these rotations reflects the imagined demands globalization has placed on American biomedicine. Biomedical educators value short-term global health experiences such as EUMS's rotation on the medical wards of Referral Hospital for their capacity to provide American medical students with the opportunity to encounter conditions they might seldom or never encounter in the course of their training but that they must be prepared to treat in a "globalized" world. Visiting Americans' ideas of what global health is, where it might be practiced, and why it is important thus carry with them implicit conceptualizations of American medical practice as well as the medical requirements of a future America (Sullivan 2018; Wendland 2012a). To this end, proponents praise such programs for their capacity to "broaden a physician's differential diagnostic skills" in the sense that they "introduce clinical entities rarely seen in the U.S." and expose students to "diseases at more advanced stages than in the U.S." (Grudzen and Legome 2007, 2).

On the other hand, proponents also argue that American students gain diagnostic skills that they cannot learn in highly technicized American medical settings. EUMS students told me that their encounters with patients in the US were governed heavily by laboratory tests and other diagnostic technologies, leaving students feeling as though decisions had been made for them. EUMS educators also expressed frustration at the ways laws and technologies kept American trainees distant from patients' bodies. Medical practice requires a "feel" that technologies could not provide, they told me, but students had few opportunities for the "hands-on" practice elementary to shaping a competent medical practitioner. In a "resource-poor setting," stripped of the technologies upon which they usually depended, students had to "rely on their history and physical exam rather than laboratory and radiologic tests as they have fewer resources" (Grudzen and Legome 2007, 4), thereby cultivating a "cost-conscious practice and back-to-basics diagnosis" (Panosian and Coates 2006, 1773) from which future (American) patients would benefit.

The technical skills cultivated through global health, in short, had implications for physician-trainees' futures as moral professionals who wielded their expertise ably and responsibly. At Referral Hospital EUMS students had "less distance, more contact" with patients than in the US, said Dr. Goldberg, thereby making "the gap between the haves and the have-nots" visible to them in ways their US-based training did not afford. At Referral Hospital, he continued, students could "get close to the humanitarian impulse that drives many students into medicine" but that was lost, he explained, in the process of biomedical education itself.[6] EUMS personnel were not alone in this assessment: Since the early 2000s biomedical educators have argued that students who have taken part in global health rotations have a better grasp of medicine's "true" mission: they are more likely to enter careers in public health, primary care, or humanitarianism; to express a commitment to underserved or marginalized communities; and to demonstrate cultural competence, sensitivity, and compassion (Evert et al. 2007; Grudzen and Legome 2007; Nelson et al. 2008; Panosian and Coates 2006; see also Drain et al. 2007; Haq et al. 2000; Ramsey et al. 2004).[7]

The day-to-day burden of teaching and supervising the constant influx of EUMS students arriving in groups of six or seven fell to a handful of doctors recruited to the "permanent" EUMS staff in Gaborone. This small group included Michael Matheson, a tall, affable American who specialized in both medicine and pediatrics, a young Australian doctor named Jonathan Frank, and a Motswana physician named Moagi Tsileng, who had trained in the West Indies and the US. These men divided their efforts among several tasks. In addition to teaching and mentoring both EUMS students and "local" doctors on the medical ward, EUMS had also committed these men to an outreach program that involved traveling to outlying district hospitals to mentor their medical officers and to staffing a specialized outpatient clinic attached to Referral Hospital. As the EUMS physicians rotated among these tasks, I sometimes found it difficult to know which physicians I would find in the medical ward from week to week, if not day to day. Even these doctors themselves were sometimes confused by their schedule.

To further complicate matters, other physicians from EUMS, often either highly specialized practitioners like neurologists and pulmonologists or physicians nearing retirement, would sometimes "drop in" for a few weeks. These new arrivals would introduce themselves to the Medical Department at the morning report that began each day, but this left them largely unknown to the ward's nursing and support staff. Over the time I was there, the medical ward's nursing staff became increasingly frustrated with their inability to identify the various *makgoa* (white people; foreigners) roaming the ward, whether EUMS students, residents, attendings, or inhabitants of a ragbag category that included the few students from other schools who had managed to attach themselves to the EUMS program, the handful of British medical students who had found their way to the ward, and a few eager Americans who had only just finished their Bachelor's degrees but who had their sights set on medical school and had found their way to Referral Hospital for the North American summer months, often through personal or family connections. The "local" MOs, interns, and some of the nurses also changed assignments, rotating among the hospital's various wards, but they did so on a much less frequent and much more predictable basis as personnel assignments at the hospital changed synchronously. The "local" attendings assigned to the medical ward had a more constant presence, but they also had their own shifting schedules for staffing the outpatient clinic, continuing education, annual leave, and other commitments that took them away from the ward for periods of time. The arrival of a new group of EUMS students every six or eight weeks only aggravated the existing fluctuation of personnel on the ward.

Not *Here*: Teaching the Terms of Global Health at Referral Hospital

Upon the arrival of each new group of students the EUMS clinical staff delivered a set of lectures designed to introduce students to Botswana's healthcare system and help them participate more effectively on the ward. These lectures covered topics such as Botswana's national regulations concerning treatment for infections commonly encountered on the ward, such as tuberculosis, HIV, and meningitis. The lectures also tried to prepare students for what were, from EUMS physicians' point of view, the ward's day-to-day challenges and frustrations. Neither before leaving the US nor upon arriving in Botswana were students briefed on popular contemporary Tswana concepts of illness or *bongaka*, Tswana medicine, a flexible and changing practice still widely used by many Batswana in conjunction with biomedicine (Haram 1991; Livingston 2004). Nor did these lectures deal with social codes concerning, for example, the body, gender, or generational relations. In the thirty-page handbook issued to students, no more than a page addressed either language or social mores. In sum, these lectures had virtually nothing to do with Botswana beyond the more or less apt application of a presumably universal medicine.[8] While Dr. Rosen maintained that these lectures were open to any Batswana physicians, especially those returning from medical training abroad to begin their internships at Referral Hospital, I rarely saw more than a few MOs or interns in the classroom.

One afternoon in September 2007 I joined the current group of EUMS students as they headed down the breezeway to the hospital cafeteria. We moved slowly through the line as the woman behind the counter filled Styrofoam containers with rice or *phaletshe* (a stiff cornmeal porridge), meat and sauce, and small scoops of cooked beets, cabbage, or greens. We grabbed plastic forks and cans of soda or fruit juice and made our way to the conference room at the far end of the female medical ward, sitting at tables or on benches along the wall. Dr. Matheson began his lecture on Botswana's public-sector pharmacy, reading from the slides his laptop projected onto a pull-down screen:

> You're probably confused right now. That's important: it reflects what it's like to work in a resource-limited setting. The pharmacy here is based on WHO [World Health Organization] guidelines, on the WHO essential medicines list, 15th edition. We work with the Botswana Essential Drug List, which is what the Central Medical Stores, or CMS, uses.[9] That's what you'll find on the ward drug cart.
>
> The main dispensary [at Referral Hospital] is near the [outpatient] medical clinics. ARVs are kept in the IDCC [infectious disease care clinic] pharmacy. If it's not on the cart, that means it's not available. "I-N-N" means the International Nonproprietary Name; the "B-A-N" is the British Approved Name.[10] Nurses and pharmacists won't know the name you know. They [the drugs] might be slightly different, but they're similar agents.
>
> Dosing notation: Many pharmacists are international, so they'll recognize your notation. As far as availability goes, when you're unsure, ask senior pharmacists, like Soumano, Adebayo, and Akbar. They seem to know what's going on, unlike a lot of people.

Dr. Matheson continued his lecture, identifying medications commonly used to treat conditions regularly encountered on the ward and explaining how guidelines set down by the Botswana Ministry of Health shaped treatment:

> We've moved away from Demerol/pethidine in the U.S., but it's a first-line drug here. We see an overuse of Phenobarbital, which has gone out of style in the U.S.—which it should; it's sedating, but it works when the others are out of stock. Penicillin: you'll be using it a lot more than you're used to; it still works here. We hope you didn't bring any MRSA [methicillin-resistant *Staphylococcus aureus*] infections with you from the U.S., ha ha! Ciprofloxacin is reserved for MDR-TB [multi-drug-resistant tuberculosis] and pseudomonas. Vancomycin: works better here than in the U.S., where it's used all over the place. Anti-malarials: the guidelines say Fansidar, but you should know this is inadequate; there's Fansidar resistance.

At this point, Dr. Frank, sitting on a bench along the side of the classroom, broke in: "Start with quinine," he suggested. "The WHO has issued new guidelines for quinine. But," he added, "you should have cardiac monitoring."

"Not *here*," Dr. Matheson responded curtly, shaking his head and dismissing the possibility of routine cardiac monitoring for patients on quinine.[11]

In his first statement Dr. Matheson laid out the conceptual geography that shaped the activities of EUMS on the medical ward of Referral Hospital. This geography was tripartite: Dr. Matheson introduced a third mediating term, a category I gloss as "international" or "global," rather than merely contrasting "the U.S." with "here." This third term marked a zone of transition—rational, standardizing, and benevolent if also distant—between the unmarked setting, resources, and guidelines that characterize "the U.S." and the marked characteristics of "here." After all, this was meant to be a "global" or "international medical experience," so it was necessary to mark how the category of "the international" structured elements of medical practice, even if its principles were ineptly implemented by the Botswana Ministry of Health.

The confusion generated by this new cartography enabled Dr. Matheson to emphasize for the students their current distance from the source of their training. They had entered the space of "global health," where the pharmacopoeia was based on guidelines from an "international" body such as the World Health Organization. Their own knowledge and practices were made "local": "they won't know the name you know." That said, they were capable of transcending this localization and communicating with "international" pharmacists: "they'll recognize your notation." Most of the pharmacists working at Referral Hospital were expatriates; many were from Nigeria or South Asia, places from which Botswana's Ministry of Health actively recruited physicians and auxiliary health professionals. EUMS students could trust these rational and benevolent "international" pharmacists who shared with EUMS students the capacity to transcend their localization. Those who could not transcend their localized knowledge, naturally, did not "know what's going on."

In his second statement Dr. Matheson, having reminded students of both the localized nature of their knowledge and practices and their capacity to transcend this localization, pointed out to the students that, however localized, their knowledge and practices belonged to a universal medicine and were thus superior to those of the "here" in which they found themselves working. By mixing acronyms EUMS students would find familiar (MRSA, WHO, ARVs) with those that require explanation (CMS, INN, BAN), for example, Dr. Matheson both highlighted the seeming specificity of their current location and emphasized the degree to which this seemingly exotic location was subsumed within the presumably universal biomedicine the students had already mastered. Their confusion indexed less students' unfamiliarity with the particularities of Botswana's health system than students' conformity to "global" standards (cf. McKay 2018, 188). The distinction between an unmarked universal and a marked subcategory of "local" was made temporally as well as spatially: Standards of medical practice "here" reflected what "we" used to do "in the U.S." before we "moved away from" such practices. Certain drugs that were used in Botswana had gone—and *should* have gone—"out of style in the U.S.," blurring the line between any use and "overuse" and marking morally suspect "overuse" as something invisible to doctors "here" but visible to doctors *not* from "here." Practicing medicine in Botswana was like going back in time. This spatiotemporal distancing was disparaging and yet also suffused with an odd nostalgia for the efficacy of drugs, like the penicillin that "still works here," for simpler delivery concepts, and for a space-time from which MRSA is excluded. This statement also points to the complexity of rendering the bodies of Batswana both "universal," that is, subject to the biomedical interventions deployed by American medical personnel, and "particular," that is, naïve to certain treatments in ways the patients imagined to inhabit American hospitals are not, thus highlighting the ironic costs and benefits of "treatment naïveté" (cf. Petryna 2005, 2009).

Moreover, "here" was a place whose guidelines and practices, however inflected or informed they might be by the "international," were "inadequate" to the task at hand, that is, effectively treating malaria. Within the scope of what "a lot of people"—that is, "local doctors"—"don't know" was that Fansidar may well be ineffective in treating malaria "here." Notwithstanding the extent to which "the WHO" informs knowledge and practice "here," such as the treatment of malaria or the stocking of the national pharmacopoeia, even if a doctor "here" were lucky enough to "know what's going on," the sign of "here" was that "international" guidelines could not be met. Throughout the second chunk of text, "global health" or the "international" was largely discarded in favor of a point-by-point comparison between "the U.S." and "here," culminating in a critique of "here" as hopelessly inferior in resources, practice, and expertise. When Dr. Frank re-invoked the "international" by mentioning WHO guidelines, it was already clear that although EUMS students required training, such as the current lecture, to move beyond their localized knowledge in order to wield the knowledge and practices of "global health," they were nevertheless in a position to judge the violation or mishandling of "global health" and things "international" by "local" doctors, whether those doctors "know what's going on" or, in all likelihood, did not. Not only was it established that the practice of medicine "here" was threatened by limited resources, inadequate guidelines, outmoded practices, and medical staff who did not know what was going on; EUMS physicians and students belonged to another realm of space-time entirely, one of unquestionable technical and moral superiority. Eerily echoing nineteenth-century missionary rhetoric of an Africa that "still lies in her blood" (Moffat [1842] 1969; quoted in J. Comaroff and J. L. Comaroff 1991, 324) while obscuring the historical conditions that have given rise to the gaps between "the U.S." and "here," the lecture framed EUMS's Global Health Program, of which the program at Referral Hospital was the jewel in the crown, as an endeavor that could only bring enlightenment and progress to this downtrodden hospital.

All this was largely accomplished through Dr. Matheson's use of the term *here*. As a deictic, *here* accomplishes two things. First, it grounds itself in and draws its referential sense from the context of its emergence, thereby "creating a shared, intersubjective representational-universe-to-hand that provides a medium for adjusting mutual role inhabitance" (Silverstein 1997, 280–81). At the same time, Dr. Matheson's use of deictics also provided a "virtual framework" within which speakers arrange nondeictic words and expressions, which carry their own senses into that framework (Silverstein 1997, 281). By means of this framework, "words and expressions that invoke the same cultural realms of belief and value are organized by grammatical arrangement and deixis into discernibly local segments of text" (281). In other words, as Dr. Matheson contrasted *here* with "the U.S.," these terms began to point far beyond themselves to senses of backwardness and inferiority on one hand, and competence and universality on the other.

This framework had implications for the subject positions inhabitable by the interactants insofar as "words and expressions used to make senses and stereotypes intersubjectively 'in play' must invoke particular cultural domains of knowledge relative to group memberships that are plausible for interactants at the particular point of interaction" (Silverstein 1997, 281). If we view this lecture as a process by which "localized" EUMS students were made practitioners of "global health," we can recognize a diagrammatic iconicity between the categories laid out by means of deictic reference and the roles laid out as inhabitable—indeed, as already inhabited—by EUMS students and their "local" counterparts.[12] In other words, the two categories of location laid out in speech—*here* and "in the U.S."— and the stereotyped meanings upon which they drew and which they recapitulated recruited students to regard themselves and others as naturalized categories of people aligned with these two locations.

The chronotopic grid of interpretability laid out using the terms of "global health" thus not only framed space and time but also laid out inhabitable moral and professional roles. In her essay examining how East Berliners locate themselves as subjects with a particular political orientation vis-à-vis the now-unified German state, Deanna Davidson argues that "the study of the sociocentricity of deictic reference aids interpretation of how East Berliners use shifters like *here* and *these times* in order both to make spatial and temporal reference and to represent themselves politically" (2007, 221). As a first-order indexical, Davidson notes, *here* might refer to "a naturalized space or 'commonsense geography' among speakers who have a shared history of orienting themselves within this space" (Davidson 2007, 221; Schegloff 1972; Silverstein 2003). The deictic *here*, when used by EUMS physicians and students, increased its scope to index not only the medical ward or only Referral Hospital as an institution but an entire genre of place glossed as "resource-limited settings"—as microspatial as the medical ward of Referral Hospital, as broad as "Africa," and many things in between. At a second order, however, "use of 'here' indexed the speaker's membership in the category of persons who knew how to use 'here' in this sense" (Davidson 2007, 221). By deploying *here* in this manner, EUMS students situated themselves as the kind of subjects who consistently recognized the contrast between *here* and another category, thereby indicating that they were not, in fact, of *here* (cf. Pigg 1992).

The global health chronotope is further marked by the capacity for EUMS students to cultivate themselves as moral medical practitioners by moving through time and space in a highly specific way. In Davidson's analysis, the use of *here*, "infused with the moral qualities of 'back then,'" may also index a third order, that of an in-group-valorized political affiliation with the former East German state (2007, 214, 221–222). For EUMS students, the third indexical order was the moral position they inhabited by being in a place they could call *here* in the sense laid out previously. They were able to travel back in time, as far as medical practice was concerned, by moving from a highly technicized space into a "resource-limited" one where they practiced medicine without the technologies they had been trained to deploy in the interest of patients' well-being and in the interest of protecting themselves and their colleagues from liability. To complete the process of constituting themselves as the moral characters they become through such movement, they had to move *back* into those highly technicized medical spaces from which they could point to what they learned *here*. The framing of a "global health experience" required students to relocalize, making a *here* into a *there*.

EUMS students, encouraged by EUMS attendings, became versed in an understanding of the medications, lab tests, and equipment unavailable to them *here* in contrast to an idealized wonderland where the labs always ran on time. As they rounded with their assigned firms, students learned to recognize the deployment of *here* with its laminated or entailed senses of inferiority, inadequacy, backwardness, and parochialism. They also learned to deploy it themselves and to recognize themselves as the budding practitioners of "global health" they made themselves through these deployments. EUMS physicians, teaching from one case to the next, recruited students to inhabit a "global health" position from which they might regard Referral Hospital (in addition to the incredibly wide range of referents that could be drawn into the sphere of *here*) as the periphery of medical practice. EUMS attendings charged the students with the responsibility both moral and professional of embodying an elevated (i.e., "global" or "international") standard, a responsibility they also viewed as their own. Discussing the risk of tuberculosis transmission and the need for infection control with students in the classroom, Dr. Matheson concluded by stating, "Hopefully EUMS students and residents can be the vanguard" in these efforts.

It follows that among EUMS personnel the most reliable index of authority was the capacity to successfully laminate, or refrain from laminating, a sense of inferiority upon things "local" that was both moral and technical. EUMS carries a reputation among medical schools for cultivating assertiveness among its students, and many eagerly took up the charge to embody the "vanguard" of biomedical practice, sometimes failing to recognize resources that were, in fact, available at Referral Hospital. Upon arrival many struggled with the fact that they could only imperfectly tell which resources, practices, and personnel were worthy of their derision. Students occasionally went too far, prompting Dr. Rosen and Dr. Matheson to defend "local" practices as "different but not wrong." One EUMS resident explained to Dr. Rosen that he was about to give a patient a particular medication orally. Dr. Rosen advised the resident to give the medication intravenously, emphasizing, "in the U.S. we wouldn't even *think* about [giving that medication] PO [per oral, i.e., by mouth]. We can do IV [i.e., give the medication intravenously] here, so why compromise on *this* point when there are so many other points of which we *have* to compromise?"

This is not to say that EUMS physicians and students always intended to portray Referral Hospital in a negative light. Indeed, Drs. Rosen and Matheson had a vested interest in helping their juniors distinguish the different-but-adequate from the inadequate inasmuch as they had a far greater interest than did their juniors in maintaining longer-term relationships with "local" doctors and with Referral Hospital. But even positive comparisons were not exempt from these dynamics, such as when Drs. Rosen and Matheson reminded their students that, whatever its faults, Referral Hospital was "not *bad* for an African hospital," causing "local" staff to bristle at the backhanded compliment. In this statement, "African hospitals" figured as places where not even Referral Hospital's standard of care was available. Like *here* and "local," "Africa" was susceptible to this kind of semiotic ordering. When several layers of distinction become laminated upon one another, the indexical values of each layer are in "dialectic competition" with one another (Silverstein 2003, 194). One could hardly use the term *here*—or similarly, "local" or "African"—without invoking these the indexical values, thereby taking a stand with regard to how EUMS's presence at

Referral Hospital was to be understood in terms of morality and expertise as well as space and time.[13]

"Local" Doctors, "African" Medicine, and Other Uncomfortable Positions

Health professionals working in Botswana's public health sector came from as far away as Bangladesh, India, Ghana, Nigeria, and Tanzania as well as Botswana. Batswana interns returned from training in places as diverse as Ireland, South Africa, Australia, and the West Indies. China and Cuba sent health professional to work in Botswana's public hospitals, where they joined a small number of European medical missionaries. Heterogeneous though their backgrounds were, many shared at least a British Commonwealth–style medical education and, if not always common practices of care, a common set of technical terminology not always shared by North Americans. They discussed among themselves variations in Botswana's health facilities, such as the district hospital in Ramotswa, forty kilometers southwest of Gaborone, which many praised for its high-quality maternity care, audiology services, and treatment for snake bites, all considered superior to what Referral Hospital offered.[14] In the course of their daily practice they became familiar with the small number of conditions, such as certain congenital heart defects and neurological disorders, that could warrant Referral Hospital staff transferring Batswana patients to hospitals in South Africa for treatment at the government of Botswana's expense.

For the purposes of EUMS as well as other partnership organizations, however, all these doctors, regardless of race, origin, or training, were "local." Through a process of iconization, "local" doctors became "local" not, or no longer, by their relative physical, institutional, or national proximity to Botswana, or Gaborone, or even Referral Hospital, but by their resemblance to one another. Distinctions that mattered among these "local" doctors became both invisible and immaterial to EUMS personnel, such as when a group of students called on Dr. Chilube, an intern, to translate between Setswana and English for them during consultations with patients. Dr. Chilube later explained to me that iKalanga was his "home" language and expressed discomfort at being asked to translate from Setswana, which he referred to as his "school language."[15] Even more awkwardly, visiting Americans sometimes called on MOs who hailed from other regions of sub-Saharan Africa to translate from Setswana with no consideration for their fluency in the language. In other words, the category of "local" only made sense in marked contrast to EUMS or another partnership, such as the

Superlative Clinic. Susceptible to the same diagrammatic effects discussed previously, "local" was imbued with all the values of "here."[16]

The positions doctors and students working at Referral Hospital took up with regard to the global health chronotope did not fall easily into two camps, with all Americans claiming Referral Hospital was "resource-poor" and all "local" doctors denying it.[17] Instead, as EUMS physicians deployed the terms of the global health chronotope during the ward teaching and clinical mentoring directed toward "local" doctors, they recruited these "local" doctors to a set of contradictory positions. On the one hand, many MOs and interns working on the ward valued the presence of EUMS personnel (students and residents as well as attendings) both for the labor they contributed and for the opportunity to learn from them. Visiting Americans offered "local" doctors an opportunity to constitute themselves as elite, cosmopolitan, and possessed of ties to distant metropoles. On the other hand, "local" MOs and interns had various reactions to the EUMS narrative of Referral Hospital as a "resource-poor" environment that ranged from joining EUMS personnel in deriding Referral Hospital to voicing anxiety about the capacity of medicine (and by extension, the doctors) in Botswana to "measure up" to attempting to reframe the social meanings their position as "local" entailed.

One afternoon over lunch, I listened to Dr. Kgosiemang tell his fellow interns a story about a German man who had been in a car accident while traveling in Botswana. The man had been treated at Referral Hospital for a leg fracture that required surgery. Dr. Kgosiemang recounted how both the man and his doctor back in Germany had been impressed with the quality of treatment the man had received. To Dr. Kgosiemang's chagrin, the other three or four interns at the table began laughing. "Why were this man and his doctor so amazed?" they asked. "What had they thought might happen? What did these people think about *African* doctors, anyway?" One intern chortled with a combination of scorn and mirth: "Did they expect they would find *a stick of wood* where they should find a rod or a pin?"

Why should Europeans have been surprised when "African" doctors did high-quality, up-to-date work, when they correctly practiced "universal" biomedicine? Dr. Kgosiemang's colleagues challenged the chronotope that situated "African" doctors temporally as well as spatially distant from "European" medical practice, what Fabian called the "denial of coevalness" (1983). In fact, they went so far as to question the necessity of his claim to such "coevalness" altogether. Similarly, when an Indian pharmacist who was visiting Botswana in conjunction with a meeting of the pediatric HIV clinics affiliated with CHAN asked Dineo Mogomotsi, an Irish-trained Motswana MO, whether Botswana's HIV prevalence rate was so high "because it's such a *poor* country," Dineo, ordinarily the picture of decorum, snapped, "Botswana is not a '*poor* country!'" Dineo's objection, I suggest, was less an assertion that poverty does not exist in Botswana than an attempt to resist an ideology prevalent in "global health" narratives about Botswana wherein Botswana's high rate of HIV prevalence reflects poverty and ignorance and points to the country's need for outside salvation.

In other moments, however, "local" doctors' speech employed a spatiotemporal configuration that resembled the global health chronotope. After all, the "local" doctors, Batswana and expatriates, had all trained overseas, and they often recognized the attitude of EUMS personnel toward technology: its geographical distribution between *here* and "elsewhere"; the prestige it conferred on its practitioners; and the presumed quality of care it enabled. Discussing the curriculum for Botswana's new medical school, for example, young Batswana MOs raised the question of whether the school would enable its students to participate in clinical research, or whether it would be "just an *African* medical school." Another small group of Batswana doctors, newly returned to the country to begin their internships, recounted with some nostalgia the MRI machines at the hospital in Ireland where they had trained. Both of Botswana's referral hospitals could perform CT scans, but these young physicians focused instead on Botswana's lack of imaging technologies.

In other instances, "local" doctors pointed out, with differing degrees of intent and subtlety, American physicians' own provinciality in ways that destabilized the spatiotemporal configurations of "global health." One morning in September 2007, Dr. Baum, an EUMS neurologist on a four-week visit, turned abruptly to Mpho Moseki, a Motswana MO, and asked, "What treats bacterial gastroenteritis?" "Flagyl or Cotrim," she responded promptly.[18] The first answer was Pfizer's trade name for the compound metronidazole. The second was Teva Pharmaceuticals' trade name, an antibiotic compound widely used in Botswana that, at the time of this exchange, was no longer sold in the US under that name. Dr. Baum gazed at Mpho blankly. "Co-trimoxazole," she elaborated, giving the name that serves as both the British Approved Name and International Nonpropriety Name of the medication and turned back to the notes she was writing. Dr. Baum continued to stare at her blankly. Looking up, she realized he was still waiting and said, "Sorry . . . *Bactrim*," giving him a trade name for co-trimoxazole he finally recognized.

In this exchange Mpho illustrated the disruption that "local" and "international" realms undergo in practice. Dr. Baum may have failed to recognize a trade name not used in the US ("Cotrim"), but he also failed to recognize the "international" name for the medication. Mpho had to work to find a trade name for co-trimoxazole that Dr. Baum could recognize, and the only name that registered for him was one "local" to the US. When Mpho shifted from a "local" trade name ("Cotrim") to an "international" name ("co-trimoxazole"), Dr. Baum should have recognized the latter—in part as a "global health" professional presumably familiar with things "international," and in part as a specialist physician in a position to supervise and correct Mpho. Instead, Mpho had to "relocalize" the drug name for Dr. Baum, a move for which she, in recognition of his supervisory position, seemed to apologize. Dr. Baum's response, however, is telling of his effort to maintain his supervisory position despite his failure to master "international" terms, let alone their "local" equivalents: "No, I should adapt," he responded, "relocalizing" Referral Hospital as a deviation from a norm, a space marked by difference.

Variations of this interaction happened frequently on the ward, largely over matters of naming conventions with regard to practices and materials. The irony lies in the fact that, while EUMS assumed that its practitioners were capable of instructing across multiple contexts and conventions while the "local" doctors were locked firmly in the "local," it was the "local" doctors who were often more versed in multiple conventions of medical practice. By virtue of the fact that all "local" doctors, Batswana as well as expatriates, had trained outside Botswana, they often had a ready grasp of multiple conventions of medical terms and practices with varying scopes, whether Irish or Indian techniques, fixed to regulatory institutions in the British Commonwealth or Europe. The medical ward, like the hospital more generally, was *already* "global"—if by "global" we only mean that its practitioners hailed from a multitude of nations and had received their professional training in a wide range of locations around the world. Clearly, though, this was not what EUMS and other partnerships meant by "global health." What did it take for a space to be "global health" enough? What happened when this failed?

Paul Farmer Would Never Stand for This!

Thus far, I have argued that EUMS medical educators had to labor to make what counts as "global health" visible and recognizable to their students, while other actors sometimes contested and reoriented its terms. Global health as practice and pedagogy is contingent not only upon different actors' efforts to maintain or redraw temporal and spatial contrasts between one site of practice and another. The flexibility of deictics and their indexical orders is a key element of the global health chronotope inasmuch as the constitution and maintenance of the terms of global health also demand that actors make commensurable the multiple "theres" in which global health can be argued to exist. Through a process of iconization similar to one through which "local" doctors were made "local,"

EUMS educators, students, and administrators had to work to make vastly different times and places, diseases and people—a six-week stint in a tuberculosis laboratory in South Africa, for example, and a summer working on HIV/AIDS prevention in Thailand—commensurable under the sign of "global health." In this sense, "global health" is an argument, a position, as much as, if not more than, a thing. In this section I return to Referral Hospital's pediatric medical ward to examine one physician's efforts to reframe the conditions in which he found himself in order to highlight global health's radically flexible cartography. I argue that through this flexibility global health acquires the characteristics of a frontier, that is, "an imaginative project capable of molding both places and processes" (Tsing 2005, 32). As "a space of desire," argues Anna Tsing, a frontier "appears to create its own demands" (2005, 32). The global health chronotope can be constituted wherever its conditions can be authoritatively argued to exist, or contested and dismantled wherever those conditions can be authoritatively questioned.[19] Thinking of the global health chronotope as a frontier reminds us of its endless capacity to be shifted even as these shifts are naturalized.

As described in chapter 1, the Pediatric Squad, upon arriving in Gaborone in August 2006 to staff the Superlative Clinic, had been dismayed to discover they were expected to work on the hospital's inpatient pediatric medical ward and to "take call," that is, remain at the hospital overnight on rotation to admit patients and tend to the needs of those already admitted. On the ward they had found themselves assigned to already established firms, requiring them to cooperate with the ward's two "local" pediatricians as well as supervise "local" MOs and abide by regulations handed down by Botswana's Ministry of Health.[20] By early 2007 many Squad members were deeply dissatisfied with the arrangement, accusing Dr. Buyaga and Dr. Amy of capitalizing on the pediatricians' labor on the ward in order to smooth relations between ward and Clinic while dismissing Squad pediatricians' criticisms of what they saw as poor medical practice on the ward.

In January 2007 Dr. James, much to his irritation, found himself assigned to the inpatient pediatric medical ward, cosupervising a firm with Dr. Sung, one of the "local" pediatricians. Dr. James, whose parents had immigrated to the US from Hong Kong, oscillated between warmth and aggravation with the older Chinese woman. Early one morning I found Dr. James tending a child with a suspected bacterial infection. He had sent a blood culture sample to the hospital's pathology lab, but the lab, whose pace of work was chronically unpredictable, had not yet returned any results. Because he did not know which infection the child had, he could not determine which antibiotic to give. A simple blood culture should not take this long, he grumbled; his patience was wearing thin. Frustrated, he ordered three different antibiotics at once, including ciprofloxacin, which, as Dr. Matheson noted in his lecture, MOH guidelines reserved for two conditions, one of which was multidrug-resistant tuberculosis (MDR-TB), a significant public health threat in a country with a large immunocompromised population.[21] Dr. Sung, seeing Dr. James' order, firmly but not unsympathetically explained that his approach was simply not possible. Dr. James stormed outside; I followed. As we stood beside the ward in the warm summer sunshine, Dr. James lost his temper. "Paul Farmer would _never_ stand for this!" he thundered. "_This_," he fumed, "is _not_ what I _came here_ to _do_!"

Once again, the lamination of social meaning onto deictics enables Dr. James to convey an enormous amount in very few words. By "this" he referred beyond the instant at hand to the problem of acting as an arm of the Ministry of Health, providing the standard—or to his thinking, substandard—of medical care he felt forced—by Dr. Sung, his supervisors, the hospital administration, the Ministry of Health—to provide. How could abiding by the Ministry of Health's regulations elevate the standard of pediatric care in the country? By "Paul Farmer" Dr. James referred to the physician-anthropologist who served as an icon of moral righteousness, or "medical culture hero" (Wendland 2012b, 119), vis-à-vis "global health" for the vast majority of American medical students and young American physicians I met in Botswana. Consciously or not, Dr. James may also have been leveraging the tense relationship rumored to exist between the Superlative Clinic's parent organization and Farmer's own organization, Partners in Health. In a few short words, Dr. James lined up "this" against "Paul Farmer," and declaring that anyone asking him to do "this" was not, as it were, on the side of the angels.

By "came" Dr. James acknowledged the temporality, in the concrete form of his contract, of his presence "here." By "do," James indicated the problem this temporality posed in the sense that Squad doctors, like most American personnel, struggled to understand how to best "make a difference" in Botswana within their limited time constraints (cf. Pigg 2013). In this moment, Dr. James, in a move I saw American medical personnel make time and again, attempted to align the temporality of his career and the temporality of the epidemic. Not only should doing "global health" now pay off later in his individual career as a morally and technically competent medical practitioner; his presence in Botswana should, ideally, contribute to the project of "building capacity" or "elevating the standard of care" in the long term through the accumulation of short-term individual actions that added up to more than a sum of their parts. Dr. James, like many others, drew upon the terms of the global health chronotope and the moral stances they indicate in order to calibrate his professional and moral transformation. The abstract language of epidemic's epidemiology, by contrast, resists narrativization as a series of "differences" made through the discrete actions of individuals.[22]

Dr. James's use of *here* best illustrates the capaciousness of this particular deictic vis-à-vis the global health chronotope. If Dr. James took his presence in Gaborone as a sign that the hospital was a "resource-limited setting"—why would he be there otherwise?—he also expected himself to intervene in Botswana's standards of medical practice. Dr. James complained that he and his fellow Squad members had been misled regarding the type of work they would be doing, that their skills were misused in Referral Hospital's wards. "We're not doing our job, we're not being *allowed* to do our job," he grumbled. "We shouldn't even *be* in the city," he told me, his vision rapidly expanding. "We should be going out into the countryside with only a nurse, identifying kids who are building resistance to ARVs." He would be willing to live in a hut, to sleep on the ground, he assured me. Dr. Paul Farmer, as the title of the biography by Tracy Kidder made famous, is "a man who would cure the world" (2003). To the extent that this suggests a one-to-one correspondence between a doctor and "the world," it contributes to medical students' and novice physicians' requirements for an ever-increasingly flexible global health chronotope as these young medical professionals go in search of their own world to cure. Referral Hospital was not a *here*, with all the values imputed to it by the global health chronotope, enough for Dr. James, for whom a *here* to which he was prepared to come needed the qualities of a frontier. Suffused with all the promise of a truly heroic medicine, the *here* of global health was just over the horizon, a fantasy, infinitely displaceable.

The Global Health Frontier

Spaces and subjects emerge in relation to one another. "Global health" and its attendant spaces, objects, and practices, I have argued, do not mark a particular institutional arrangement of biological threats and expert practices so much as they index subject positions and trajectories and the stances these make tenable. The "global" in the "global health" of American medical education points to a configuration of space and time, technology and morality, movement and fixedness that characterizes contemporary American imaginations of what medical education and medical practice ought to be. There can be no doubt that "global health" is remapping the currents through which medical experts and expertise flow, but we should recall that there are significant material as well as moral stakes in the designation of spaces as "here" and "elsewhere," in the description of people and practices as "global" and "local." The ability of American medical personnel to continue to work in "global health" and to transform themselves by means of this work is contingent upon their capacity to continually redraw temporal and spatial contrasts between the technologies and moral stances that characterize "international" or "global health" against an unmarked "there," to make commensurable the multiple "heres" in which they practice this "global health," and to maintain and police the boundaries of these categories and their inhabitants.

This argument has three major implications. First, linguistic anthropologists and medical anthropologists tend to work at a distance from one other, but to leave language out of the analysis of medical education is to risk falling into the very claims that biomedicine makes for itself, namely, that there is something transcendent, ineffable, and universal about it. Attending to how experts and trainees construct their objects of expertise opens up the possibility of examining the strange and multifarious institutions, claims, and stances "global health" makes possible, letting these experts demonstrate to us how one knows "global health" when one sees—or says—it. Second, while "the globe" as much as any other space must be made recognizable, it remains seductive to both scholars and activists. Yet we risk much if we take the "global" of "global health" as

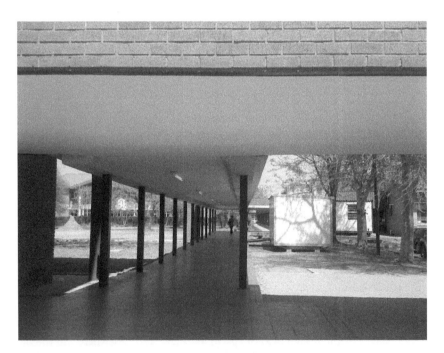

FIGURE 4.   Referral Hospital breezeway, Superlative Clinic in the background (photo by the author)

self-evident, however much we might agree with the political impetus behind doing so. "Global health" is an object of technoscientific knowledge and value production just as much as "development" or "biomedicine," and requires as much labor and "purification" (Latour 2000) as they do. Anthropology's great strength lies in criticizing the taken-for-granted—in asking what makes "global health" so self-evident, and so generative, and what ways of imagining and acting in the world it eclipses or forecloses.

Last, uncritical approaches to "global health" obscure the highly unequal power relations that are revealed when we examine competitions over its terms. While the seductiveness of "global health" lies in its vanishing horizon, at once totalizing and elusive, this flexibility also makes possible the naturalization of politics, the making of a "global" that facilitates spatial, temporal, and moral claims even as it erases the conditions of its own production. Having demonstrated how American medical trainees attempt to establish themselves and their practices as "global health," the next chapter turns to how global health emerged as a site for American medical trainees to stage moral and affective transformations and the uneven conflicts engendered by this practice.

EXPERIENCING AIDS IN AFRICA

One afternoon I shadowed Molly, an EUMS student who had just arrived for her six-week rotation at Referral Hospital, as she moved from patient to patient through the female medical ward. She was following up orders that had been placed during the green firm's mornings rounds, taking samples of blood and sputum for lab tests, moving from bed to bed with the unwieldy cart that contained empty phials, laboratory request forms, sputum cups, and the hard, yellow plastic "sharps" box with red biohazard markings on the sides in which to deposit used needles. One of Molly's fellow students had recently taped a sign on the cart that warned the ward's staff: "Keep me neat or I will practice my cannula [i.e., intravenous needle] skills on you." As I followed her on her slow, meandering trek down the ward, Molly explained to me that most of her global health work up to this point had taken place in Latin America. She had found the short periods of time she had spent there rewarding and felt a connection to the region. She was studying Spanish and wanted to pursue further opportunities to work there. Nevertheless, she had avidly pursued the opportunity to come to Botswana despite, as she put it, "the line out the door" at EUMS. When I asked why she had made such an effort, she replied: "I don't think I can say I *really* understand global health without experiencing AIDS in Africa."[1]

Two days later, while working with the green firm, Molly stuck herself in the forearm with a needle that she had removed from the vein of an HIV-positive patient only moments before. The firm knew that the patient in question had developed resistance to the medications that composed Botswana's first-line ARVs at that time. Molly's chances of contracting the virus from the stick were thus arguably higher in other instances of exposure.[2] As she recounted to me later, she washed her hands and, pricking her own finger, gave herself a rapid-test for HIV and documented the results. Dr. Frank, who was on the ward, called Dr. Rosen on his cell phone to report the incident and, after consulting him, prescribed Molly a twenty-eight-day postexposure prophylaxis (PEP) regimen of four ARVs, rather than the two-drug or even three-drug regimen that might be prescribed in other instances of exposure.[3] Molly hurriedly took her first dose and retreated to the set of apartments EUMS maintained for its medical students.

Molly remained in good spirits after the incident, a remarkable feat given the anxiety and embarrassment that needlesticks provoke in Botswana, as elsewhere, and that often lead to underreporting of such injuries.[4] Molly did admit to me that she was disappointed: Her injury took place the week before the Superlative Clinic's week-long camp for HIV-positive children at which she and the other EUMS students had been invited to volunteer (Brada 2019). Once she began experiencing the side effects of her PEP regimen, including stomach cramps and diarrhea, she grew concerned about whether she would be able to participate in Camp at all. Indomitable in spirit if rather green around the gills, Molly attended Camp intermittently, returning to the EUMS apartments when she felt too ill to continue. But Molly found a silver lining in her predicament: While she found the side effects of her ARV regimen unpleasant and uncomfortable, she assured me that taking the medications "helps me feel closer to my patients."

This chapter examines the ideological framework that grounds the fantasy of transformative encounters that global health pedagogies promise to students like Molly. In this fantasy, embodied experiences such as a needlestick injury simultaneously confirm and constitute an affective orientation, a biomedical expertise grounded in and shaped by the "humanitarian impulse" identified by Dr. Goldberg in the previous chapter. How does global health make such transformations seem possible? Anthropological and historical scholarship has amply shown that biomedicine is a violent enterprise both in its approach to the human body (Bosk 2002; Good 1993a; Kleinman 1995; Prentice 2013) and in its long entanglement with colonial racism (Anderson 2006, 2008; Arnold 1993; J. Comaroff 1993; Packard 1989; Vaughan 1991). For African bodies to serve as sources of value in deeply unequal and often off-shore regimes of scientific and medical knowledge production is hardly new (Geissler and Molyneux 2011; Graboyes 2015; Molyneux and Geissler 2008; Tilley 2011). Moreover, a number of scholars have shown how global health programs, whether oriented toward research or treatment, depend on and perpetuate the very inequalities they seek to ameliorate, at best ignore and even undermine local experts, and have dangerous and even lethal consequences for patients (Crane 2013; Feierman 2011;

Geissler 2013; Sullivan 2018). At Referral Hospital EUMS students fought with nurses and matrons, took sheets and other supplies from other wards without permission, routinely ignored and disparaged "local" medical professionals, and performed medical procedures beyond their level of training with little to no supervision and little to no censure. How, then, did students learn to regard their time on the medical ward as confirmation of their own and one another's beneficence?

To speak of ideology or fantasy is not to cast Molly's claim as disingenuous. It does, however, work against a trend in medical anthropology toward approaches that privilege first-person accounts of embodied experience. Such an account might explore how, by virtue of the lived experience of nausea, diarrhea, and the temporal constraints of her regimen, Molly gained an embodied, even visceral understanding of ARVs that contrasted sharply with a biomedical framing of them as neutral technologies. Such an account might propose that taking ARVs, like all embodied practices, held the capacity to shape not only Molly's view of the world but the ways she inhabited it. But such an account would obfuscate the extent to which it reflected a commitment shared between the overlapping fields of American biomedicine and American medical anthropology to the morally transformative potential of embodied suffering. Instead, I use Molly's statement as an entrée into a different set of questions: What did Americans expect from the ward, and why? How did these expectations shape EUMS students' time on the ward? How were transformative encounters recognized as such—both by those who aspired to them and by those enlisted to ratify them? Last, what transformative potential, if any, did interactions with patients hold for the hospital's "local" practitioners?

My concern is with the semiotic scaffolding within which medical professionals and trainees labored to recognize themselves and others in terms of these anticipated transformative embodied experiences. This scaffolding becomes apparent in contrasting registers, that is, sets of "entextualized techniques" (Urciuoli 2008, 213) by means of which medical professionals and trainees at Referral Hospital aligned aesthetic experiences of their own and others' bodies with expressions of their emotional states. By means of these registers, medical professionals and trainees attempted to cast what might have been mere physical proximity into moments where moral subjectivities were both constituted and revealed. Chapter 4 focused on how actors positioned themselves and one another with regard to space, time, and expertise; this chapter examines the moral stakes of those positions, that is, actors' efforts to frame embodied experiences as morally transformative, and particularly what I call the register of heroic American medicine. Whether any American medical trainees and practitioners were truly transformed by their time on the ward is the wrong question. What requires explanation is how and why these stances of having been transformed were longed for, asserted, and occupied by actors relative to their different social positions through a set of deeply unequal, even violent encounters.

I begin by asking how embodied experiences figure in the fantastic transformations promised by global health pedagogies. Next, I explore why American medical education makes such transformations seem necessary and desirable. I then analyze a series of stance-taking exercises wherein EUMS personnel discursively mark themselves and others as imbued with the "humanitarian impulse" that global health is understood to confirm in those who are open to its transformative powers. I draw attention to the register of heroic American medicine, that is, the entextualized techniques at play as EUMS personnel narrate their own transformations and ratify the transformation of others, techniques that both anticipate off-stage transformations and evaluate them *ex post facto*. The ideological framework of the global health fantasy becomes discernable when the narratives of EUMS personnel about the ward are contrasted with those of the ward's medical officers. These junior Batswana physicians narrate a very different fantasy of transformation that aligns them and their encounters with patients in terms of Botswana's national progress. This contrast helps pinpoint the terms of the ward's ongoing tensions, that is, how each group came to regard the other as undermining care on the ward, and how each responded in such a way as to reinforce, rather than ameliorate, this conflict. Moreover, this contrast helps us see the promised transformations of global health pedagogies *as* fantasy, that is, as lying not in the actions themselves (i.e., caring for HIV patients) or even the context in which these actions took place, but in the claims made about them, claims grounded in profound institutional and national inequalities. I conclude with a story of another needlestick injury that illustrates how seemingly similar alignments of bodies and technologies lend themselves to radically different accounts of experiencing AIDS in Africa.

The Problem of Anesthesis and the Register of Heroic American Medicine

Why are embodied experiences so central to global health's promises of moral transformation? In addition to presenting opportunities for the acquisition of technical skill, short-term global health programs, like study abroad programs more generally, are imagined to create the conditions for Americans to encounter "a transformative otherness" (Urciuoli 2013, 7; cf. Cramblit 2017; Stewart 2013). Such transformations reveal the influence of philosophical pragmatism's prioritization of the experiential aspects of learning; more specifically, they draw attention to an assumed relationship between mediation and affect in the cultivation of a moral orientation in novice experts. In this ideological framework, "knowledge is most fully or usefully internalized if it derives from experience" (Keane 2008, 317), and the body holds a unique position as a site of immediate experience, a commonsense epistemological primacy and authenticity.[5] This affective and aesthetic pedagogy is threatened by improper mediation with terrifying consequences. For example, as nuclear weapons scientists shifted from above-ground to underground testing and, eventually, to computer simulations, Joe Masco argues, they grew anxious about the ability of the new tests to shape their own and other scientists' affective orientations. Simulated nuclear explosions, they worried, mimicked the sublime pleasures of unsimulated ones but failed to cultivate the fear of the bomb trainee weapons scientists needed to do their job properly (Masco 2006, chap. 2). Similarly, Rachel Prentice argues that while surgical simulators make a powerful promise of an ever-available body that can be reset whenever trainees make mistakes, these simulators do not incorporate the affective and ethical dimension of surgical training. This "acculturation," she argues, "entails lessons that go far beyond the technical skills a simulator can teach" (2013, 253), leaving her wondering "whether the imperative to do no harm can be embodied in a situation in which one truly can do no harm" (2013, 266). In these accounts, novices' ethical formation is imperiled when their objects of expertise fail to engender the affective and ethical dispositions expert practice demands. What medical trainees and their educators confronted, in short, was the problem of anesthesis, a fear that novice experts lack the moral dispositions that ought to guide the deployment of that expertise *as a consequence* of their newly acquired expertise. The problem of anesthesis and the anxieties it engenders drives a search for a pedagogical object that precipitates a morally transformative encounter. This chapter draws particular attention to the register of heroic American medicine as a site wherein biomedical professionals and trainees articulated fantasies of overcoming anesthesis through transformative embodied experiences.

By bringing attention to the language of biomedical socialization, this analysis departs from established analytical trends in medical anthropology that privilege physicians' bodies. While such analyses reflect long-standing anthropological interest in the naturalization of corporeal pedagogies (Bourdieu 1977; Mauss 1935), they also mirror biomedicine's own epistemological framework.[6] While biomedical training may be transformative of medical students' bodies and subjectivities, these transformations must be made recognizable and ratified through the stories students and educators tell about them. Encounters with doctors and doctors' bodies can be profoundly transformative of patients' subjectivities (Cooper 2015; Nations and Rebhun 1988; Smith-Oka 2012; Yates-Doerr

2012). This chapter focuses on the inverse, that is, the narratives of moral transformation that trainees and practitioners produce from their encounters with patients. Enregisterment, that is, "the process and practices whereby set of performable signs become recognized (and regrouped) as belonging to distinct, differentially valorized semiotic registers by a population" (Agha 2007, 81; see 2003, 2005) is useful insofar as it highlights the social distribution of ways of speaking and the subjectivities indexed by these ways of speaking, and it emphasizes that the distinctiveness of these performances must be maintained through ongoing processes of differentiation.

As an engagement with the problem of anesthesis, the register of heroic American medicine echoes broader neoliberal trends that integrate emotional reflexivity and expressivity into late-capitalist forms of labor rather than excluding them. "Discursive self-reflexivity, especially expressing feelings through talk," argue Bialostock and Aronson, "is one of the techniques of self-disclosure emphasized in late capitalism" (2016, 99; cf. Gershon 2011), part of a shift toward the cultivation of an entrepreneurial self that can respond to demands for emotional labor and that is reflected in pedagogical institutions as well (Bialostok and Aronson 2016; Bialostok and Kamberelis 2012; Hardt 1999; Hochschild 1983; Illouz 2007; McWilliam and Hatcher 2004; Muehlebach 2011; Rose 1999; Taha 2017). If American medical trainees, like other workers in the neoliberal marketplace, "have come to be seen as personally responsible for skill acquisition, to the point of self-commodification" (Urciuoli 2008, 212), then we might read narratives such as Molly's as the anxious performance of the skill of "being humane," an overcoming of the anesthesis induced through her training (cf. Vinson and Underman 2020). This quality of "being humane" must be ratified and naturalized even as it defies quantitative measurement or even direct observation.

The register of heroic American medicine as the site of the fantastic solution to the problem of anesthesis, moreover, partakes in a broader sentimental politics, one with distinctly American contours. Tracking "the place of painful feeling in the making of political worlds" (1999, 53) across a wide range of American texts, literary scholar Lauren Berlant argues that sentimental politics recasts political relationships in terms of a shared universal suffering and relocates the site of injustice and its amelioration to intimate domains; it reframes them as a question of "having the right feelings about what is wrong" (2008b, 54). It entails a double-move in terms of scale: first, the political is recast in terms of personal suffering; and second, "emotional justice" at the scale of interpersonal relationships "figures the pre-experience of its resolution" beyond the interpersonal (2008b, 37). Sentimental politics admits that "personal stories tell of structural effects," but its commitment to universal suffering means that disparate accounts "can become all jumbled together into a scene of the generally human," with the result that "the ethical imperative toward social transformation is replaced by a passive and vaguely civic-minded ideal of compassion" (41). This is, I suggest, why a claim to "feeling closer" and the register of heroic American medicine more generally are at once so powerful, so deeply desirable, and yet so difficult to pin down (cf. Ticktin 2017).[7]

This compassion, Berlant continues, by scaling toward a general humanity appears as more than "just a feeling" insofar as it bound up in a fantasy of "the transformation of unjust social institutions through the production of new mentalities" (41). In sentimental American texts, Berlant argues, "the act of enraptured consumption" of testimonials of suffering "becomes inextricable from the moral act of identification" (45), creating "a space of deliberate dis-interpellation or self-misrecognition" (47), wherein another's pain becomes the means to "a better self" (56), and the universality of pain underwrites both its imaginative availability and the possibility of a universally recognizable and transformative empathetic response. In an assessment that begins almost like a pitch for those embarking on short-term global health rotations, Berlant argues that "the possibility that through the identification with alterity *you will never be the same* remains the radical threat and the great promise" of the affective aesthetic of sentimental politics (47, emphasis added). The difficulty, in short, in analyzing the ideology grounding the fantasy of global health as transformative embodiment is that it is grounded in a broader politics that misrecognizes the pleasure of transformed sentiments as justice (Berlant 2008a, 2008b).

Making American Medicine Heroic

As a pedagogic tool in biomedical education, global health is a historically and politically specific answer to a more general problem: the *affective* dimension of biomedical education, that is, the cultivation of practitioners with a particular moral orientation toward their work in addition to technical proficiency. Scholars of biomedical education have frequently characterized it as a dehumanizing discipline in which students learn the protocols of encountering bodies and subjects in deeply invasive, even violent ways that would be at least criminal, if not also pathological, outside the bounds of formal medical practice (Bosk 2002; see Beagan 2000; Becker et al. 1961; Sinclair 1997). "Research in medical schools and residency programs," Claire Wendland observes, "has demonstrated the premiums placed on reductionism, on technological intervention, and on an emotional detachment construed as essential to the objectivity a new doctor must have" (2012a, 756). "Medical trainees," she continues, "learned quickly that medical thinking (and speaking and writing) required them to strip all social, emotional, and biographical material from patient narratives in order to understand the patient as biological being: bare life readied for technical intervention" (756). Yet biomedical education is also charged with creating practitioners who possess a proper affective orientation of "detached concern" toward their patients and their well-being.[8] Biomedical educators must thus determine how best to cultivate students' affective orientation as well as their technical skills. Examining the historical trajectory of solutions to this problem in the late twentieth century, Renee Fox argues that US biomedical educators have tended to put their faith in "magic bullet" solutions, expecting targeted coursework—psychiatry and community health in the 1950s and 1960s and bioethics in the 1970s and 1980s—to produce humanist physicians (1999). But if the solutions have varied, the problem has remained essentially the same: What will transform technical skill into moral practice?

While anthropological literature tends to present the challenge of cultivating medical trainees' affective dispositions as a problem inherent to biomedical training itself, it has specific dimensions in the contemporary United States. For one thing, the question of what form an affectively transformative encounter for American medical trainees might take runs up against the political history and postcolonial realities of biomedicine in the United States. American biomedicine shares with other postcolonial settings a historical reliance on the use of poor, Black, enslaved, and colonized bodies, both living and dead, as its pedagogical objects, and a blurring of the lines between treatment, training, and experimentation, and even more sinister activities (Owens 2017; Rothman 1991; Washington 2006; cf. Anderson 2008; Arnold 1993; Graboyes 2015; Tappan 2014; White 2000). The bodies that populate American biomedical training reveal not only the violence at the heart of the biomedical encounter but also the social dynamics that make some bodies more available to the medical gaze and that have tended to legitimate violent encounters in terms of the specific qualities of racialized and gendered subjects, such as naturalized differences in the capacity to perceive or endure pain (Livingston 2012, 134–38; Martin 1987). In the US, lingering ideas regarding the suitability of some subjects as objects of biomedical pedagogy reinforced deep suspicions among people of color, women, and other vulnerable populations that their well-being may be secondary to other priorities in healthcare settings (Byrd and Clayton 2002; Friesen 2018; Gamble 1997; Thomas and Quinn 1991).

If the potential for individual and institutional violence and the anxieties this potential engenders lie close beneath the surface of American biomedical pedagogy, educators and trainees must also contend with the increasing politicization of healthcare over the past three decades. Since the 1990s debates over how to price healthcare services and manage their costs, over the role of the state in these processes, and over citizens' entitlements and obligations have moved healthcare toward the center of an increasingly polarized national political landscape, culminating in the rancorous debates over the Affordable Care Act (Beaussier 2014; Morgan and Campbell 2011).[9] These debates, alongside grassroots movements that advocated for healthcare reform, have arguably increased the visibility of inequalities in access to and quality of care as well as outcomes while also going some distance toward undoing their naturalization (Hoffman 2008; Pescosolido, Tuch, and Martin 2001). The result is an ever-narrowing possibility for medical trainees to frame their work as unquestionably beneficent or to divorce their work from the broader framing of healthcare as a pressing national political problem. Biomedical training demands bodies that can be encountered by novices with at least impunity if not beneficence, but the potential for American trainees' actions to index violence at multiple interpersonal and institutional scales has, arguably, only increased in recent years.

Moreover, studies of North American medical students show that trainees, confronted with the limitations of biomedical treatments and the realities of clinical failure, respond by directing their cynicism and anger toward patients (Wendland 2012, 771; cf. Good 1995; Hojat et al. 2009; Wear et al. 2006). The more intractable a patient's problems are and the greater the possibility of clinical failure, the more likely the patient is to become the object of trainees' antagonism (Feudtner, Christakis, and Christakis 1994). Wendland observes that medical trainees in both Malawi and North America reported feelings of disillusionment, demoralization, and eroded ideals as they moved from a basic science curriculum into clinical work. But the similarities ended there: Rather than the hostility toward patients observed in North American students, Malawian trainees directed their anger toward Malawi's political system (2012a, 771). "None described patients as noncompliant or irresponsible," Wendland continues, "they were just poor and sick" (771). Malawian trainees learn to read even the most difficult cases as signs of state failure that engendered a heightened political consciousness and an awareness of the social determinants of health and disease, but American patients seem unable to offer similar lessons for American trainees. Instead, American students come to regard caring and technical competence as mutually exclusive, and prioritize the latter.

In an effort to reintegrate moral orientation and technical competence, some American medical educators in the 1990s and 2000s began to advocate for "teaching empathy," culminating in the reframing of empathy as an essential learning objective by the American Association of Medical Colleges (AAMC 1998; cf. Stepien and Baernstein 2006).[10] This turn toward empathy has paralleled the incorporation of the humanities and social sciences into biomedical curricula, including the introduction of a section of the Medical College Admissions Test (MCAT) focused on social and behavioral sciences, the emergence of pre-med programs for students majoring in the humanities, and coursework, including medical anthropology and the anthropology of global health, that promises to orient students toward patients' experiences and offers students opportunities to align themselves with such valorized concepts as structural violence and the social determinants of health. Yet biomedical training ultimately relies heavily on the shaping of bodily hexis, that is, the coordination and manipulation of the bodies of both trainees and patients. Faced with fears that medical trainees and even qualified practitioners simply did not touch patients' bodies enough and growing concerns regarding cultural insensitivity in biomedicine, educators grappled with the problem of how to structure trainees' encounters with patients so as to engender empathy, dulled in the course of their training, while occluding the violence these encounters threaten.[11]

Short-term global health rotations promise an experience that precipitates moral transformation through the acquisition of technical skill, rather than sacrificing students' "humanitarian impulse" to the demands of competence and the anger that American patients inevitably provoke. On one hand, students viewed their time in Gaborone as perhaps their only opportunity to learn to handle patients' bodies in ways their future careers demanded. Some complained that even as the growing litigiousness of American medicine multiplied the number of tests and procedures any given patient underwent as a preemptive counter against malpractice suits, students themselves felt increasingly restricted handling patients' bodies despite the premium placed on doing so. In the US, they explained, they would only perform these procedures with careful supervision. And because a different burden of disease resulted in less demand in the US for some procedures, such as lumbar punctures, medical students in the US found themselves competing with the residents and interns supervising them for the opportunity to practice these procedures. Moreover, the increasingly fine division of labor in American healthcare also contributed to students' feelings of restriction. In many American teaching hospitals, they told me, phlebotomy teams drew patients' blood, leaving students without an opportunity to practice this skill. Dr. Goldberg concurred: "There's so much support in the U.S., and so much lab information that students are restricted to just managing patients' care while someone else is making the relevant decisions," he told me.[12] Medical practice requires a "feel" for which technologies could not substitute, several EUMS educators confirmed, but opportunities for these embodied pedagogical practices were dwindling, and they feared that students lacked the hands-on practices elementary to shaping a competent medical practitioner.

On the other hand, EUMS personnel aligned students' need to acquire technical skill with their perception of Referral Hospital as a space of emergency. The demands of this "resource-poor setting" and of Botswana's epidemic more broadly could be marshaled to defend students against accusations of violence, including moments when they overstepped their level of training, ignored or outright challenged local clinicians, or flouted hospital and even national regulations. Beyond the pervasive stereotypes of Africans' suffering and gratitude that have endured across centuries (J. Comaroff 1993; J. Comaroff and J. L. Comaroff 1991; Wainaina 2005), EUMS personnel recapitulated two racialized tropes that inform global health representation and practice more broadly: (1) the assumption that African practitioners lack professionalization simply by virtue of being African; and (2) that any care visiting Americans provide is not only "good enough for the poor" (Feierman 2011, 172), who have no grounds to complain about technical inadequacies, but also superior to any care that is locally available (Sullivan 2018, 312).[13] In other words, the occlusion of the violence of short-term global health rotations as pedagogical encounters relies on a perceived congruence between students' need for clinical experience and patients' need for care, a congruence that reflects a sentimental fantasy wherein subjects "share the same sense that the world is out of joint" (Berlant 2008a, 21). "Do procedures," one outgoing EUMS student urged a newly arrived group of fellow trainees: *Do all the procedures you can.* This alignment offered EUMS students an encounter with patients' bodies that insulated them from biomedicine's enduring associations with violence, racism, and colonialism and from more recent framings of American biomedicine as the minimization of expenditure and the maximization of social capital and profit, confirming instead students' "humanitarian impulse" by means of presumably humanitarian actions (Brada 2016).

The fantasized pedagogic value of students' encounters with Batswana patients, then, lay not only in an increased responsibility for patients' care or in the challenges presented by a different and presumably defective working environment but in the power of these encounters to *both* endow students with the technical skills a biomedical career demanded *and* confirm that they possessed the moral dispositions that had guided them toward medicine and would continue to guide the deployment of their technical skills in the future, all in the process of offering presumably superior care (cf. Hanrieder 2019). Students learn to diagnose and treat an unfamiliar range of diseases and conditions while interacting with patients in ways less governed by laboratory results and imaging technologies and less supervised by attendings and residents than in the US. In this manner, students would learn to economize their use of laboratory results and imaging technologies, lessening their reliance on them while better appreciating their value. Even a short time working in a "resource-poor" or "resource-limited setting" such a Referral Hospital, Dr. Goldberg said, would make them better appreciate the resources available in the US. Their encounters with patients at Referral Hospital prefigured the competent and humane interactions with patients they and their supervisors could anticipate upon their return to the US: "We'll be great residents for doing this."

"Something So Completely Different and Disturbing"

"Real isn't how you are made," said the Skin Horse. "It's a thing that happens to you."
"Does it hurt?" asked the Rabbit.
"Sometimes," said the Skin Horse, for he was always truthful. "When you are Real you don't mind being hurt."

Margery Williams, The Velveteen Rabbit (1922)

Insofar as Molly and her educators considered empathy within an Euro-American ethnotheory of emotion, Molly's transformation from a student whose "humanitarian impulse" was presumed but unconfirmed to one who could authoritatively claim "closeness" to her current and future patients was a private ritual encounter, an unobservable event bracketed on one hand by "anticipatory shaping of a person's anxious ritual-readiness" and, on the other, by signs that she and those around her could read *ex post facto* as evidence that a transformation had, in fact, taken place (Silverstein 2009, 271). Private rituals, argues Michael Silverstein, pose a puzzle to analysts and a source of anxiety to participants for similar reasons: the reflexive poetic (Jakobson 1960) or metasemiotic "density" that makes rituals efficacious is manifest in private rituals "only before- or after-the-fact, in this way producing their *worried expectation of being* or their *certainty of having been* 'performative,' in the sense of well-formed and therefore effective entextualizations of all their ritual conditions of possibility and co-organized sign manifestations that go into such an event" (2004; 2009, 273, emphasis in original; Stasch 2011). Private rituals thus entail, Silverstein concludes, "a metasemiotic moment of self-transformation by self-recognition" (273). This transformation is one for which participants are "primed" (288): there is, in other words, "anxious denotational metasemiosis in the form of orienting discourse about what such ritual events are, in general, all about, allowing people to have heightened sensitivity to the possibility of such private, solitary ritual encounters having happened or potentially happening"

(288). While they are private, these transformations are nonetheless consequential for those who undergo them and those who ratify them insofar as "characteristics of vital importance to how individuals function in society emerge from such an event" (288).

The fantastic transformation promised by global health pedagogies is precisely this self-transformation by self-recognition, a "feeling of rich continuity with a vaguely defined set of like others" (Berlant 2008a, 7). Not only did Molly articulate her capacity for empathy; she enacted her capacity to recognize and prioritize these feelings of empathy in the first instance. And these claims, when efficacious, offer the possibility of retrospectively regimenting past events (Silverstein 2009, 273): that is, they offered to Molly, newly endowed with the capacity to recognize empathy, and to her audience confirmation that she had, in fact, never lost her "humanitarian impulse." Her empathetic response following her needlestick did not so much engender the affective dispositions Molly needed as a humane practitioner as it drew her attention, and the attention of her educators and classmates, to the dispositions that had always been there, progressively obscured but not eroded by her training. Her response brought all past patient encounters into alignment as evidence of the empathetic subject she had always been even without always recognizing it. Moreover, it offered a frame within which to read all subsequent patient encounters in light of this transformation, that is, as encounters with a humane practitioner. Molly used the register of heroic American medicine to situate herself within a global health fantasy as the always already humane and empathetic practitioner she had once thought she needed "AIDS in Africa" to become (Silverstein 2005; Tambiah 1985).[14]

And while such ritual transformations are private, taking place "at the very edge of empirical ordinariness" (Silverstein 2009, 281), their ratification is anything but. As "metasemiotic indexical signage" (273), Molly's claim was both recognizable and anticipated with macrosocial order of American biomedicine, that is, it lined up with a set of conventions by which Americans biomedical trainees assessed among themselves the possibility for moral transformations by virtue of encounters with African patients and subjected them to *ex post facto* ratification. The felicitousness of the act of self-recognition that Molly and other EUMS personnel undertook required other "metasemiotic indexing" as interdiscursive "confirmatory regimentation" (274). In other words, any such act had to be brought into conformation with other instances of fantastic moral transformation by a community of participants authorized to recognize such transformations—transformations modeled, as Dr. James reminded us in chapter 4, by global health's heroic figures, against whom trainees' sought to position themselves in terms of iconic resemblance and devotional consequence (Citrin 2011).

The register of heroic American medicine also highlighted the specificities of African patients as the catalysts for these acts of self-transformation by self-recognition. Dr. Jackson, who had set the EUMS rotation on the medical wards in motion, recalled how the "suddenness and fierceness of death" at Referral Hospital had "stunned and shocked" him. He continued:

> [During residency in the US] I don't think I really witnessed anyone, especially someone so young, die in my presence. Of course, I had been present at "codes" . . . but that experience was more similar to a drill—a bunch of people in a room carrying out different tasks in a generally organized fashion. The patient seemed almost irrelevant and completely dehumanized. This was *something so completely different and disturbing*.[15]

In this account, Dr. Jackson frames witnessing a death "in the U.S." and witnessing a death at Referral Hospital as qualitatively distinct, with different moral values imputed to each: regularization and distance, in the first case, and humanization and shock in the second. If the former resembles a simulation of events in which the fact of the patient's humanity seems occluded and the doctor remains emotionally uninvolved, then Dr. Jackson casts Referral Hospital as a space where patients—and by fantastic extension, the physician himself—were humanized and made relevant, where suffering and death are palpably *more real*. Likewise, a story published in Eastern University's alumnae magazine on the program in Botswana noted that, its educators' best efforts notwithstanding, EU "can't prepare [EUMS students] for . . . the deaths they will witness." Using the register of heroic American medicine, EUMS personnel cast AIDS in Africa and its deaths as experientially distinct from those in the US, morally transformative in a way that deaths, even deaths from AIDS, in the US are not. The qualitatively distinct shock of African death provided Americans with an opportunity to awaken humanitarian sensibilities dulled by the routinization and dehumanization of American medical practice, that is, to be humanized through their recognition of a particularly African suffering.

This example illustrates how American trainees and their educators built associations between students and the patients they encountered at Referral Hospital, and how they evaluated these encounters in terms of assumptions about the trainees and patients involved. In her study of Chinese art schools, Lily Chumley argues that quantitative evaluation regimes amenable to standardization and anonymization (grades, licensure exams, etc.) exist in tension with and reinforce the need for a second, personalizing regime, with the consequence that "a productive dialectic relationship" exists between the two (Chumley 2013, 173; see Chumley 2016). In biomedical training, this tension is evident in claims that qualities like compassion are indispensable features of physician-trainees while also insisting that such qualities cannot be measured quantitatively and cannot be inculcated except through embodied practices. Chumley contrasts standardized tests with "a rhematizing regime," that is, a process of evaluation wherein "the qualities of objects and individuals are iconically and indexically made to serve as figures of one another" (Chumley 2013, 171; Gal 2002, 2005). In the performance of rhematizing evaluation regimes, Chumley argues, groups of individuals build associations between subjects and objects in terms of the qualities each is recognized as embodying or possessing (Chumley 2013; see Chumley and Harkness 2013; Munn 1986). In the context of global health, these performances confirm in practitioners such as Molly and Dr. Jackson the qualities of African diseases (realness) and African patients (humanity, relevance) and ratify their capacity to recognize those qualities in themselves and evaluate them in others (Chumley 2013; Harkness 2013; Silverstein 2003, 2004).

What emerges is a connoisseurship of suffering oriented toward the performance of having overcome anesthesis. Vague yet emotionally laden terms such as *stunned, shocked, close, real* are entextualized techniques tied to personalized processes of credentialization and professional performance from medical school applications to residency and beyond (Urciuoli 2003, 2008). In keeping with American sentimental politics, these performances highlight consciousness as the site of transformation (Berlant 2008b, 64).[16] The enregisterment of these terms makes the transformative ritual discernible *ex post facto* to those who have a stake, either as participants or as audience, in its ratification. The ability to authoritatively perceive and comment on the distinctions mapped out by the register of heroic American medicine rested on "multiply voiced" utterances (Bakhtin 1984) evident in the contrasts Dr. Jackson diagrammed between merely *being present* versus *witnessing*, with all its moral entailments (Fassin 2008; Redfield 2006), and between *codes* and *drill* as opposed to *die*. Such discernment served as an ongoing alibi of EUMS personnel's sensitivity and compassion.

The fantasy of moral transformation in global health thus rests on the imputation that if American patients can only make American medical trainees angry and cynical but African patients awaken their humanity, then the difference lies in the qualitative distinctiveness of the suffering of Africans, who do not, as Dr. Jackson reveals, even have to be alive for these transformations to transpire. Yet the transformative capacities of Africans' suffering did not lie in a perceived *cultural* difference. I was struck in my encounters with American medical trainees in Botswana by the extent to which their desire to wield biomedicine as a tool of justice had been shaped by an insistence on the primacy and universality of suffering and a skepticism toward culture as a potential alibi for that suffering (see the Introduction). As I shadowed an EUMS student on the wards, we began discussing Tswana medicine, or *bongaka*, a category that, while hardly a fixed tradition, is locally salient; as a predominant focus of the "long conversation" of the colonization of the southern Tswana (J. Comaroff and J. L. Comaroff 1991, 171), *bongaka* has historically been juxtaposed to biomedicine as well as to Christianity and other cultural institutions at the heart of the colonial encounter (Jean Comaroff 1985; J. L. Comaroff and J. Comaroff 1997a; Livingston 2004, 2005; Schapera 1933, 1940, 1947, 1971). Eager to learn more, the student suggested I give the EUMS students a short talk—only for Dr. Rosen to object that I would promulgate cultural stereotypes. I recount this not to reify ethnographic authority but to illustrate the extent to which knowledge about culture was devalued *prima facie* as reification by American biomedical experts for whom culture was at worse suspect and at best an afterthought.

As we saw in chapter 4, EUMS personnel positioned themselves as enacting a universal expertise in contrast to what they saw as the parochial and deficient practice at Referral Hospital. In this case, the deficiency was primarily one of moral perception. Americans' perception of the distinctive qualities of African death and subsequent expressions of horror called into question whether any practitioner who failed to perceive this aesthetic did so due to their deadened sensibilities. Americans could locate this distinction even among themselves: For example, EUMS students contrasted their activities on the medical wards and the patient encounters of other Americans professionals. As I followed Jessica, an EUMS student, around the ward, she explained that she had heard from her fellow students that Harvard "isn't here for the people, they're just here for the research, for getting papers out." Dr. Rosen later concurred, adding, "all their [Harvard's] patients are trial subjects. They don't do rounds; they only have a research mandate. EUMS is working on clinical treatment. *We're* here to help the people in the wards." The register of heroic American medicine and its attendant moral subjectivities mapped a contrast between the "help" offered by EUMS students that might precipitate the promised transformations of global health and the activities of those who were "just here for the research." Such evaluations, structuring and structured by the fantasies figured in Molly's and Dr. Jackson's stories, reflect how actors used this register to both ratify ritual transformations *ex post facto* and narratively structure their anticipated unfolding even as these transformations transpired off-stage, as it were, in the presumably invisible world of sentiment.

But while, in the eyes of EUMS students, some Americans might refuse the transformations that EUMS personnel anticipated, sought, and ratified in one another, such transformations were generally unavailable to "local" doctors. At first glance, this might seem contradictory: If encounters with African patients held the fantastic capacity to transform American biomedical experts and trainees by precipitating a novel self-awareness in the midst of the acquisition of technical know-how, then Referral Hospital's medical officers, by virtue of their everyday labor and even the seemingly natural similarities of nationality and race, ought to be suffused with the capacity to recognize suffering. In general, however, EUMS students tended to regard "local" personnel as incapable of recognizing the qualitative distinctiveness of African suffering. While EUMS trainees' narratives traced a mutually reinforcing enactment of moral disposition and acquisition of technical skill, for "local" personnel, deficient in technical skill and thus unable to "help" their patients, encounters with suffering could only coarsen their capacity for empathy and deaden their moral sensibilities. Recall Evan's bitter question: *Don't they care about their own people?* That "local" doctors did not engage EUMS personnel's' narratives of horror and transformative shock, that they did not act as though an emergency was unfolding around them, served, in the eyes of EUMS students, as a confirmation of "local" insensibility and apathy, reinforcing for EUMS students the necessity of their own moral example. Thus, for Mpho, whose children were very young, to yawn during rounds or for the ward's nurses to adhere to a daily schedule of tea breaks could incite a startling degree of contempt and even anger and bitterness among EUMS students and residents insofar as these actions tended to assume and reinforce the set of social identities that Evan's question had done.

At the extreme end of this fantasy of heroic transformation is the trope of the plague doctor. Plague doctors are an iconic index of their patients' suffering: that is, they resemble their patients insofar as they share their patients' condition, but the plague doctors' manifestation of illness is a consequence of their efforts to assuage that suffering. Their illness is not a tragic mishap nor a logical consequence of either pathological essence or poor decisions, but a consequence of their professional practice, their service to their patients. Their sacrifice lies in their willingness to share a feature with their patients in a way that accentuates the distinction between patient, whether hapless or guilty, and self-negating expert. Squad pediatricians told me over and over how Dr. Mark, the first of the Squad doctors assigned to work on the inpatient pediatric medical ward, lost twenty-five pounds in just a few weeks because, Dr. Rachel said, "things were so bad on the ward." Dr. Mark's efforts to provide what he and his American colleagues considered standard treatment had literally cost him his body. As Squad pediatricians struggled to define the scope of their labor and the Superlative Clinic's intervention, Dr. Mark's diminished body served for his colleagues as a warning of the limitlessness of the demands of Botswana's epidemic and the unwillingness or inability of Batswana to meet those demands. For the Squad, Dr. Mark had done was what necessary for his patients, but this obligation had extended so far that it consumed the physical substance of his body. In an iconic recapitulation of the hallmark "slimming" of HIV infection, his body served as a reminder of the corporeality (Boyer 2008) of global health expertise and a benchmark of heroism.

Squad pediatricians felt keenly the possibility for bodily damage driven by their own compulsions to rectify what they saw as local deficiencies in care. But while this bodily sacrifice for the sake of heroic medicine might come with its own pleasures, the danger of self-destruction in the face of the seemingly limitless sacrifice was just as potent. Dr. Mark began, and other Squad pediatricians continued, a protracted conflict with the nurses on the pediatric inpatient ward over the placing of intravenous cannulas. The conflict hinged on whether nurses could and should place these cannulas with a doctor's supervision. Many Squad pediatricians were fresh from their residencies, newly promoted to the role of attending physician, and eager to defend the privileges of rank. They regarded procedures, including those that involve sharps, such as blood draws, the duty of the ward's MOs, interns, and nurses, not of specialists such as themselves for whom such work was demeaning. The nurses, protesting that they lacked the necessary training, maintained that they could not be required to place cannulas.[17] Most nurses at Referral Hospital rotated among different wards and did not receive specialized training. A survey of nurses in an Emergency Department in Botswana revealed that only one had undergone specialized training in emergency medicine (Chelenyane and Endacott 2006, 150). All the nurses participating in the study expressed a fear of contracting HIV/AIDS or other diseases in the course of their work, and many feared endangering their families; fifteen of the twenty-two respondents had been injured via needlesticks or splashed with blood or other bodily fluids (152). The anxieties of the nurses on the pediatric medical ward should thus be read in terms of trends in training and hospital staffing, rather than as personal moral failures. Yet for Squad pediatricians, the nurses' objections to handling sharps on behalf of "their people" confirmed Dr. Mark's sacrifice, pointed to its necessity, and prefigured their own.[18]

"It's As if They've Been Told, 'You're Going There to Save the Africans'"

The medical ward's MOs and interns did not generally fault EUMS students for wanting to touch patients. All had studied medicine overseas, often in Ireland, Australia, or the West Indies, but many had arranged their training to conduct some of their clinical rotations in hospitals in Botswana or South Africa in order to avoid the sort of distance from patients' bodies that prompted EUMS personnel to complain. For these junior physicians, the novice's thrill of handling bodies rather than merely observing and discussing them was easy to recall. Even more experienced clinicians deeply valued this aspect of patient care. Mma Kgosietsile, head nurse of the Superlative Clinic, put it this way: "When you are a manager in a big hospital, it's not possible . . . to follow up to the letter to see if what you had said has been done. [. . . Here] I'm very close to the floor, to where things are happening, and I see things happening and I can actually even make a difference . . . in *actual* patient care. Not just talking about theory, management, whatnot, but [thumping her hand on the table] *hands-on.*"

Yet Batswana medical professionals tended to frame the transformative potential of these encounters as a contribution to a national effort, a slow yet perceptible amelioration of the epidemic's toll. Individual patients pointed beyond themselves to the idealized nation they composed as citizens. Neo Baatlhodi, a young, soft-spoken nurse at the Superlative Clinic, told me: "I've found I'm obligated to fight against HIV for my country. That's why I like working with HIV patients, because I believe . . . I can make a difference in someone's life."

Neo was in her mid-twenties. Her adolescence and early adulthood had been shaped by the peak of Botswana's epidemic in the years before the treatment program began. Other young Batswana professionals also spoke of studying nursing or medicine with the desire to respond specifically to Botswana's epidemic. Mpho Moseki had completed a Bachelor's degree in the US and had been about to begin a doctoral program in biology when a visit home in 1997 caused her to change her plans, opting to attend medical school instead. Like many young medical professionals I met who had come of age in Botswana's pretreatment era, the state of Referral Hospital in the late 1990s had made a lasting impact on her. She told me, "You think the medical ward is full *now*? *Jo!* The medical ward was *overflowing* back then. . . . So, when I came back as a doctor, for me, things were so much better. But if you hadn't seen it when it's bad and you come here, you'd think, "This is terrible."

Like Mpho, other Batswana practitioners also scaled patients relative to the nation, reading individuals' improvement as an index of the progress of Botswana's treatment program more broadly. In this they resembled Malawian medical students, who approached "the body politic as a worksite" (Wendland 2010, 205). Malawian students, Wendland argues, "tended to move from a vision of rather abstract sacrifice . . . to one of greater engagement, a feeling of shared identity or political purpose" (181) and viewed medical training as "a step toward development for themselves and for their country" (83). For young Batswana, moral medical practice consisted of contributing to the national project of HIV treatment one citizen-patient at a time, acting as agents of the state in a country where citizens expected the state to act in their collective interest and to judiciously redistribute public goods (Gulbrandsen 2012; Livingston 2012). From this point of view, patients might not receive everything they needed, but the care they receive should be no less than any other citizen would receive. Indeed, heroic efforts on one patient's behalf could threaten this moral economy of care.[19]

The ward's MOs were thus distressed to find EUMS students approaching everyday life on the ward as an ongoing emergency that warranted students to act on their own authority. Lesego Balebetse, an MO who had worked at Referral Hospital since completing medical school in 2006, emphasized the contrast between EUMS students, who acted without seeking guidance or approval and who did not anticipate supervision, and her own experience as a trainee on the wards. EUMS students, she told me, wrote prescriptions in patients' charts without consulting anyone, an act that, for Lesego, violated both Referral Hospital's standards and what she perceived as the standards of American biomedical education. "When I was a student, I came here on vacation and . . . whatever I did, I had it countersigned [by one of the ward's physicians]," she explained. "So why should they be different because they're from the States?" She continued: "In [the] X-Ray [Department], they'd go there and just start charting people's x-rays [i.e., going through the Department's files and taking the films of patients under their care] without even saying hello. They'd go to ICU [the Intensive Care Unit], they want to change the settings on the ventilators even though there's somebody [i.e., a Referral Hospital physician assigned to the ICU] who is in charge of those patients."

"They're not qualified doctors," she emphasized with mounting frustration. "They don't have the degree, they're not registered." Imagining the danger students posed to patients, she added: "They can't be prescribing dangerous poisons to patients and no one knows what they've prescribed." This perspective was not universally shared on the ward: "They have to learn sometime," shrugged Dr. Manisha, one of the ward's attending physicians. But even Dr. Chilube, a mild-mannered intern whose habitual business attire, including a necktie, under his white coat drew gentle teasing from his peers, confided that he had seen EUMS students doing things he knew he was not authorized to do without supervision, adding, "And *I* already *have* my medical degree." Moreover, many of the MOs concluded that EUMS students had been primed for a heroic encounter in a way that precluded any interpretation of their actions as violent, dangerous, or even questionable. Wary of painting all Americans with the same brush, Mpho nevertheless found EUMS students' attitudes consistent enough to speculate that they had received explicit instructions to this point: "They come here with the mentality that they're saviors of Black people," she told me. "[It's] as if they've been told, 'You're going there to save the Africans.'" Lesego separately arrived at a similar conclusion, saying, "I honestly think they're pulled aside and told, 'Listen, you're going to Botswana. This is how you're going to behave when you get there: Don't listen to anybody. Do what you want to do. You know it all.' They're not overtly disrespectful," she added, "We sorta get along. But there's this subtle . . . *thing* going on."

The trope of the plague doctor emphasizes a physicians' humanization through suffering as the *consequence* of expert enactment. Young Batswana health professionals, by contrast, tended to frame their expertise as the moral and practical *outcome* of Botswana's epidemic.[20] The sense that young Batswana nurses and physicians made of their work and of the epidemic and its potential for moral transformation positioned them as citizen-experts whose professional formation enabled them to respond to the threat of national extinction. This framework emphasizes their contiguity with the nation while highlighting their ability as professionals to evaluate and intervene in it in a way their fellow citizens could not. Moreover, like some Malawian students, some young Batswana were sensitive to the ways their status as health professionals signaled a rejection of colonial and apartheid policies that had kept African practitioners subordinate to white supervisors and limited professional advancement and mobility (Wendland 2010, 83; cf. Iliffe 1998; Marks 1994). It is not surprising, then, that their accounts tended to balance a recognition of the epidemic's devastation with an account of its incremental amelioration at their hands. To the extent that Batswana health professionals saw themselves as contiguous with Botswana as a nation, to read the epidemic only or even primarily in terms of suffering threatened to cast all Batswana as powerless to remediate it regardless of expertise.

This identification by Batswana health professionals as both of the nation and empowered to intervene on its behalf and the register they employed was no less ideological than EUMS students' perspectives on Referral Hospital.[21] But they contrasted sharply with those of EUMS personnel, revealing discrepant understandings of their circumstances and what was demanded of them. As the ward's MOs perceived their own minimization and erasure in EUMS students' efforts to ratify heroic transformations, relations between the two groups became increasingly discordant as the range of inhabitable social positions narrowed and solidified over time (cf. Silverstein 2003, 2004). Mpho explained:

> A lot—a *lot* of the doctors [i.e., physicians staffing Referral Hospital], *ga ke re* [you see] . . . they *hate* . . . I mean, if an American goes to ICU and asks for a bed, he's not getting the bed. If *I* go to ICU to get a bed, Dr. Murewa [the head of the ICU] will give me one just because I don't walk in there saying, "Oh, *I* know more than you and *I'm* the best there is." I don't order him around, saying, "You'll give me a bed because *in America* a patient like this needs to be in ICU."[22]

These contrasting yet interlocking ideologies illuminate the heart of the ongoing acrimony I observed on the ward, a mutually reinforcing dynamic wherein each group's efforts to morally transform themselves, to solve the problem of anesthesis, actually *reinforced* their anesthesis in the eyes of the other. That "local" doctors did not join them in their perception of the ward as a site of emergency was seen by EUMS students as further evidence of "local" doctors' callousness, lack of training, and disregard for their patients, thereby necessitating even more vigorous and unrestrained intervention by EUMS students and further justifying their presence on the ward. What students saw as necessary acts of "taking charge" of patients' care confirmed the MOs' suspicions that students held little regard for the authority of Referral Hospital personnel and that, lacking the moral sensibilities entailed in a long-term engagement with the epidemic, they were insensible of their capacity for violence toward patients, good intentions notwithstanding. The orders of indexicality that constituted these contrasting ideological frameworks shaped practice in ways that reinforced these social distinctions.

"Fifty Times on the Same Patient!"

Where were patients in all this? One June morning I joined Dr. Julie, an EUMS resident, and an EUMS student named Adam in the procedures room, a small room off the male medical ward, where Adam was preparing to perform his first lumbar puncture. Kenosi, a sturdily built man in his early forties, was suffering from an excruciating headache, a possible sign of meningitis. The procedure had two purposes. The first was diagnostic: to assess the intracranial pressure that was causing Kenosi's headache and collect cerebrospinal fluid so that the hospital's lab could investigate a possible infection. The second purpose was to relieve Kenosi's pain by draining excess fluid. The four of us crowded into the procedures room, hemmed in by filing cabinets and other equipment. Adam explained to Kenosi, who had been conversing haltingly with him in English, that the test would let them see what was causing the headache so that they could give the correct medication.

Adam asked Kenosi to lie on a vinyl-covered table on his right side; Adam positioned himself on a stool facing Kenosi's lower back. Julie stood behind Adam; I squeezed against a filing cabinet. Adam pulled on latex gloves and asked Kenosi to bend his knees toward his chest. "Tighter," said Julie to Adam, who stood and moved Kenosi's knees, increasing the tension in his spine. Adam swabbed the Kenosi's lower back with dark antibacterial ointment and began palpating his vertebrae, asking him to remain as still as possible while he tried to find the separation between the bones. Picking up a hollow needle with a removable internal stylet, Adam began inserting it between Kenosi's vertebrae. His goal was to guide the needle past two of the membranes that cover the brain and the spinal cord and into the spongy tissue containing cerebrospinal fluid. As he moved the needle slowly and uncertainly, trying to feel his way, Julie reminded him that he should feel a "give" or a "pop" as the needle moved past each membrane.

Kenosi had clenched his jaw and was breathing noisily. Adam struggled with the needle as he attempted to maneuver it into place. Julie encouraged him to withdraw it for a second attempt. It was a cool winter day, but we were all dripping with sweat. Adam moved with more confidence the second time, but when he removed the stylet, no fluid flowed. Kenosi was whispering, *Jo, jo, jo,* and there were tears on his face. Not knowing what else to do, I asked him the question to which everyone in the room, including me, knew the answer: *A go botlhoko, rra?* Is it painful? *Ee, go botlhoko!* he whispered. "He says it's painful," I said. No one responded. Adam was still working the needle back and forth, and this time, when he moved the stylet, drops of a clear liquid began to fall to the floor. Adam attached a gauge to the hollow needle to measure the pressure of the fluid. He and Julie noted the pressure, then she handed him a few phials, one after the other, to fill with fluid to be sent to the lab. Adam then replaced the stylet and, placing his left hand against Kenosi's back to steady his right hand, slowly withdrew the needle.

The training of American students in procedures such as lumbar punctures as Referral Hospital reflected an economy of available bodies, as noted previously. Moreover, the increasingly fine division of labor in American healthcare also contributed to students' feelings of restriction. In many American teaching hospitals, for example, specialized teams draw patients' blood and conduct other invasive procedures, leaving students without an opportunity to practice these skills. Second, these encounters reflected EUMS personnel's perception of Referral Hospital and of Botswana more broadly as a space of emergency wherein students contributed to patient care as they practiced technical skills, remedying local technical and affective deficits. But the encounter was also shaped by culturally specific conceptualizations of pain and language, a subject Julie Livingston addresses in her writing on oncology care in Botswana. Livingston argues that for Batswana, "pain may be spoken of, but rarely screamed or cried over" (2012, 124) noting that, "people from approximately age five and up are expected to undergo all but the worst pain in silence" (128). Batswana nurses on the oncology ward, she tells us, were "intensely aware of and sensitive to [patients'] pain" (131) and that onlookers frequently found ways of responding to and even voicing for those in agony (128, 131). But she also observes that Americans clinicians visiting the oncology ward frequently implied that "African staff are callous" toward patients' pain while "other non-African staff are not" (134), reflecting the legacy of a colonial racism that paints Africans as both lacking sensitivity to pain and indifferent toward the pain of others (133).

For EUMS personnel, such encounters were shaped by their perceptions of patients' need for care, but also by an ignorance of—in fact, a cultivated disregard for—the ways Tswana people conceive of pain and its expressions. Reiterating the common clinical logic of "see one, do one, teach one," Lesego told me that EUMS students could competently perform some procedures, like routine blood draws, and some could even do lumbar punctures if they had seen one and had been supervised doing a few more. "You've seen lumbar punctures being done," she continued, adding drily, "It's not the most pleasant thing. But you'll see them [EUMS students] trying to do one, like, *fifty times* on the same patient!" I heard in Lesego's exaggeration a fear that the clinical logic governing experiential learning was giving way to violence, that students had moved from a mode of pedagogy embedded in the course of providing treatment to a situation wherein treatment is secondary, even incidental, to pedagogy such that treatment approaches injury. Yet, in the face of what they saw as inadequate and unsympathetic local forms of care, the pain EUMS students inflicted in the course of learning procedures could *feel* beneficent—and as importantly, could be anticipated *a priori* and narrated *ex post facto* as beneficent—even as these feelings depended on students' insensibility to patients' attempts to manage their own pain, an insensibility bolstered by white American trainees' doubts regarding the capacity of Black bodies to feel pain in the first instance (Hoffman et al. 2016). Students frequently contrasted the gratitude patients at Referral Hospital expressed for treatment with the suspicion and truculence students perceived among the patients at EUMS's urban teaching hospital. But expressions of gratitude and the absence of any remonstration at Referral Hospital were shaped by a locally normative model of the clinical encounter (Livingston 2012, 76). Adam might have lacked technical skill at the beginning of the encounter but, using the register of heroic American medicine, he and his colleagues could reframe his clumsiness in terms of the global health fantasy of embodied transformation, that is, as a gesture of care toward Kenosi—treatment as good as, if not better than, anything Lesego, Mpho, or the ward's other MOs could provide. Adam's acquisition of technical skill could thus serve as the grounds for self-transformation by self-recognition. Kenosi's pain, to the extent that EUMS personnel could discern it, was expunged through anticipations of "local" gratitude taken at face value. Referral Hospital's MOs, by contrast, would never undergo such transformations no matter—or perhaps because of—how many lumbar punctures they did.

"Now I Have to *Really* Not Get HIV"

> *The Rabbit . . . longed to become Real, to know what it felt like . . . He wished that*
> *he could become it without these uncomfortable things happening to him.*
>
> Margery Williams, *The Velveteen Rabbit* (1922)

This chapter has analyzed the ideological framework that grounds the fantasy of transformative encounters that global health pedagogies promise. By contrasting the registers EUMS personnel and the medical ward's MOs used to narrate their embodied experiences, this chapter has elucidated the semiotic scaffolding within which medical professionals and trainees labored to recognize their own moral subjectivities and to evaluate the moral subjectivities of others in terms of the transformations these embodied experiences seemed to offer. The register of heroic American medicine EUMS personnel employed to assert and ratify self-transformation through self-recognition reflected both the specific challenges that the problem of anesthesis poses to contemporary American biomedical training as well as a broader sentimental politics. This register and its attendant moral subjectivities contrasted sharply those of the ward's MOs, who positioned themselves as citizen-experts motivated by the threat of national extinction to intervene in Botswana's epidemic. Once again, we see the scale-making—and ideological—work of stance: The ward's Batswana MO's scaled themselves relative to a national epidemic, grounding their moral subjectivities in expertise deployed in the service of the nation one fellow citizen at a time. For EUMS personnel, the moral subjectivities they sought to ratify were portable, durable dispositions acquired through a connoisseurship of suffering, scalable relative to a world that needed saving wherever they happened to be. If global health partnerships perpetuate the very inequalities they propose to remedy, this is no less true with regard to the capacity to position oneself as a moral biomedical practitioner than with regard to funding or equipment.

One afternoon my friend, Tumelo, a nurse at the Superlative Clinic, and I were chatting as we leaned on the counter in the Clinic's reception area. It was the end of the day; only a few families were waiting to pick up their medications from the Clinic's pharmacy. I told Tumelo about Molly's needlestick, and Tumelo responded that she, too, had recently pricked herself and was taking PEP. I was surprised: in her day-to-day activities Tumelo ordinarily had little contact with sharps, though she was more willing than many nurses to handle them and expressed a great deal of interest in and comfort with pediatric nursing. She had once called me from the hospital on her day off, where she had been placing a baby's cannula, a difficult task due to the small size of an infant's blood vessels. The nurses who had called her, she had explained to me, were too scared to place the cannula, fearing their lack of dexterity might harm the patient, themselves, or both. While Tumelo did not share these fears, she sympathized with the nurses, saying that she could see no reason why they should be compelled to carry out orders they regarded as dangerous to their patient and potentially self-destructive.[23] Given their personal and collective historical experiences of the epidemic, including leaving their shifts at the hospital only to care for ailing kin at home, and their cognizance of their lack of specialized training and the limitations of the materials at hand, refusing to handle sharps looked to Tumelo less like shirking and more like a form of care.

Tumelo told me that on the occasion of her most recent needlestick injury, she had been standing in for Mma Molefi, the clinic's phlebotomist. Mma Molefi, clad in latex gloves and a translucent plastic apron, handled needles day in and day out. I asked Tumelo whether Mma Molefi had ever stuck herself. Tumelo said she didn't know. The government provided PEP for its health workers, she explained, but one had to test for HIV before beginning the regimen so that anyone who was already HIV positive could receive treatment rather than risking the drug resistance that short-term PEP might induce. The rapid test used in Botswana tested not for the virus itself but for the antibodies to HIV. Even if a nurse tested negative, she still had to take the PEP regimen for twenty-eight days and then retest to confirm that she had not contracted the virus. If she tested negative, she could she discontinue taking PEP. For a nurse testing for HIV before beginning PEP, the best-case scenario could only be discovering that she had not seroconverted *yet*. Faced with the requirement to test, Tumelo continued, some of her colleagues simply didn't report needlestick injuries. Mma Molefi, Tumelo speculated, had probably "pricked herself so many times that she doesn't even *want* to test." But reported or not, injuries still took place. Tumelo told me that Duduetsang, one of the Clinic's lab technicians, had been spattered in the eye with blood two years earlier. Dudu, Tumelo continued, had been on medications ever since, leading to speculation among the nurses as to whether Dudu had acquired HIV from the injury or whether the injury had simply facilitated the revelation of an already existing infection.[24] Fiddling with the gauzy hairband belonging to her daughter that she had wrapped around her own long plaits, Tumelo confided that this most recent injury was her third needlestick in three years and thus her third round of PEP. Giving me a wry smile, she concluded: "Now I have to *really* not get HIV because I'll be resistant to the medications in the prophylaxis."[25]

Fetishizing anesthesis as a problem entails forgetting that people in pain may actually want and sometimes desperately need anesthesia. Tumelo's statement casts into stark relief the point where a desire for transformative closeness gives way to the terror of ineluctable destruction. Compare Mma Molefi's fear of testing to Molly's pleasure at the closeness that taking ARVs for four weeks might impart—or at very least, the frame available for Molly to recast terror as an opportunity for a particular form of pleasure, a moment of emotion pedagogy (Wilce and Fenigsen 2016), wherein she both enacted and recognized her capacity to care. Tumelo engaged the fantasy of the plague doctor with more ambivalence. On one hand, she recognized her vulnerability vis-à-vis Botswana's national epidemic, a vulnerability her professional practice increased. On the other, it was her status as a trained health professional that allowed her to assess the danger of drug resistance she faced. By pointing to the ironic fact that treating patients with HIV might increase her own chances of contracting the virus, Tumelo mitigated the terror of too much closeness, the moment when the ideological ground for her expert enactments, that is, shared citizenship and a shared experience of a national disaster and the distance conferred by specialized training, gave way as she became indistinguishable from those she treated. For Molly, by contrast, the capacity of her needlestick injury to transform her, and her claim, however provisional, to feeling close to her patients at Referral Hospital were made possible by contemporary American biomedicine's neoliberal affective pedagogies, by the ideologies that made Kenosi's pain both unrecognizable and unimportant to Adam, by the "melodramatic conventions of individual historical acts of compassion and transcendence . . . adapted to imagine a nonhierarchical social world" made possible by "good intentions and love" (Berlant 2008a, 6), and finally, by the unlikelihood that she might ever become a patient there.

PEDAGOGY AS DISPOSSESSION

Dr. Sibanda and I gradually became acquainted as we moved through the same small circuit of Gaborone's biomedical and public health professional institutions. We exchanged greetings at the tea table at the monthly meetings of the Botswana branch of the Southern African HIV Clinicians' Society (SAHIVCS). We found ourselves seated next to one another at the Superlative Clinic's weekly journal club. But I found him difficult to place. He did not seem to be affiliated with the Superlative Clinic or EUMS or with any of the other US-based partnerships, such as the Botswana Harvard Partnership (BHP). He lacked the relaxed stateliness of Batswana physicians in private practice, who tended to be somewhat older. But neither did he fit the bill of Ministry of Health personnel, who were treated deferentially by Batswana health professionals, at least in public, and by most Americans health professionals with a stiff formality mingled with a marked wariness that at times bordered on hostility.

When I finally introduced myself in May 2008, I learned that he was a biochemist trained in Zimbabwe and the UK and was currently teaching at the Institute of Health Sciences in Gaborone (IHSG). The Institute, located next door to Referral Hospital, offered diplomas in nursing and midwifery as well as training for allied health professionals such as pharmacists and laboratory technologists (Seboni 2012; Seitio and Newland 2008). The roots of the IHSG lay in the National Health Institute, founded as a nurse training facility in the early 1970s as Botswana began emphasizing preventative public health in rural areas (Høgh and Petersen 1984). The Institute eventually decentralized, opening campuses in major towns around the country; in 1985 these facilities were brought into affiliation with the University of Botswana, which assumed responsibility for accreditation (Parsons et al. 2012, 43; Seitio and Newland 2008). The University of Botswana also granted bachelor's and master's degrees in nursing, a program that had evolved from one initially designed to train nursing instructors (Seboni 2012), but the vast majority of nurses in Botswana trained at an IHS.

Having grown accustomed to the overwhelming focus on physicians and physician training that characterized the Superlative Clinic and EUMS, I was embarrassed to admit I knew little about the IHSG. Dr. Sibanda explained that EUMS had initially sought a partnership with IHSG and BOTUSA, the US CDC field office in Gaborone but, shaking his head and smiling ruefully, "The big people at UB [the University of Botswana] got involved." IHSG, he continued, had subsequently been sidelined from the partnership with EUMS and had struggled for recognition as an institution with a vested interest in clinical training and practice in Botswana. And even though the tall, glassy building that housed the Botswana Harvard HIV Reference Laboratory (BHHRL), which conducted the polymerase chain reaction (PCR) tests used in HIV diagnosis and treatment as well as laboratory work for the BHP's ongoing clinical trials, was only a stone's throw from his own office, he had never even been inside. "When I call my friends who work there to ask if they can show me around," he told me, "They say, 'Well, what can I say you want to be shown around *for*?'" "With all this interest coming in," he said, shaking his head in disappointment, "Botswana is in a position where it should be making the calls, calling the shots." Instead, despite calls from the MOH for IHS staff to generate research oriented toward shaping national health policies, the Reference Laboratory remained out of bounds to him and to other health and science professionals working in Botswana's public sector, and this exclusion left Botswana continually dependent on foreign expertise: "If Harvard left today," he demanded with regard to the laboratory, "who would run it?"

A few months later this discontent took a more public stage. In September 2008 the Ministry of Health's Health Research Unit (HRU) held a workshop to solicit input as it began drafting a national health research agenda. The attendees were largely American and Batswana. Almost all of the Americans were employed by US-based institutions, including EUMS, the Superlative Clinic, and BHP; the Batswana were split fairly evenly between the partners and government institutions, as were the small number of non-American expatriates. Mma Modise, a much-respected senior nurse who managed the Superlative Clinic's ongoing clinical trial, pointed out to me in a whisper that beyond the staff of the HRU, only a handful of MOH employees were present, as evidenced by the empty chairs in front of the placecards for "Food and Nutrition" and "Drug Regulatory Unit." "BOTUSA and ACHAP are here," she noted, "but NACA is not," indicating to her the extent to which the event implicitly catered to "the partners," as she called them, and had been recognized by Botswana's civil servants as such.

The organizers distributed a list of priority research areas for discussion, but the attendees quickly dispensed with the question of what should be researched in Botswana and why. They turned instead to matters of infrastructure, that is, the need for Botswana to invest in validating laboratory equipment, training laboratory technicians, and standardizing laboratories in accordance with WHO guidelines, thereby facilitating adherence to "international" benchmarks, the standards to which American institutions adhered. The partners rapidly arrived at a consensus: Botswana needed to build research capacity. The partners were already pursuing that goal, but more capacity was needed, particularly more research governance. The response was anxious muttering among the other attendees. An HRU staff member acknowledged the need for more robust research governance, observing that with the increasing number of clinical trials in the country, Batswana were asking more questions about risks and benefits, about ownership of samples they provided and their stake in any profits that might derive from them. At this point Dr. Sibanda stood up and, with the air of one gesturing to the obvious, declared: "You say you're building capacity. The problem with 'building capacity' is that it means just preparing specimens to be sent overseas for processing. We are all," he concluded, gesturing to an audience stunned into silence, "just specimens."

Pedagogy as Capacity Building, Capacity Building as Dispossession

Global health partnerships in Botswana frequently touted "capacity building," particularly related to clinical care and clinical research, as one of their primary objectives, one they valued, as Dr. Alison did in chapter 1, over the mundane task of "just seeing patients." This goal fell in line with broader trends both in global health and in international development more generally. "Partnerships between African and non-African institutions," notes Claire Wendland, "are increasingly justified by their impact on capacity" (2016, 416), framed in terms of not only practical benefits to Southern research and treatment infrastructures but also Northern institutions' ethical commitments (Crane 2013; Minn 2015; Street 2014). With regard to global health, "there is," observes Bronwen Poleykett, "almost universal agreement that capacity building is necessary in order to build a fairer, efficient and more locally embedded system of research and service delivery" (2018, 277). Much like global health itself, capacity is presented as "an undisputed good" (Geissler and Tousignant 2016, 350).

This chapter analyzes clinical pedagogies framed in terms of capacity building as a key "rhetorical strategy" (West 2016, chap. 2) of global health in Botswana. Specifically, this chapter is concerned with the ideological frame that made it difficult to pinpoint the *extractive* dimension of the clinical pedagogies American institutions offered or to articulate this dimension in anything other than the type of shocking outburst depicted earlier. In her study of tourism, conservation, and development in Papua New Guinea, Paige West draws an explicit connection between rhetorical representations of Papua New Guinea and their material effects, arguing that that rhetoric lays the ground for material dispossession and the reinforcement of structural inequalities. Drawing on geographer Neil Smith's work on gentrification, which illustrated how investors "depressed the market for a site so that they can profit from investing in it themselves" (West 2016, 79; see N. Smith 1979, 1996), West emphasizes the rhetorical and ideological conditions of possibility for the constitution and recognition of value, potential, capacity, or their absences. Ideologies, West reminds us, "are meant to persuade," to "guide people's actions," to "serve as a logic and means by which people justify their actions" that reinforce relationships of power (2016, 6). Rather than focusing on the extradiscursive (i.e., nonlinguistic) forms of dispossession that threatened to accompany clinical research in Botswana—that is, the specimens Dr. Sibanda feared he and some of those around him had already become—this chapter focuses on the rhetoric of clinical capacity building as "the discursive beginnings of structures of dispossession" (West 2016, 12).

Capacity building gained traction in development programming in the 1990s before global health solidified as an organizing principle for interventions in the Global South. As structural adjustment programs reduced state institutions, capacity building emerged as a neoliberal development strategy designed to address the failures of development's technological fixes, failures attributed not to the fixes themselves but to the "capacities" of those receiving them. And while capacity development schemes, as Paige West notes, were directed at multiple scales—"individuals, organizations, and whole societies" (2016, 71), the locus of intervention is the individual framed in terms of a lack that recapitulates and reinforces a trope that framed colonized peoples in similar terms. This trope, West notes, had long informed development interventions, "but the term 'capacity building' smuggles it back in as a modern rhetoric" (2016, 72). What capacity building imagines, in short, is transformed individuals who bring about a promised future (Douglas-Jones and Shaffner 2017; LaHatte 2017, 19; cf. Ferguson 1999; 2006b): "the ultimate goal" of capacity building "is to produce new kinds of persons" and "it is assumed that new kinds of institutions and societies will follow" (West 2016, 73; LaHatte 2017). In the process, structural inequalities and their histories are erased while individuals are called on to recognize their own insufficiencies and enact social transformations through practices tied to new forms of social reproduction and new social networks.

The overwhelming focus in capacity building on technical interventions targeted toward individuals, interventions that are themselves amenable to enumeration and audit, dovetails with the orientation of global health partnerships toward the unidirectional transfer of technologies and expertise from North to South. In her review of representations of capacity building in recent medical literature, Claire Wendland notes that capacity is consistently framed as something "non-material and usually cognitive, highly specific, something that can be counted, something that is transferred from a teacher to a student, and something that flows from North to South" (2016, 416). "The single most common goal of clinical capacity-building projects," she observes, "was to teach a particular diagnostic or therapeutic intervention" (417). These interventions were oriented "globally," that is, toward a generic incapacity rather than addressing local epidemiologies or specific infrastructural constraints (Feierman 2011). The "targets," she continues, "were black boxes . . . their already existing capabilities and weaknesses were set aside as irrelevant to the task at hand" (420). And while some "local" doctors may enthusiastically embrace trainings and workshops for the professionalization and networking opportunities and even funds they offer (cf. Scherz 2014, chap. 5; Smith 2003; Watkins and Swidler 2013), these activities nonetheless draw attendees away from clinical work (Wendland 2016, 421).

Moreover, clinical capacity is frequently entangled with research capacity. Geissler and Tousignant note that, "reinforcing research capacity . . . has played a key role in garnering support for global health as a morally unambiguous but fundamentally apolitical enterprise" (2016, 349). Scholars of sub-Saharan Africa have emphasized this entanglement, illustrating how transnational clinical research collaborations have "filled in the gap" of public health systems dismantled under structural adjustment policies, creating the conditions of possibility for treatment programs in the absence of state support (Crane 2013; Geissler 2011; Nguyen 2011; Whyte 2014). Accounts of East Africa in particular highlight a long legacy of professionalized biomedicine and the establishment in the early postcolonial era of the expertise and infrastructure clinical research required (Mika 2021). This lay the groundwork for future research partnerships as the HIV epidemic unfolded despite the neglect or underfunding of these infrastructures due to political instabilities (Iliffe 1998; Mika 2016; Okwaro and Geissler 2015; Poleykett 2018). Hospitals, as these and other studies have shown, have increasingly become laboratories as the lines between treatment and experimentation have become increasingly blurred (Nguyen 2009; Petryna 2005; Street 2014, chap. 8). Yet building research capacity, Wendland argues, generally entails increasing capacity in terms that facilitate the commensuration of practices and findings across settings, including research governance mechanisms such as institutional review boards and laboratory certifications, thereby facilitating the involvement of Northern partners and reflecting their priorities (2016, 418).

That the purported beneficiaries of these efforts to enhance research in the Global South experience them as extractive, then, is unsurprising.[1] From Senegal to Uganda, "local" researchers fear being relegated to "blood-senders" (Crane 2013, 105; Fullwiley 2011, 190). My focus in this chapter, however, is less on clinical research itself than on ideological struggles over the pedagogies directed toward the tangle of treatment, training, and research. Botswana's particular assemblage of these overlapping activities provides a contrasting perspective on the relationship between global health science and the HIV epidemic in sub-Saharan Africa. The prioritization of primary healthcare in the postcolonial era and the absence of a medical school through the first decade of the treatment program left clinical research largely in the hands of US-based institutions; the challenges of treating HIV lay less in a lack of public health funding and infrastructure than in a lack of trained healthcare professionals and the facilities to produce them. Clinical research, while entangled with treatment from the very beginning, did not, at least in the mid-2000s, dominate treatment, but instead hovered on the horizon, figuring largely as the sort of promise and threat Dr. Sibanda articulated. This chapter asks how clinical pedagogies *themselves*, not just the research they enabled, figured as a mechanism of extraction, as "a vessel for external investment, which will provide high rents to investors" (West 2016, 83), and how the broader ideological framework of global health constrained efforts to articulate this point.

I begin by examining the clinical research infrastructure in southeastern Botswana that predated the treatment program, tracing the ways that clinical research preceded and gave shape to the emergent treatment program and how the treatment program, in turn, shaped clinical training. I then examine efforts on the part of Superlative Clinic and EUMS personnel to build capacity on the wards of Referral Hospital, efforts that reveal ambivalences structured by the "sedentarist metaphysics" of global health (Crane 2013, 157; cf. Malkki 1992), that is, the logics of mobility and morality that chapters 4 and 5 made apparent. Efforts to expand clinical research at Referral Hospital promised to enhance clinical training for "local" doctors; instead, I argue, it tended to either detract attention from training or reinforce existing social and professional hierarchies. I turn then to the anxieties around clinical research in Botswana in order to illuminate how the entanglement of treatment, training, and research shaped clinical capacity building into a pedagogy of extraction, one that called on Batswana to imagine themselves in terms of the offshore production of knowledge and value.

From Research to Treatment, Treatment to Training: 1995–2005

In the years before Botswana's treatment program began rolling out, clinical research had been largely in the hands of BOTUSA and BHP, both founded in the mid-1990s. Established in 1995, BOTUSA was initially a partnership between the Ministry of Health and the CDC's Division of Tuberculosis Elimination (DTBE). It was initially, some people told me, just a field office oriented toward improving Botswana's existing TB Control Program and conducting operational research. For example, BOTUSA developed an electronic tuberculosis register and, through research on causes of death in HIV-positive Batswana, found that cotrimoxazole, an antibiotic prescribed prophylactically before ARV treatment became available, was inadequate for preventing lethal opportunistic infections.[2] In 1999, however, BOTUSA's mandate began to shift as the CDC expanded its own mandate to include direct support for HIV-related programming. BOTUSA gained a separate HIV Prevention Unit (HPU), and in 2000 institutional oversight was transferred from DTBE to the CDC's Global AIDS Program (GAP). When the disbursal of PEPFAR funds began in 2004, BOTUSA was tasked with administering funds within Botswana as the nearest USAID field office was located in Pretoria, South Africa. Over the course of my research, a number of BOTUSA staff members referred to ongoing tensions and even resentments over the amount of money earmarked for HIV-related activities and the extent to which the HPU's mandate was steering the entire institution, diverting attention away from the disease that was its *raison d'être*. More concretely, the HIV Prevention Unit, rebaptized as the HIV Prevention *Research* Unit (HPRU) to distinguish its work from less prestigious prevention programming, moved away from BOTUSA's earlier focus on operational research geared toward improving country-specific tuberculosis surveillance, diagnosis, and epidemiology to participating in a transnational network of HIV-related experimental research that produced the kind of knowledge that could be freed from context and circulate "globally," that is, among other sites in the Global South via connections to research institutions in the Global North (cf. Biruk 2018; Feierman 2011; Street 2014, chap. 8).

BHP was founded in 1996, one of many research and treatment initiatives led by the Harvard AIDS Institute, itself founded in 1988. Unlike BOTUSA, however, BHP never had a mandate for the type of country-specific operational research that characterized BOTUSA's early work on tuberculosis. By contrast, in 1999 HAI received a US$2.5 million grant to support basic research, including genomic analysis, vaccine development, and, perhaps most programmatically, the evaluation of different PMTCT regimens, including variations in antiretroviral medications and infant feeding practices.[3] On December 1, World AIDS Day, of 2001 BHP, with financial support from the same pharmaceutical philanthropy that supported the Superlative Clinic and the Pediatric Squad, officially opened the Botswana Harvard HIV Reference Laboratory (BHHRL), though Rebecca, the administrator whose comments open chapter 3, told me the laboratory only became functional in April of the following year. As the national treatment program unfolded, BHHRL provided the laboratory services the program required, running viral load tests and CD4 counts on the same machines that were used for research projects. As Rebecca led me through the hushed building, past the enormous padlocked freezers in the basement used to store samples, she explained that since the BHHRL had opened, BHP's leadership had leveraged research grants from the NIH, pharmaceutical philanthropy, and ACHAP to support the institution as a whole, that is, both its research endeavors and the key role it played in the treatment program. And while BHP's researchers, like the staff of the HPRU, presented their findings as knowledge that could circulate globally, its research staff also insisted that BHP studies could be readily used to shape the country's domestic health policy (Harvard AIDS Initiative 2005).

Neither BOTUSA nor BHP were directly responsible for developing or administering the ARV treatment program, and while both institutions made efforts to recruit and train Batswana scientists, neither institution made building capacity among medical practitioners an explicit part of its mandate. That said, the treatment program's history is thoroughly entangled in Botswana's emerging research apparatus and the forms of training it made available. Pediatric HIV treatment in Botswana, as I explained in chapter 1, had begun under the aegis of a clinical trial that was halted once ARVs became publicly available. Adult treatment began under similar circumstances: BHP staff had begun preparing to launch a similar trial, hiring nurses and outfitting a small room off Referral Hospital's Accident and Emergency ward. Faced with a delay in gaining approval from Harvard for the study, they began screening patients to see if they would qualify for the ARV treatment program once it began, recruiting EUMS physicians who were rotating through Gaborone, such as Dr. Jackson, to the cause. "There was nothing," Rebecca recalled. "No Tebelopele [Botswana's public HIV counseling and testing service], no routine testing, nothing. Patients had CD4 counts of 2." The team tested patients for HIV, added them to a wait list if they qualified, and referred very sick patients to a sympathetic private practitioner, who provided medications at reduced prices. Word of the ersatz clinic's existence spread. As the number of patients increased, Referral Hospital's superintendent offered the use of the hospital's then-unused isolation ward. This building, during my research, was sometimes referred to as "the old IDCC" to differentiate it from the prefab "new IDCC" at the back of the hospital; it had since returned to its original purpose as cases of first multidrug-resistant and then extensively drug-resistant TB emerged in Botswana (WHO 2008). The old IDCC thus became operational before the treatment program formally began. Moreover, it emerged as a model of clinical care for HIV, Elise Carpenter argues, "both for its combination of clear protocols, written at a time when the ARV program was starting, and for its being the first working HIV clinic in Botswana where other doctors came to observe" (2008, 79).

This observational mode of clinical pedagogy was reinforced by clinical preceptors, foreign HIV experts posted to hospitals around Botswana to mentor clinicians through the first six months of providing ARV treatment and who, over time, became key in integrating HIV treatment into the existing bureaucracy of clinical care in Botswana (Carpenter 2008, chap. 3). It ran parallel, however, to a more modular, classroom- and lecture-based mode of pedagogy oriented around a standardized and presumably universal set of "best practices." This approach was epitomized by KITSO, a training program developed by BHP to support HIV clinical training.[4] "Underpinning the KITSO program," argues Carpenter, "was the idea that scientific, universal, research-based knowledge ensured good clinical care" (2008, 92). Early versions of the program assumed physicians as their audience and focused on the technical aspects of HIV treatment rather than the managerial ones; the scant attention given to adherence relied on research conducted in the US as though those findings were unproblematically generalizable (Carpenter 2008, 96). KITSO's inattention to local context, Carpenter argues, was less an inadvertent omission than a sign of "good development work" insofar as it was standardized, portable, and measurable; moreover, Carpenter speculates, it offered a way of insulating Botswana's treatment program and the Americans supporting it from accusations that public ARV treatment in Africa would lead to drug resistance (2008, 104). The practitioner imagined by KITSO was also standardized and thus innocent, prepared to treat HIV regardless of context and oriented toward research problems of global import, not the specificity of national programming. KITSO offered its ideal physician-researcher-trainees a way to scale science—a way, in short, out of Botswana. That many of the physicians trained by KITSO or working within

BHP—including, during my fieldwork, the director—were expatriate Africans working in Botswana, not Batswana themselves, did nothing to dispel this impression. Clinical training via KITSO could look like American experts preparing expatriate Africans to conduct research in places *like* Botswana, not improving clinical practice *within* Botswana.

Clinical Pedagogies in Everyday Practice

In contrast to BOTUSA and BHP, the Superlative Clinic and EUMS explicitly committed themselves to building clinical capacity in Botswana. This generally translated into two activities: classroom teaching for MOs and, to a far lesser extent, nurses; and mentoring for MOs, particularly during ward rounds. Both EUMS physicians and Squad pediatricians were deeply troubled by the lack of opportunities for specialized training, particularly residencies, available to the MOs. They frequently commented on the small number of Batswana physicians in the public health system, reminding one another that there were no Batswana physicians outside the country's two referral hospitals and that the physicians staffing the country's primary and district hospitals were largely expatriate Africans (cf. Carpenter 2008, 30). The government of Botswana had been sponsoring citizens to study medicine overseas since the 1990s in an effort to decrease this marked reliance on expatriate physicians, but only a small number had returned.[5] Both Dr. Amy and Dr. Rosen explained to me at different moments that although the Ministry of Education held a financial lien against the students it sponsored to study medicine, the Government had difficulty enforcing this lien and that those who failed to return to Botswana had little difficulty paying it off, earning far more in the countries in which they had earned their medical degrees than they could in Botswana, particularly in the public sector. In the best of circumstances, those working abroad could use their salaries to support their extended families and still retire to Botswana in relative comfort.[6] Furthermore, many Batswana medical professionals eventually left the public sector for private practice or, increasingly, for one of the "partners."

The capacity that the Superlative Clinic and EUMS sought to build, then, was oriented toward keeping Batswana physicians firmly in Botswana. That said, these American physicians tended to approach this project with a great deal of ambivalence. While American physicians and medical trainees sometimes seemed to suggest that Batswana health professionals could and perhaps even should seek professional training or experience "somewhere else," they also frowned on the idea of Batswana health professionals actually leaving Botswana. On one hand, some Squad pediatricians, resentful of what they perceived as the failings of Botswana's health system, expected that *any* physician working within it would axiomatically want to leave. Early in 2007, for example, the Squad pediatricians began offering a series of lunchtime lectures reviewing aspects of pediatric advanced life support (PALS) for the staff of the pediatric medical ward. Nurses tended to outnumber the MOs at these lectures, but the lectures themselves, while ostensibly open to all ward staff, tended to focus heavily on the skills and responsibility of MOs. One afternoon I joined the group seated on benches in the ward's small conference room, where Dr. James was reviewing the management of respiratory distress. Frustrated by what he perceived as the group's unresponsiveness to his questions, he added, "If you go somewhere else, and take a test, these are test questions you might see."[7] The purpose of the lecture was ostensibly to improve the clinical skills of Batswana clinicians on the assumption that the ability to offer a higher quality of care, that is, care on par with "somewhere else," would motivate them to stay in the country. But by framing the elements of PALS as skills and knowledge clinicians would be expected to demonstrate "somewhere else," Dr. James drew explicit attention to the increased and presumably desirable mobility PALS training offered clinicians who mastered those skills and knowledge. Such standardized trainings, opined Dr. Frank on another occasion, were "good to have on your *c.v.* [curriculum vitae] wherever you are in the world." These statements implied that, unlike Botswana, "other places" would demand and foster a standardized set of clinical proficiencies as a matter of course.

On the other hand, American physicians disparaged Batswana physicians who did leave the public sector, framing these decisions as the morally suspect pursuit of financial gain or political acumen over fulfilling a moral and professional duty to their country. Moreover, some American physicians expressed doubt as to whether "local" health professionals had the moral and technical capacity necessary to work "somewhere else." When Dr. Mark presented one of the PALS lectures, he described, with the assistance of overhead slides, a hypothetical situation involving a child in respiratory distress. He then presented the room of MOs and nurses a multiple-choice question regarding the management of the child, reading each option aloud. Each option began with the words, *Do you . . .* ; one option was, *Do you take a break for lunch?* This drew a low murmur from the group; it fell into a general pattern of Squad pediatricians' complaints about the pace at which care proceeded on the ward and their resentment of the conventions that governed staff breaks at Referral Hospital and that extended to the public health system more generally (Brada 2016). Using his slides, Dr. Mark continued to work through the hypothetical scenario, eventually arriving at another question he posed to the group: "Your orders were not noticed until now [i.e., 2 hours after they were placed]. What would you do?" The room went very still, a tension that recalled the proverbial knife. This question was ostensibly directed at the MOs who, presumably, would have placed such orders. But it clearly laid blame on the nurses for failing to notice, let alone follow, a physician's orders, and recruited the MOs to the position of recognizing this mistake as though their credibility as professionals lay in the execution of a suitable rebuke. Increased capacity for the MOs, this line of questioning suggested, lay in emulating Dr. Mark in his disparagement of the ward's nurses, who stood in for Botswana's health system in their presumed immobility relative to physicians.[8] As if blaming poor clinical care on a failure of empathy and offering remedial instruction, Dr. Mark, speaking to an audience in a country where it is not hyperbolic to suggest that the epidemic has left no one, least of all health professionals, untouched, admonished them: *"You should think, 'What if this were my child?'"*

Even when American medical educators were less starkly ambivalent about Batswana physicians' clinical acumen or moral subjectivity, clinical pedagogies did not unfold as intended. Emphasizing EUMS's commitment to improving training for "local" physicians, Dr. Rosen told me that he made all his clinical interactions into "teaching moments" by always having "local" interns or MOs present. Likewise, Dr. Goldberg, recounting the mentoring Dr. Jackson had done in the old IDCC as the treatment program got underway, recalled that, "Every time I saw him, he had someone there as a learner." What I observed on the medical wards, however, presented a different picture. The MOs generally received Dr. Rosen's contributions with a respectful silence.[9] One morning as Lesego Balebetse was presenting a case during morning report, Dr. Rosen interjected; Lesego stared at her notes so long that Dr. Rosen eventually began answering his own questions as if they were rhetorical ones, at which point Lesego returned her gaze to him and listened attentively. Dr. Rosen backtracked, metapragmatically reframing his interjection as though Lesego might have felt chastened: "It's just advice," he almost consoled her. "I'm not correcting you." The MOs' silence stood in marked contrast to the eager responses of EUMS students to Dr. Rosen's questions; those responses tended to lead to far more dialogic interactions. As he rounded that morning with Lesego's firm, Dr. Rosen posed a question to the group, which included an EUMS student named Jessica, two British medical trainees, and two American undergraduate students. Regarding the first patient, who was anemic and showed signs of liver disease, he asked us, "Do you have an approach to hepatic anemia? What's the algorithmic tree regarding hepatic anemia: intrinsic, extrinsic, etc.?" Jessica jumped in, and Dr. Rosen amiably interrogated her as he sketched an algorithmic tree and drew pictures of hepatic cells while Lesego stood silently by and the rest of us scribbled in our notebooks.

The MOs' contributions to these interactions frequently consisted of identifying aspects of care specific to Referral Hospital or to Botswana rather than contributing to a differential diagnosis or discussing the merits of different approaches to treatment. That morning, as we turned to the second patient, who had been admitted with chest pain and shortness of breath, Dr. Frank, who had joined our firm, turned to Jessica, asking, "In the States [i.e., the US], what's your investigation of choice?" Jessica suggested an MRI, shrugging as she acknowledged that Referral Hospital lacked the necessary equipment, and a clotting test. "Should we—can we," Dr. Rosen said, turning to look at Lesego and then turning back to Jessica, "get that test here? Would it be useful?" Dr. Rosen explained that the first step would be a spinal CT, which was available in Botswana, but that patients often couldn't hold their breaths long enough for a clear image.[10] He continued, "I think I'd . . ." but trailed off and turned again to Lesego, asking, "What would you do?" Lesego turned to the nurse who was rounding with the firm and asked a series of questions about the patient in Setswana. As if to while away the time, Dr. Rosen turned again to Jessica, saying, "Regarding tests . . . it's important to think about why you want them, but even more so because of limited resources," as Lesego arranged the patient's course of treatment.

Time and time again, EUMS physicians posed open-ended questions to groups composed of both "local" junior physicians and EUMS trainees and yet, whatever their intentions might have been, they ended up conversing almost exclusively with EUMS trainees. This reflected dissimilar, if implicit, norms regarding the division of speaking labor across social hierarchies both inside and outside formal instructional venues, as numerous examples from previous chapters have illustrated. Moreover, when we spoke in private Lesego positioned herself *outside* the group of individuals toward whom these pedagogies were directed, saying of the EUMS students, "They're still learners." She did not imagine, in other words, that Dr. Rosen and his colleagues directed their teaching toward her; as a qualified physician, she imagined little gain from the type of dialogic exercise in which Dr. Rosen engaged Jessica and would even have usurped the time and attention the students needed. Far from the primary target of Dr. Rosen's teaching, Lesego regarded herself at most as a neutral bystander or a source of essential insider information. At stake in these interactions was not just the question of whether EUMS was, in fact, transferring skills and knowledge, but broader political questions regarding EUMS's activities in Botswana. In early 2008 I arranged to interview the head of BOTUSA about the office's clinical research. Very rapidly, however, I found myself in the hot seat: As the institution charged with managing PEPFAR grants in Botswana, BOTUSA administered funds EUMS had received to "improve" clinical training for "local" clinicians on Referral Hospital's medical wards. Aware that I had been spending time on the wards, my would-be interviewee quickly turned the tables, pumping me for information about EUMS, her mounting irritation obvious as my halting attempts at neutral and anonymous descriptions nevertheless seemed to confirm her suspicion that EUMS students derived more benefit from EUMS's presence on the wards than did Referral Hospital's own medical staff.

In some instances, such as outreach visits to southeastern Botswana's district hospitals, "local" physicians were more easily identified as the subjects toward whom EUMS personnel directed clinical pedagogies. Yet these interactions were far from neutral. Dr. Frank explained to me that EUMS had begun an outreach program at one of the district hospitals consisting of a series of lectures regarding the general medical care of HIV-positive patients. Dr. Frank had been excited to work with the MO who ran the hospital's renal clinic and who, Dr. Frank said, was developing a specialist's level of knowledge. The hospital's chief medical officer (CMO), however, had put a stop to the program. Dr. Frank described the CMO's objections as "ideological": "She's convinced we're a vertical HIV program," he grumbled. In conversation with me, however, the CMO stoutly defended her decision, telling me she knew EUMS thought her unreasonable but that she could not spare her staff to listen to lectures. Moreover, she explicitly reframed EUMS's activities as *removing* health professionals from the national health system rather than fixing them in place or even enhancing clinical care. By hiring a particular Motswana physician to lead their partnership, she told me, EUMS had deprived Botswana's health system of the only physician in the entire country trained in a particular specialization. "But," she shrugged, "people go where the money is." When I repeated what Dr. Goldberg had told me, that the specialist would continue see patients, the CMO dismissed this as "illusory." "Once you're in the office, you stay in the office," she said drily. "When is she going to see patients, at 12 midnight? Once you take people out of the clinical area, you can't go back. You lose your clinical chops." This extractive redistribution of personnel extended, in her view, to other "partners" as well: The laboratory technician she had hired fresh from training in the US had been "poached" by BHP, as had the hospital's pharmacist, losses felt acutely in a small district hospital. Later I told Tshepo Kokeletso, a young MO who I knew from the adult medical wards, about my exchange with the CMO. Tshepo sighed deeply and said, "Well, you can't *blame* them [i.e., staff who left for positions with "partner" institutions]. And it's not like they're *really* leaving. But . . . you're taking people out of government service. You're taking people away from the very system you're claiming to strengthen."[11]

Even when efforts at building clinical capacity seemed more expressly directed at individual Batswana, their outcomes could be disappointing. MOs often had little control over their assignments, but Tshepo had applied for and received from the MOH a transfer to the Superlative Clinic, where he could develop his interest in family medicine without resigning from government service, thereby retaining his status as a civil servant and the benefits it entailed. And when I heard in early 2008 that the Clinic's parent organization, CHAN, would be sponsoring two MOs, including Tshepo, to do residencies in the US, I had assumed that they meant the MOs would be accepted into residency programs at the elite medical school with which CHAN was affiliated. I was very pleased on their behalf: The process of applying for sponsorship from the Government of Botswana for advanced training was lengthy and complicated, never mind the obstacles MOs faced in actually being accepted into American residency programs or the difficulties such training entailed (Chen et al. 2011; Crane 2013, 158).[12] That said, I was also a little surprised: Promises of support for specialization often seemed largely ephemeral: Mma Mokento, leaning over Clinic's reception counter, had quietly opined: "They [the Clinic's administrators] are cheating us—calling us pediatric nurses but not sending us for training [i.e., specialized training in pediatric nursing]. They say they have a training plan. But when I ask to see the training plan, they won't show it to me."

In April I ran into Tshepo at a meeting CHAN was holding at one of Gaborone's resorts. An annual event that rotated from one CHAN site to another, these meetings brought together personnel from CHAN's network of affiliated clinics in Africa and Eastern Europe and its US headquarters. The meeting in Gaborone was attended by members of Botswana's public and private medical sectors and representatives of affiliated NGOs, private foundations, and the other "partners." After greeting Tshepo, I observed that he looked tired. He explained that the CHAN meeting, by drawing the Squad pediatricians away from the Superlative Clinic, had increased his patient load. He was also dealing with bureaucratic troubles related to his visa and his contract with the hospital that housed his residency program—which, it turned out, was not the school affiliated with CHAN but one affiliated with EUMS. As his departure date approached, however, Tshepo's troubles were multiplying. He and Dr. Mokwele, the other MO whom CHAN was sponsoring, had been asked to resign from government service. "When government sponsors you," he explained, "you go on leave, and they pay your full salary for the first year and half salary for any year thereafter." This policy, Tshepo acknowledged, was "wasteful" if one received a salary in conjunction with training, as he and Dr. Mokwele would be doing. But he was nonetheless unhappy to be relinquishing his status as a civil servant and with it his job security and any seniority he might accrue while abroad.

In the meantime, Tshepo continued glumly, CHAN was meant to have assisted with his relocation expenses, as the government did when it sponsored training overseas, but he and Dr. Mokwele had had to pay out of pocket for their plane tickets. Dr. Buyaga had hinted there might not be funds to reimburse them. Tshepo was despondent: The head of CHAN had been on the radio saying CHAN was sponsoring people, he told me, but where was the sponsorship? At this moment, Mma Modise approached us, greeted me and, staging a version of a popular joke in which elders exaggerate the social status of their juniors to a third party, gestured to Tshepo with exaggerated deference and said to me, "That's my boss." Shaking his head ruefully, Tshepo replied, "I'm not even my own boss."[13]

Dynasty Building

That clinical training in Botswana was supported by medical schools located within elite American research universities gave a particular emphasis to the role clinical research played vis-à-vis clinical care and those who provided that care. Participating in "good" research—that is, standardized knowledge production practices, the results of which were universal and portable—scaled the activities of elite physicians and their trainees from the needs of individual patients to findings of global import (Carpenter 2008). But despite this instance that familiarity with clinical research was foundational to good clinical practice and that, ideally, clinical practice itself constituted a form of inquiry (Feierman 2011, 192), efforts to increase clinical research at Referral Hospital, rather than informing or augmenting the clinical pedagogies directed toward "local" physicians, seemed instead to detract from them. In the course of my fieldwork, EU struck out in a number of new directions as groups of nurses, undergraduates, engineering students, business students, and even EU's President joined the throngs of medical students and residents rotating through Gaborone. The number of clinical research projects based at Referral Hospital seemed to mushroom overnight. This expansion was driven largely by Dr. Caffrey, a researcher in EUMS's Division of Infectious Disease, whose brusque and overbearing manner during his periodic visits tended to unravel whatever cordiality existed between EUMS personnel and the Referral Hospital staff among whom they worked and the civil servants whose approval and cooperation EUMS required. Unaware of articulating a self-fulfilling prophecy, Dr. Caffrey's research assistant, an EU undergraduate named Heather, told me that the "endless criticism" Dr. Caffrey encountered in Gaborone was "one of the reasons [he] doesn't spend much time here."

Amanda, an EUMS student, caustically reflected on this "dynasty building," as she called it. Amanda was spending a full year between her third and fourth years of medical school on Referral Hospital's medical wards conducting research on diagnostic techniques for tuberculosis. One of a very small number of Black American women to come to Referral Hospital under the aegis of an American partnership, she had made a concerted effort to get to know the ward's MOs and nurses and to try to see the ward from their perspectives. In mid-2008, toward the end of her year in Gaborone, she observed that as Dr. Goldberg had grown more invested in making the partnership between EUMS and Referral Hospital into a selling point for the medical school and expanding the involvement of EU beyond just EUMS, Dr. Rosen had spent less and less time teaching on the wards and more time in meetings oriented toward, on one hand, "putting out fires," that is, repairing the relationships trampled by a seemingly endless procession of unsuspecting students and imperious senior researchers alike and, on the other, expanding the scope of EU's activities in Botswana. For example, Dr. Goldberg and Dr. Rosen were concerned about finding a research institution in Botswana that could administer the US federal research grants they wanted to support the partnership. The Institutional Review Boards (IRBs) run by Referral Hospital and University of Botswana, they worried, were ill equipped to review their clinical research protocols, and they saw the ethical review process overseen by the MOH's Health Research Unit as too politicized to be acceptable to US federal agencies (and perhaps also to themselves). Research capacity, in this instance, meant the type of IRB that would satisfy the demands of a US institutional Federalwide Assurance (FWA), thereby allowing the University of Botswana to administer grants from the US National Institutes of Health (NIH) on behalf of the EUMS partnership.[14] As Dr. Rosen's priorities had shifted, Amanda continued, the other EUMS physicians had effectively abandoned morning report as a teaching venue. "The MOs and I really wonder where those guys are all the time," she added.

If efforts to establish clinical research sometimes undermined clinical pedagogies, in other instances research was simply off limits, its hierarchies aligned with and reinforcing already existing racial and geopolitical divisions of biomedical labor (Brada 2017; cf. Benton 2016; Geissler 2013; Okwaro and Geissler 2015; Street 2014; Wendland 2016). In 2003 the Superlative Clinic, with the support of pharmaceutical philanthropy and with Dr. Buyaga as the principal investigator, reorganized its clinical research program and launched a study of interrupted therapy: researchers withheld ARV medications from children who met certain criterial with regard to stable CD4 counts and suppressed viral loads and good general health, reintroducing the medications if those children could not maintain the criteria. The virtue of such a protocol if successful, the study protocol suggested, lay in its lower costs, its alleviation of the burden of daily medications, and its reduction of risks of side effects and drug resistance.[15]

The research team was divided between the US and Botswana, though half of the Gaborone team, including Dr. Buyaga, were expatriates. Mma Modise coordinated the study at the Clinic; as it unfolded, it acquired its own team of nurses, laboratory technicians, and pharmacists, many of whom, though not all, were Batswana. Dr. Amy joined the study, as did some of Squad physicians; a young East African physician was hired directly by the Clinic to work on the study. But no Motswana physician was part of the original study team or had a hand in its design.

The politics of the study, its exclusions, and the deep resentments it engendered crystalized for me at the meeting where I had chatted with Tshepo. In the morning each pediatric HIV clinic was given time to present an account of their treatment and research activities and their accomplishments for the year. The Superlative Clinic's leadership had spoken enthusiastically about the trial, inviting participants to tour the study's facilities in the afternoon. One of the Squad pediatricians whispered to me aside that when the presentations ended, staff from the Clinic and CHAN were holding a meeting about the trial. As the session broke up, I tried to follow her to this meeting, but Dr. Amy, a look of determination on her face, herded me, along with Tshepo and another MO, Dineo Mogomotsi, into a room where two child-sized manikins lay on a table crowded with what looked like disembodied doll parts. A white American woman welcomed us to a training in WHO guidelines for pediatric emergency triage, assessment, and treatment (ETAT).[16] As the trainer began discussing strategies for injecting medications into a child's bones, I looked around the room and realized that the attendees were a collection of the Clinic's nurses, pharmacy technicians, MOs, and me, with Dr. Amy—the only white person besides the trainer and me—keeping a watchful eye on us. The concentration of the Clinic's Batswana staff in a top-down, standardized training oriented toward patient care and *not* in the research meeting did not escape notice. Tumelo walked up to me, took my hand and, holding her head high, marched me out of the training, past Dr. Amy, and over to a nearby ATM where she withdrew a large sum of cash in order to repay money I had lent her, whispering gleefully as she did, "Did you *see* how Amy was staring?" Tumelo and her colleagues were well aware of how supposedly professional boundaries in the Clinic between those who did research and those who "just saw patients" mapped very readily onto racial and national ones as well as distinctions between donors and recipients. In her public display of casually handing me a thick wad of banknotes, Tumelo subverted these boundaries for the benefit of Dr. Amy who, Tumelo surmised, could not imagine a Motswana who had more to give than she had to receive.

A Living Experiment

If the expansion of clinical research could undermine EUMS's claims to bolster clinical pedagogies and, in the case of the Superlative Clinic, harden lines of exclusion, the involvement and inclusion of Batswana health professionals did not necessarily alleviate these problems. Botswana was one of the sites of a set of controversial clinical studies of pre-exposure prophylaxis (PrEP), studies that examined whether daily ARV medications could reduce rates of HIV infection in HIV-negative populations at "high risk" for exposure to HIV. Researchers with BOTUSA's HPRU began laying the foundation for the first trial in 2005, but the trial was halted before researchers began administering the study drugs as PrEP trials in other countries were suspended in the face of mass protests (J. M. Grant 2016; Peterson and Folayan 2017, 2019; Peterson et al. 2015; Singh and Mills 2005). In early 2007 HPRU staff began enrolling subjects in another PrEP trial with a slightly different study drug.[17] Around that time I began hearing rumors that the trial involved deliberately infecting Batswana with HIV. The study design included counseling in HIV prevention and free condoms for participants, but the study also assumed that *some* participants would nonetheless engage in behavior that exposed them to HIV, enabling researchers to determine whether prophylactic ARVs reduced the rate of infection. Indeed, the study design *required* that Batswana expose themselves to HIV. That the exposure of Batswana to the virus, moreover, presented an opportunity for American researchers, even offering a benefit to them, was regarded with apprehension.[18] In 2008 a senior Motswana researcher in the HPRU told me softly that a member of the *Ntlo ya Dikgosi* (House of Chiefs), which serves in an advisory capacity to Botswana's Parliament, had said to him: "We know you, and we know your family. Because of this, we will not contest the trial. If it were not you, we would not allow it to continue."[19]

At the heart of the matter lay an anxiety among Batswana that, to the extent that Americans recruited Batswana to conduct clinical research, they did this so that Batswana researchers could make their fellow citizens more available as objects of US-driven investigation. Building clinical research capacity, in other words, mirrored the offshoring of risk onto Batswana, obscuring both the liabilities that research entailed and the value it produced. The "capacity" of this Motswana researcher, from his chiefly interlocutor's point of view, lay in the researcher's potential to mitigate this threat, in his loyalty to this *kgosi* [chief] and to his fellow citizens, not his knowledge or skill as a researcher.[20] Yet EUMS personnel seemed to regard these anxieties as matters of misunderstanding to be solved by insisting on the *clinical* virtues of the PrEP trial and of clinical research in general. Around this time, Dr. Frank, giving a presentation to the Gaborone SAHIVCS on the state of research on microbicides for HIV prevention, suggested

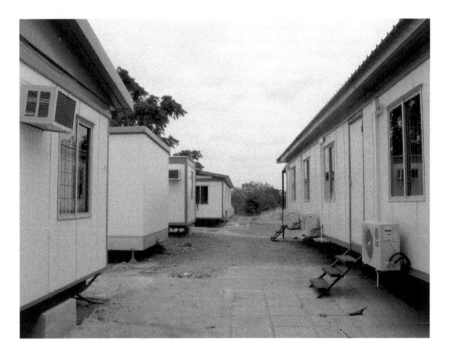

FIGURE 5.   The built environment of clinical research in Botswana (photo by the author)

that the trials should not have included counseling and condom provision because participants' efforts to avoid acquiring HIV caused the trial to take more time, as researchers waited for enough data to draw conclusions, than it would have done if participants took fewer steps to avoid infection. The MOs in the audience looked dismayed. Was it not, one MO objected, a physician's duty to do all he could to help his patients stay healthy? On what ethical grounds could one refrain from helping a person avoid infection?

This mismatch of anxiety and enthusiasm came to a head in September 2008 at the 2nd Botswana International HIV conference. Sponsored jointly by Botswana's two branches of the Southern African HIV Clinicians Society, it was, like the CHAN meeting, held at one of Gaborone's resorts and attracted a similar mix of public sector health professionals, civil servants, physicians in private practice, policymakers, representatives of local NGOs and advocacy groups, and the "partners." As the first panel began, an American microbiologist affiliated with BHP explained that because various biomedical prevention measures such as vaccines and microbicides had failed to produce substantial results, BHP was preparing to launch a multidimensional project in Mochudi, a large village about forty kilometers from Gaborone, capital of the BaKgatla kingdom and home to about forty thousand people. The aim of the study, the speaker explained, was "to screen everyone [in the village] that is willing to be screened, to then do a viral load as rapidly as possible on everyone who's positive, and to provide [ARVs] to those whose viral load is 100,000 or more, regardless of CD4, as a way of preventing or reducing transmission." The study would use genome signature tracing, making it possible to trace the virus along the paths of its transmission. It would promote other prevention programs, such as male circumcision, voluntary counseling and testing, condom use, and partner notification, in order to see which elements worked best in combination with one another. The village of Mochudi, he explained, would serve as a model for HIV prevention as researchers, using all the tools at their disposal, figured out what worked and what did not.

The ballroom filled with whispers as the speaker began taking questions. Was it a study? An intervention? Its scope was staggering: The *whole village* of Mochudi? How could a whole village give consent? Would the study, one Motswana physician asked, require Batswana to be exposed to HIV like the PrEP trial? As though reasserting the PrEP trial's legitimacy, the speaker identified the senior Motswana researcher mentioned previously, then assured the audience that the Mochudi study, by contrast, sought to identify and treat HIV-positive individuals with high viral loads but did not require anyone to be exposed to HIV. Would the study, Dr. Sibanda pressed the speaker, treat these individuals only long enough to lower their viral loads? No, the speaker assured him, the ARV treatment would be the same as that provided by the national treatment program. The speaker and another BHP researcher seated on the stage emphasized the importance of having "good scientific data" on mortality and on long-term survival in order to accurately model the epidemic and determine the relative efficacy of different prevention measures. These efforts at mollifying the audience, however, came crashing down when the third panelist, an eminent American behavioral scientist who had last visited Botswana nine years earlier, jumped into the fray: "Since we don't have very much randomized controlled evidence for what works in HIV prevention—male circumcision and prevention of mother-to-child transmission are the only two areas where we have randomized controlled trial evidence—I think it would be very helpful for those of you in Botswana to think of this country as a living experiment."

The Gift That Keeps on Taking

Can it be any surprise that at the meeting to discuss a national research agenda for Botswana, just days after the 2nd International HIV conference, Dr. Sibanda should conclude that, "We are all just specimens"? Rather than a set of pedagogies that would give "local" health practitioners and scientists the knowledge and skills to alleviate the suffering around them, global health partnerships offered them an opportunity to imagine themselves and those around them—indeed, the entire country—primarily in terms of the value they provided to outside observers, a "vessel for external investment," in Paige West's words. The Mochudi Study promised "to slow and eventually stop the spread of HIV/AIDS in one village in Botswana," true, but its "ultimate goal" was to identify "prevention interventions that could be scaled up."[21] Even as they extolled the project's virtues, its American advocates seemed to forget where they were or who was in the audience as they reminded one another that, "Africa is really quite heterogeneous" or that "If you work in HIV, Botswana is one of those places that you quote. You quote it all the time." Make no mistake: this was a global health pedagogy; it was also a pedagogy of dispossession. The American researchers in the audience might have imagined an unfolding utopia of integrated prevention, care, and training that, at least implicitly, offered opportunities for professional advancement to "locals." But some Batswana at least, understood that what was being "scaled up" was their ability to render themselves and their fellow citizens—indeed, the entire country—as points of someone else's data: a living experiment.

Accusations that American researchers were in Botswana to convert its people into data, to steal the country's value out from under its citizens' feet and give nothing in return, could seem exaggerated, the stuff of paranoid fantasy. Yet the number of American personnel in Gaborone continued to swell as every interaction seemed to acquire its own research project and Botswana's needs seemed to multiply.[22] *Makgoa a mantsi!* [so many white people], I heard more and more frequently both at the hospital and around Gaborone. My point here is not how many samples changed hands, how many papers published, how many grants acquired, or how many research assistants recruited. Instead, my objective in this chapter has been to focus on clinical capacity building as a rhetorical strategy, one that argues for and promises a particular vision of the world and guides us toward that vision. And given the powerful moral valence of capacity building in addition to its political and material stakes, it should not surprise us that the response in southeastern Botswana, with the rare exception of denunciations such as Dr. Sibanda's, consisted largely of silences, pointed questions, muttered anxieties, whispered complaints, and careful, even covert, alliances. These are not simply "weapons of the weak" (Scott 1985); as I argued in chapter 3, they reflect an enduring set of political strategies in Botswana that, while not foreclosing outright criticism, emphasize absorption, incorporation, and hierarchically inflected consensus building over overt conflict. By means of these strategies, "local" health professionals grappled with an ideological framework that obscured capacity building's extractive aspects, that is, the devil whose hand they shook in engaging US-driven clinical pedagogies.

In the meanwhile, EUMS personnel kept rotating through the medical wards as though doing so was at least mutually beneficial, if not beneficent. When I asked Lesego if she benefited from the teaching that EUMS physicians did on the ward, she replied: "Don't get me wrong; we learn a lot from them. But . . . sometimes you get a feeling that they think they're just here to do us a favor. And I think the [EUMS] students and the residents—they benefit more from the attendings than we [the MOs] do."

"What are the students getting out of it?" I asked her.

Her voice cracked with frustration as she replied, "What are they getting *out of it*? All the experience and exposure that they get, all the things they get to do that they don't get in their own country on their own patients, they do *here*, you know? And we *let* them do that."

Lesego's gesture toward collective self-recrimination illuminates thornier questions: Had Batswana, through partnerships such as that between Referral Hospital and EUMS, committed themselves to being the ground upon which Americans produced valuable knowledge and constituted themselves as experts in exchange for the resources that these partnerships provided? Had entering into these relationships given rise to a set of circumstances wherein Batswana could no longer dictate their terms? Had the act of requesting assistance, while preserving the nation from extinction, deprived Batswana of the very control of their country and its destiny they had sought to retain? *We let them do that.* These questions help us understand the relief in Mpho's voice as she, conversely, imagined a moment when Referral Hospital ceased to be a site of global health: "Pretty soon . . . [EUMS] are gonna find a greener pasture somewhere in some poor, backward African place. And that's where they'll go because they need to feel like they're saviors. Here [at Referral Hospital], we'll be like, "Yeah, you don't really *do* much." And they'll go."

As much as Mpho's fantasy reflects anxieties about global health pedagogies as a form of dispossession, it also highlights the instability of global health as a pedagogic object. It thus returns our attention to the pedagogic labor entailed in learning to save the world. What changed in Mpho's account was not Referral Hospital or southeastern Botswana or the epidemic, but the fantasies of transformation engaged by those who sought a world to save. *You don't really do much.* The seemingly mundane tedium of "just seeing patients" and helping others learn to do so remained to be done—tasks that, even as American global health partnerships imagined them as the very grounds for their existence, rarely actually seemed worth doing.

This chapter has explored how global health pedagogies themselves, not just the research they facilitate or forecast, figure as a mechanism of extraction. I focused

on the ideological frame that made it difficult for African professionals working in Botswana to pinpoint how clinical capacity building functioned as a rhetorical strategy of dispossession. Together, the scalar stances that American
trainees and practitioners and their institutions learned to assert in Botswana
were that they were "global" as opposed to merely "local" doctors, no matter the
details of their respective itineraries; that they were transformed into humane
practitioners through clinical practice in Botswana while "local" doctors engaged in the same practice remained locked in drudgery, ineptitude, and cru-
elty; and that they could understand and intervene in Botswana's epidemic in
ways unavailable to Batswana themselves. These lent themselves to a view of the
world in which clinical pedagogies could only ever flow one way and wherein
Botswana figured as an ineradicably "local" stage for Americans' "global" endeavors. Such a view obscured the extractive dimensions of capacity building,
adding to global health's erasures and forms of violence. The seeming practical
and moral straightforwardness of capacity building, like global health more generally, is a sign of powerful ideological purchase: Who wouldn't want to save
the world? What kind of person could possibly object? Yet this book has shown
it is more fruitful to approach this seeming straightforwardness as the contingent outcome of scale-making projects and the moral stances that compose them,
projects that are deeply embedded in global health pedagogies.

   This book has focused on the fantastic promise global health seems to hold
to transform its participants and those around them, assigning them roles, positions, and expectations in this vast scale-making project. Across the book's
chapters I have shown how the language of global health pedagogies offers insight into the ideological dimensions of this process as individuals wrestle over
the legibility of places, activities, materials, and people, including themselves,
as global health. Anthropologists, increasingly drawn into constituting an anthropology *of* global health, are no more immune than our interlocutors to these
dilemmas. It is to the task of undoing global health's rhetorical grip on anthropology that my concluding chapter turns.

UNDOING GLOBAL HEALTH

Somewhere between Lesego's fears and Mpho's fantasies, time marched on in Gaborone. As I was wrapping up my fieldwork in late 2008 and getting ready to leave, a senior administrator at the University of Botswana invited me to lunch. In a nearly empty restaurant, he very quietly told me that complaints that EUMS students were "practicing" on patients and that EUMS's PEPFAR-sponsored training was largely benefitting their own students had reached the ears of powerful individuals, crossing what in Botswana can be highly permeable boundaries between academic affairs, matters of state, and chiefly influence. Not long after I returned to the US, I heard rumors of a major shakeup of EUMS's programming in Botswana. EUMS had not exactly been asked to leave, I heard, but they were told such a directive was under serious consideration by the government. This was no idle threat: As I noted in chapter 3, during my fieldwork the government had told the American NGO called PACT to leave Botswana. Other US-based institutions would have gladly stepped into a breach left by EUMS's departure. EUMS knew this; the government knew they knew this. Conditions were set: Dr. Rosen was asked to step down; Dr. Caffrey was given to understand that his attitude was so intolerable as to threaten the program's continuation. The number of trainees in each rotation was markedly reduced, the rotation's academic credit was removed, and the supervision of students was shifted toward "local" staff. Efforts were made to break up American cliques by forming smaller cohorts of more advanced trainees and assigning them to district hospitals. Some things were changing.

This story illustrates the politics of capture that is featured in chapters 3 and 6, whereby Batswana tend to prioritize the reworking of social and political relationships through absorption, incorporation, and evasion over confrontation. The warning to EUMS, however indirect, had the broader effect of putting other American partnerships on notice. Yet, when I returned to Gaborone in 2012, it was clear that the thorny questions of Botswana's place vis-à-vis "the global" and EUMS's place vis-à-vis Botswana—of who was global and who was not, with all their moral and material entailments—remained unresolved. The focus of these questions, however, had shifted away from the medical wards to the University of Botswana's new School of Medicine. This shift had been presaged by the uncomfortable question one of the MOs posed, mentioned in chapter 4: whether the School would—or could—be more than "just an African medical school." But that is a story for another time.

During that trip in 2012, I met Tumelo at the Clinic on a slow day late in the afternoon. I wanted to take pictures of the facility, something I had never felt comfortable doing when it was filled with patients and families. Cartoon voices echoed through the reception area; only a few families were still waiting for pharmacists to fill their prescriptions. Many of the nurses I had known had rotated away to other posts, but a small handful, including Tumelo, had stayed on, acquiring specialized skills in pediatric HIV nursing through daily practice. Those who had stayed were supervising stable patients, doing more direct care and far less translating, supported by a small cadre of Batswana physicians who had obtained specialized training. American specialists were still present, but in smaller numbers. Dr. Mokwele had returned from his residency and was rising in the Clinic's administrative ranks. Both he and Dr. Motlhabane, who had also completed advanced training in the US, were beginning to have a hand in the Clinic's research program. Tshepo, on the other hand, had stayed in the US after completing his residency. The other MOs were taking different paths forward: One had left government service for private practice. Another was rising in the ranks of hospital administration. A third left Botswana for graduate training in public health and subsequently took a job in South Africa that combined policy and clinical practice.

As we wandered the empty hallways, Tumelo explained to me that the Clinic staff faced a new problem. Many patients were reaching their early twenties, young adulthood. Having grown attached to the Superlative Clinic, however, and accustomed to its way of doing things, they objected to being transferred to adult IDCCs. In an ironic twist, the Clinic that had fought so hard to define and retain pediatric subjects now balked at treating them once they exceeded that category. Rather than drilling young children in the disclosure catechism, the Clinic staff found themselves concerned with "transition," that is, finding ways to convince their former child-patients to trust the same national health system that Squad pediatricians had so distrusted and disparaged, an attitude they had modeled for "local" staff with varying degrees of uptake. "They [young adults] don't want to leave," Tumelo told me almost apologetically, as if she could not fault these former children for their reluctance to give up the identities they had acquired and the privileges the Clinic had extended to them, particularly in adolescence (Brada 2019; cf. Dahl 2014, 2016). To whatever extent the Clinic's patients had transformed themselves into the kinds of subjects who could reliably demonstrate their own affective self-transformations to American pediatricians, they now confronted the loss of the venue and audience for these performances.

Pedagogic practices, I have shown, offer a key perspective into global health's enactment. By means of patient pedagogies, American pediatricians in the Superlative Clinic recruited children and their families to inhabit a global epidemic, one where children were scaled relative to the medications they took, the viruses they carried, and the futures they promised or threatened. By means of patient pedagogies, pediatricians taught children to work on their emotional worlds, forestalling an apocalyptic future by reshaping words and thus affect, affect and thus behavior, scaled from child to nation to a global epidemic. Thus could the Clinic justify withholding from Karabo the very medicines that kept him alive. In the process, pediatricians worked on their own emotional worlds, constituting themselves as arbiters of truths about the epidemic while shielding themselves from the apocalyptic visions they attributed to children damaged by harmful lies and harsh revelations. Such was Dr. Natalie's insistence that she had to dispel stigma through brutal honesty. If the scaling of the epidemic and the recruitment of subjects to inhabit it were starkly visible in consulting rooms, these dynamics also exceeded those small rooms, shaping the broader management of the epidemic, making the epidemic into a thing that structured relations of known and unknowing, of expert and object of expertise, making global health something that emerged within and by means of these relations. Thus could Valerie conclude that her employees' accounts of their infections, like the government of Botswana's account of its own epidemic, were, in a word, bullshit.

Global health's coherence and its transformative promises, furthermore, rested on the labor of those who had a stake in inhabiting its fantasies. On the medical wards, EUMS physicians and trainees who would "do" global health, and who would recruit a select group of other individuals to do so likewise, struggled to differentiate themselves, their institutions, and their work spatially, temporally, and morally from something lesser, something "local," a category always already surmounted by the global. Such was Dr. James's insistence that anything less than heroic medicine was "not what I came here to do." On the medical wards EUMS physicians and trainees strove to recognize the moral transformations they hoped to undergo by virtue of encounters with suffering Africans discernible to their peers and supervisors, seeking the ratification of a "humanitarian impulse" in conjunction with broader neoliberal trends toward the incorporation of emotional expression into late-capitalist labor forms. Such was Molly's claim to feeling closer to her patients. But these labors took on strikingly different meanings in the eyes of so-called local practitioners, rendering well-intentioned Americans parochial, violent, and insensible to the pain of those for whom they claimed to care. These "local" health professionals, recruited toward a quintessentially neoliberal mode of development, wrestled with a frame of clinical capacity building that promised the improvement of selves and institutions but threatened to create the conditions for them to facilitate the offshore extraction of their own value, making Botswana, in Dr. Sibanda's words, a living experiment.

In this concluding chapter, I turn my analysis of the fantasies of transformation of self and others that animate global health back onto that argument's generative field, examining the fantasies that animate anthropology's own global health pedagogies. When I began fieldwork, the highly scripted way Tswana children learned to talk about their HIV infections was striking in its own right, a performance, I have argued, that sought to bring about a longed-for moral transformation for patients and practitioners alike. Over time, I came to see American medical students' descriptions of their encounters with Tswana patients in a similar light. For both groups, narrative emerged as a means to reflect and enact a new moral way of being in the world; the stories they told adhered to a narrow set of conventions while attesting to and precipitating an individual, even unique, affective transformation. Once I returned to the US and began teaching in an undergraduate global health program, I was struck by the generic similarity between how (a) my interlocutors in Botswana had relied on narrative to both describe and bring about longed-for moral transformation and (b) the demands my students faced to narrate a four-week summer internship as an event that had profoundly reworked their interiorities and to scale this state of having been transformed in terms of its contribution to a project of global salvation. Their stories more closely resembled EUMS students' stories in their fierce desire for an encounter with a "transformative otherness" (Urciuoli 2013, 7) than they did Tswana children's scripts. But like both sets of narratives I knew from my fieldwork, the anthropology of global health also seemed to offer an affective pedagogy, a site wherein novices could constitute themselves as subjects of true feeling (Berlant 1999, 2008b). But this tightly scripted genre was not of the students' invention. Where did it come from? What made its performance and circulation so powerful and so necessary yet so formulaic?

An analysis of global health pedagogies thus requires us to interrogate the intertwined histories and pedagogical approaches of medical anthropology and global health and to consider anthropology's role in constituting the category of global health and the moral stances it assumes and reproduces. What unites the global health pedagogies that are this book's subject and the anthropological pedagogies that have shaped it and in which it is entangled is a particularly *neoliberal* subjectivity, that is, a self that is anxious to demonstrate its own ongoing affective self-transformation. Studies of neoliberalism and health in Africa have tended to focus on political-economic phenomena, that is, structural adjustment policies, financial reforms, the privatization of once-public services, the opening of markets to a pharmaceutical industry based largely in the Global North, and the expansion of foreign investment and influence, particularly the proliferation of NGOs and other trappings of humanitarian intervention (Keshavjee 2014; Peterson 2014; Prince 2014; Whyte 2014; cf. Ferguson 2006b). To these analyses, studies of Botswana have seemed to have little to say, recapitulating the impression that Botswana, with its diamond wealth and its relatively stable system of political compromise, cannot be scaled—that it is always an outlier, never significant with regard to the continent as a whole (but see Livingston 2019). Yet I have shown that neoliberal subjects do not emerge only when patients are thrown back upon the rough mercies of market and civil society. US-driven global health produces neoliberal subjects through pedagogies of discursive self-reflexivity characteristic of the absorption into capitalism of emotional labor. Dr. James, Dr. Jackson, Adam, Molly, and others sought ways to confirm that they had undergone a moral transformation by reference to those around them, whether catechized African children or callous African practitioners. Neoliberalism is about constituting a certain kind of interiority and ratifying such performances in others. Like innocence, global health has created "a class of saviors" (Ticktin 2017, 583); what is remarkable is the extent to which their efforts are oriented toward saving themselves. These performances, I have argued, entail significant material effects; it is the cultivation of this subjectivity that grounded and gave shape to the terrors and desires bound up in the idea of Botswana as a living experiment. That these longings are grounded in a fantasy of heroic transformation in no way makes them less affectively and politically powerful.

In what follows, I briefly recapitulate the book's broader argument before turning to an intellectual genealogy that demonstrates how the anthropology of global health as a practice became a site for the cultivation of moral stances, scalar projects, and ethical subjects. I then show how global health operates as a site of moral professionalization for anthropologists as well as novice medical experts. I argue that, like biomedical trainees and their educators, medical anthropologists and those we train face a problem of anesthesis and our critical attention needs to be oriented toward the moral and affective transformations anthropologists demand of one another and our students. I end with a discussion of what this self-reflexivity offers us in an era of unfolding global pandemics.

Crisis of Expertise, Experts of Crisis

Over the past few decades, disparate approaches in medical anthropology and allied fields have crystallized in the emergent field of critical global health studies.[1] This field synthesizes three interrelated analytic approaches that have dramatically reshaped medical anthropology since the 1980s: (1) Foucauldian analyses of health interventions; (2) the primacy of suffering; and (3) the reorientation of science and technology studies toward the global South. My objective in presenting this genealogy is to illuminate the deep investment of the anthropology of global health, and medical anthropology as its key subdiscipline, in constituting the very object it seeks to analyze and using that object as a moral barometer by which medical anthropologists evaluate ourselves and others. In short, I show how for many medical anthropologists, as well as for many of our informants, global health is the ground on which we perform as ethical actors and recruit others to recognize us as such.

The overall picture presented by studies of health interventions that rely on Foucauldian concepts, particularly biopolitics, is one of suffering and political abandonment borne predominantly by the poor. These studies highlight the surveillance to which populations are subjected by both state and, increasingly, nonstate actors, such as local and transnational NGOs, churches, humanitarian organizations, and even universities based in the Global North (Biehl 2009b; Decoteau 2013; Whyte 2014; cf. Foucault 1975, 1977, 1978, 1985, 1998). These new forms of surveillance require those who live and die under these forms of governmentality to develop the capacity to articulate their conditions through "confessional technologies" that produce "an inner self . . . as a substrate that must be worked upon" (Nguyen 2009, 2010, 39–40; Robins 2006; Zigon 2011). Survival itself may be at stake in these performances: a number of scholars have shown how patients' access to care depends on their capacity to represent themselves and their conditions in contexts ranging from clinical interactions to support groups to interpersonal connections (Nguyen 2009; Robins 2006; Zigon 2011).

This emphasis on self-knowledge and self-representation, and the linking of material resources to the production and maintenance of social identities has emerged as part of a broader emphasis on how biological identities ground contemporary forms of political belonging, a phenomenon glossed as "biological citizenship" (Petryna 2002; Rose and Novas 2005; cf. Rabinow 1992; Ticktin 2006). Moreover, scholars argue, even as greater numbers of people have access to ARVs, the focus on getting "drugs into bodies" has effectively depoliticized treatment, shifting emphasis away from the broader social, political, and economic forces that drove the epidemic, and emphasizing personal responsibility for survival instead (Biehl 2009b; Kalofonos 2010; Kenworthy 2017; Marsland and Prince 2012; Parker 2000). As one high-ranking official in Botswana said in a meeting in 2008: "Those who die choose to die."

The AIDS epidemic might seem to logically demand close attention to suffering and abandonment, yet the story might readily be told the other way around. Medical anthropologists of the 1990s and early 2000s were primed to consider suffering, above all conditions, a human universal and the object par excellence of anthropological analysis. First, as the discipline grappled in the later decades of the Cold War with what might serve as its object of analysis in the face of both shifting geopolitics on the ground and postcolonial critiques, medical anthropologists rejected earlier trends that had framed healing as the enactment of fixed traditions within closed systems, highlighting instead the historical contingency of both bodies and healing practices (Cohen 2012, 85). Second, medical anthropologists engaged a strand of phenomenological philosophy that located the site of ethics and politics in the individual and a strand of pragmatism that prioritized moral interpersonal relations and actions above a totalizing system of ethics. These engagements intersected with and reshaped so-called critical medical anthropology, a more explicitly Marxist approach that brought a political economic analysis of illness and disease to bear on their amelioration (Baer, Singer, and Johnsen 1986; Scheper-Hughes 1990; Singer 1989; Singer and Baer 1995). The result was a radical reorientation from "an epistemology and methodology of analytic distance and critical comparison" (Ticktin 2014, 246) to an all-out rejection of cultural relativism as moral relativism, an assertion of the "primacy of the ethical" (Scheper-Hughes 1995), and a reframing of medical anthropology centered squarely on the suffering body. The focus on cross-cultural difference, however problematic, that had driven previous generations of scholars was incorporated into this frame as the "enculturation of suffering" (Nguyen and Peschard 2003, 454) as suffering emerged as the predominant anthropological object.

The result was a subdiscipline reframed as an explicitly ethical project. Rather than rejecting the medicalization of culture, anthropologists instead attacked the deployment of culture as an alibi for structural violence (Farmer 1992, 1996; Scheper-Hughes 1993; cf. Cohen 2012). Medical anthropology emerged as a technique for illuminating parts of the world most in need of succor, exposing the "everyday violence" and "social suffering" of the poor, countering arguments justifying their abandonment and advocating practical solutions framed as the humane expansion of biomedical technologies and services. Portraits of the "suffering slot" highlighted the social, historical, political, and economic forces that gave rise to particular forms of suffering, framing them in terms of a common humanity shared by sufferer, ethnographer, and reader, letting us "feel in our bones the vulnerability we as human beings all share" (Robbins 2013, 455; cf. Ortner 2016; Ticktin 2017).[2] Capturing an urgency that, Lawrence Cohen observes, has long been a feature of medical anthropology's awkward relationship with both biomedicine and international development, this approach "both contracts into the immediate present of masses or persons who will suffer and die" and expands into "the infinite time of the moral," thus recasting the "moral value" of medical anthropology and its practitioners in terms of a capacity to recognize and respond to this suffering (2012, 89; cf. Herrick 2017).

At roughly the same time and in parallel with the transformations outlined previously, anthropologist and historians responded to a range of postcolonial critiques by shifting the geographical focus of science and technology studies to the global South, emphasizing how the subjects of European colonies had long been participatory in scientific and biomedical knowledge production, not merely its objects or beneficiaries (D. Arnold 1993; Tilley 2011; Vaughan 1991; cf. Harding 2008). This scholarship emphasized the ways colonialism and postwar geopolitics have enduringly shaped the politics of treatment in the contemporary moment, making some conditions and the concepts that undergird them visible and valuable through their transnational circulation while immobilizing others or rendering them imperceptible (Adams 2002; W. Anderson 2008; Langwick 2011; Pigg 2001; Street 2014). In the wake of neoliberal policies that sought to open markets and free capital (if not bodies) for movement, a focus on "postcolonial technoscience" (W. Anderson 2002) highlighted processes of knowledge production and concomitant transformations in how patients, conditions, and treatments were recognized and brought together (Ong and Collier 2005), asking what counts as evidence, who is authorized to produce it, and how value accrues in the process (Adams 2005; Benton 2012; Biruk 2012; Craig 2011; Erikson 2012; Hayden 2003; Sangaramoorthy 2012; Sangaramoorthy and Benton 2012). Indeed, the value of bodies made available in new ways for scientific knowledge production has emerged as a dominant theme, driving studies on the rapid expansion of clinical research in both postcolonial and postsocialist contexts (Abadie 2010; S. Epstein 2008; J. M. Grant 2016; Montoya 2011; Petryna 2009; Rajan

2006), drawing attention to the ethical as well as the political-economic dimensions of scientific and biomedical practice and the production of expertise (Crane 2010b; Geissler 2013, 2015; Geissler and Molyneux 2011; Nguyen 2005; Sullivan 2016, 2018; Wendland 2010, 2012b).

Critical global health weaves together these strands, that is, it combines an interest in the lived experience of health interventions as biopolitical and disciplinary phenomena with questions about how individuals and communities become not simply targets of intervention but sites for the creation of scientific knowledge and value, all framed by a broader concern with universal human suffering.[3] Critical of approaches that assume a unidirectional and benevolent transfer of knowledge and expertise, this approach pushes back against the dominance of biomedical sciences in both the conceptual and programmatic aspects of global health. At the same time, sensitive to critiques that an overwhelming focus on suffering has "situated whole communities within a discourse of victimization" (Panter-Brick, Eggerman, and Tomlinson 2014, 439; cf. Butt 2002b), proponents aim to "people" global health (Biehl and Petryna 2013, 2014), arguing that the observations of supposed beneficiaries with regard to the interventions that target them are as valuable as those of the experts who design and implement these interventions (Biehl 2016; Briggs and Mantini-Briggs 2003, 2016). Anthropologists who position themselves within the emerging field of critical global health studies approach ethnography as a strategic means of "getting to the core issues of how evidence is produced, and for whom, and what claims about efficacy it serves" (Adams 2016c, 191).[4] It explicitly engages the ultimately practical question of "what kinds of interventions are actually workable, desirable, or ethical" (Biehl 2016, 131),[5] and prizes engagement, that is, self-reflexivity with regard to the anthropologist's ethical position vis-à-vis her interlocutors and the effects of anthropological research and representations on the lives of their interlocutors. In this sense, critical global health is line with the turn toward suffering outlined earlier: the anthropologist's professional credibility lies in her ability to perform as an ethical actor.

The Problem of Anesthesis in the Anthropology of Global Health

One afternoon in 2007 I had lunch with Michael, an EUMS student who was spending a full year between his third and fourth years of medical school conducting research at BOTUSA. Michael spent most of his days at BOTUSA's offices, and BOTUSA had provided him with a small apartment. Like Amanda, the student who, as mentioned in chapter 6, criticized Dr. Goldberg and Dr. Rosen's "dynasty building," Michael was somewhat distanced from the activities of his fellow students on the medical wards and from their evening and weekend recreation and had different opportunities to participate in Gaborone's networks of health professionals. As we discussed the tensions on the medical ward, EUMS's increasingly negative reputation at Referral Hospital, and the rumors circulating in Gaborone that patients' families had discovered, to their dismay, that American students were "practicing" on their loved ones, Michael reminded me of an article in a recent issue of EU's alumnae magazine detailing EUMS's activities at Referral Hospital. A photograph accompanying the article featured two white-coated EUMS trainees beaming shyly at the camera across a hospital bed in which rested a thin, young African man, who gazed at the camera with an expression that suggested, at best, apprehension. Disgusted, Michael complained, "It looks like Abu Ghraib."[6]

Within an ideological framework shaped by a connoisseurship of suffering, claims to moral transformation are subject to fractal recursion (Gal 2002; Irvine and Gal 2000) with regard to their stances they engender. In other words, if the sign of moral transformation was the capacity to authoritatively claim moral transformation in oneself and in others, then one could solidify one's position as an audience of and potential participant in such transformations by participating in their ratification, including questioning their authenticity. Rather than breaking the ideological framework, then, questions regarding the sincerity of a given transformation reinforced it by seeming to transcend it (cf. Silverstein 2004, 644). If EUMS personnel employed the register of heroic American medicine in efforts to humanize themselves and one another through their recognition of a particularly African suffering, Michael's statement engaged in a one-upmanship of this humanization by establishing a critical stance toward his colleagues' efforts. In a similar manner, an American student working in a pediatric nutritional rehabilitation ward in Malawi who described her activity as "feeding starving children" (Wendland 2012b, 117) could counter accusations of insincerity by demonstrating her awareness of the stereotype she threatened to fulfill without actually undermining the stereotype's capacity to index medical heroism. Indeed, performing this kind of multiply-voiced self-awareness could actually enhance her connoisseurship within this ideological framework.

What, then, is the project of critique in global health? In chapter 5, I argued that in American regimes of expert formation, novices' ethical formation is imperiled when their objects of expertise fail to engender the affective and ethical dispositions expert practice demands. The problem of anesthesis, a fear that novice experts lack the moral dispositions that ought to guide the deployment of that expertise as a consequence of their newly acquired expertise, and its consequent anxieties engender a search for a pedagogical object that precipitates a morally transformative encounter. Heroic American biomedicine, I showed, partakes in a broader sentimental American politics that recasts political relationships in terms of a shared universal suffering and relocates the site of injustice and its amelioration to intimate domains (Berlant 2008a). Compassion stands in for social justice; a generic suffering humanity obviates the need for political details; the presumed universality of pain underwrites both its imaginative availability to American trainees and the possibility of a universally recognizable and transformative empathetic response.

If the sort of critical work that Michael and I engaged in seems disquietingly familiar to medical anthropologists, it is because it is echoed in our own modes of professionalization. Indeed, American biomedical personnel's fear of their own anesthesis is articulated in and, arguably, has been amplified by medical anthropologists' own commitment to suffering as a universal human experience and to the proper perception, depiction, and amelioration of that suffering, particularly as the two fields have become further entwined both institutionally and through a shared "chain of mimetic virtue" (Scherz 2013, 112; cf. Rabinow 2003).[7] In a powerfully influential essay that, in hindsight, reflects deep uncertainties about anthropology's object of analysis in a post-Cold War, postcolonial world as well as anxieties about new forms of mass mediation, Arthur and Joan Kleinman—the former a leading physician-anthropologist—bemoaned the deadening effects of representations of violence on the viewer:

> There is too much to see, and there appears to be too much to do anything about. Thus, our epoch's dominating sense that complex problems can be neither understood nor fixed works with the massive globalization of images of suffering to produce moral fatigue, exhaustion of empathy, and political despair (1996, 9).

Rather than advocate disengagement, however, the authors called for a highly specific form of engagement, one that turns a diagnostic gaze on "the cultural processes through which the global regime of disordered capitalism alters the connections between collective experience and subjectivity, so that moral sensibility, for example, diminishes or becomes something frighteningly different: promiscuous, gratuitous, unhinged from responsibility and action" (1996, 18).

The conundrum is this: How can novice anthropologists and physicians bear witness to suffering without risking its deadening effects? How can we demonstrate that our moral sensibility remains undamaged? Yet how can we demonstrate that we do, in fact, possess an intact moral sensibility *except* by purposefully encountering suffering as such and responding with "responsibility and action," making ourselves professionally recognizable to ourselves and our colleagues as "responsive, reflexive, and morally committed" (Scheper-Hughes 1995, 419)?

What I am tracing, in other words, is how anxieties about anesthesis have shaped anthropological registers as well as biomedical ones, that is, the conventionalization and professionalization of a mode of self-reflexivity specifically oriented toward reflecting the ethnographer's moral sensibility, her capacity to authoritatively and nonviolently bear witness to suffering. Writing about the moral and political economies of metrics in global health, Vincanne Adams highlights the "affective power" of stories and their symbiotic relationship with the seeming objectivity of numbers: "By being ostensibly excluded from the regimes of truth making that are tied to mathematic figuring," she continues, "stories are left to carry a nonneutral moral certainty" that quantitative forms of evidence disavow "but are, in fact, haunted by as a spectral display that they need" (2016a, 48). But stories are not the only thing that can index this moral certainty: In anthropological accounts of suffering, data become indexical not only of the circumstances of their production (that is, a claim, however provisional, to represent an empirical reality) but of the moral subjectivity of the ethnographer who collected them. In this chain of mimetic virtue, life stories of suffering individuals become indexical icons—that is, simultaneously diagrams and consequences—of a moral engagement with an informant (now an interlocutor); anthropologists' accounts of others' suffering point back to the anthropologists' capacity to recognize that suffering, an affirmation of humanity that generates a cascade of moral transformation (cf. Silverstein 2003, 194). To borrow an example from Joel Robbins (2013, 455–56): If, as Arthur Kleinman claims, João Biehl's *Vita: Life in a Zone of Social Abandonment* (2005), a book of excruciating detail focused on a single woman's affliction, affirms that woman's humanity and if, as Robbins argues, the book calls on readers in turn to reaffirm this humanity, then the book also calls on readers to affirm *in the ethnographer* the capacity to recognize and be transformed by that humanity even in the midst of suffering. And it does so through a register of "gut feeling" and "human contact" (Biehl 2005, 11), culminating in a "finely-tuned aesthetic of misery" (Csordas 2007) that beatifies both the ethnographer who renders it and the reader who is moved by it, shielding both from accusations of voyeurism, let alone violence, of the kind that troubled the discipline of anthropology in the late Cold War.[8] The register of having overcome anesthesis is the site wherein we anthropologists ratify one another's moral transformations.

Moral transformation and the anxieties entailed in its enactment are thus not limited to our interlocutors. These modes of self-assessment and self-monitoring have become heavily entrenched at multiple forms and dimensions in pedagogical institutions, including colleges and universities (Fraser and Taylor 2016; Hyatt, Shear, and Wright 2015; Shore and Wright 2000; Urciuoli 2010, 2018). Tracing parallel transformations in biomedical education and graduate training in anthropology across the second half of the twentieth and early twenty-first century, Janelle Taylor observes that, in line with broader neoliberal trends, both disciplines have come to approach "education and research . . . as something to be carefully planned, controlled, policed, documented, and accounted for" (2014, 529). Across fields, she argues, "working with people as a means of learning how to work with people . . . is increasingly understood to be inherently risky," a development that, on one hand, signals recognition of the inequalities undergirding research and the forms of abuse these inequalities foster, and on the other, places the onus on novices to demonstrate the extent to which the activities they undertake as part of their training are beneficent, that they have moral and practical value beyond their pedagogical import (530). The moral stances global health assumes and generates and the transformations it promises, then, are positions that medical anthropologists have helped make and in which they are deeply implicated—not only through a disciplinary focus on suffering and structural violence but also by the forms of professionalization that have emerged in the past two decades demanding that we perform our capacity to care as an alibi for the value of our work. Confessional technologies, in short, are not only for patients; they are modeled by physicians and anthropologists and taken up by trainees of both disciplines as the sign that they themselves are engaged in this project of constituting a moral self and building a new moral biomedicine and a new moral anthropology.[9]

All this helps us see why, despite their commitment to reflexivity and engagement, medical anthropologists tend to write from within global health, or "in and of global health" (Biruk 2018; McKay 2018, 197) inasmuch as we formulate projects intended to dovetail with global health's ideals, if not its execution, and our professionalization rests on the articulation of our engagement with this moral project. Even as it resists precise definition, global health calls on anthropologists to orient ourselves ethically, historically, institutionally; even its most clinical iterations implicate and powerfully interpellate anthropology as a discipline. Moral transformation is at stake for the child who learned to narrate her HIV infection in a manner that, in the eyes of an American pediatrician, ensured not only her survival but the manageability of the epidemic. It is at stake for Molly who, in chapter 5, narrated her needlestick injury and subsequent exposure to HIV as a source of pleasurable proximity to her patients, framing suffering Batswana as well as future patients as beneficiaries of her newly embodied compassion. But it is also at stake in the near-obligatory convention in medical anthropology for ethnographers to cast ourselves as imbued through our professional formation with a special capacity to recognize and intervene in evil—lest we be hailed as kin to the neutral angels of Dante's Inferno, damned for refusing to take sides.

Michael read the scene in the photograph as an implicit claim to moral transformation by virtue of an encounter with a suffering patient, and reframed it as torture. This move entailed a claim to perceive the difference between the two. In this interaction, Michael called on me to engage in a process of mutual ratification as the kinds of people who could read the violent encounter behind the seeming moral transformation. In contrast to Dr. Jackson, who claimed for himself the capacity to discern and be moved by real death in Botswana when local doctors could not, Michael claimed for himself, and recruited me to mutually ratify, the capacity to discern unacknowledged violence, even torture, where other EUMS personnel saw only dedication, even sacrifice. It should surprise no one that Molly, too, recruited me to this process of ratification. I was a trainee medical anthropologist, someone who presumably had a stake in undergoing, claiming, and ratifying in others encounters with transformative otherness. It was my job to find and engage "raw forms of connectedness" (Biehl and McKay 2012, 1212), to collect "stories of transformation" (Biehl 2013, 592) that are axiomatically accounts of suffering and abandonment whose depiction of "local moral worlds" would call on readers to recognize "what really matters" (Kleinman 1992, 2006) in my account, thereby affirming their sentimental transformations alongside my own. A desire to confirm our moral sensibility and a fear of revealing our own anesthesis were aspects of professionalization Molly, Michael, and I shared. At the intersection of biomedicine and anthropology, we engaged in a mutually recognizable ritual interaction that relied on qualities of our patients/informants to confirm our already-present sensibilities, that relied on distinctive registers to distinguish our ratification of those sensibilities and to differentiate ourselves from the uninitiated, and that made us into neoliberal workers capable of performing, teaching, and evaluating realness and closeness in biomedicine and anthropology. This is how global health did *us*. The extent to which we internalized it—that is, whether we actually care—is simultaneously the heart of the matter and missing the point entirely (Urciuoli 2008).

The task that remains, then, is to analyze what is at stake in global health for anthropologists as well as for our interlocutors. If those engaged in critical global health studies want to "do" global health better, my objective is different: In this book I have tried to undo global health, to short-circuit its moral and professional claims long enough to see what it looks like when I am no longer tethered to it by the obligation to offer an account of suffering that confirms my own capacity to recognize that suffering. I have focused instead on how my interlocutors learned to enact a moral transformation in terms of global health for themselves, for one another, for me, and as I illustrated previously, sometimes with me. But I have consciously tried *not* to attempt such a transformation in the act of narration. This is not to disavow suffering nor to claim a view from nowhere, but to refuse the redemptive narratives offered by both global health *and* the anthropology of global health: "To wish for a redemptive narrative," argues Beth Povinelli, ". . . is to wish that social experiments fulfill rather than upset given conditions, that they emerge in a form that given conditions recognize as good" (2006, 25).[10] In contrast to the dominant generic conventions of contemporary medical anthropology, this book does not offer the consolation of a shared vulnerability; indeed, it has striven not to. Instead, it invites medical anthropologists to reconsider the ground beneath our own feet, that is, our relationship both to global health and to our own pedagogies.

Undoing Global Health

Global health, I have argued, is a stance, a position, an assertion. Rather than a category of institutions or orientations waiting to be filled more or less successfully, it is an argument that must be made and renewed as its contingencies become apparent from one instance to the next. What makes global health *global* is the outcome of a pragmatics of scale; what makes global health useful is its capacity to transform people, institutions, relationships by scaling them, by creating or asserting moral positions relative one to the other. Global health is iterative; it is contingent. It must be asserted and it can be refused or dismantled. From consultation rooms to international funding agencies, I have shown how individuals and institutions grappled with the labor that the enactment of global health demands. Global health is, in short, performative, a means of calling a certain form of social action into being and ratifying it with all its entailments and subject positions. No wonder it is so frequently framed as something you "do" (Pigg 2013; cf. Carr 2010a). But it is no less powerful for all this. If anything, the reverse is true.

Thinking about global health as performative calls on anthropologists to reconsider our approaches to language. Too often, anthropologists of global health take language as the external expression of the internal truth of suffering, a suffering we are, I have argued, professionally predisposed to hear. This type of listening, an earnest performance of a highly particular form of sincerity, tells us as much about the linguistic ideologies that shape the anthropology of global health as it does about the lived experience of global health itself. To give up on this performance is to run the risk of looking like one is at least failing to recognize, even actively refusing to acknowledge, the suffering that promises twenty-first century anthropologists a moral redemption of their very own. An analysis of the pedagogical languages of global health, by contrast, orients us toward the power of words to do things beyond articulate inner truths without accusing our interlocutors—or ourselves—of bad faith in the process. Scale and stance, both necessary elements of any anthropological investigation, can help us diversify our analytic approaches toward our interlocutors' words without claiming an "outside"—in the sense of a position of disinterest—on which to stand.

The languages of neoliberal pedagogy at the heart of global health thus draw our attention back to anthropology's own pedagogic strategies. This book raises questions about the role anthropologists play not just in determining what counts as global health but in enacting and validating moral stances that limit the scope of criticism of global health and the forms of accountability to which institutions and practitioners can be held. HIV-positive children in Botswana are not the only ones who learn scripted ways of talking; American physicians and medical trainees and anthropologists alike describe emotional encounters with suffering others in ways that emphasize redemptive affective and moral transformations. For all three groups, narratives are imagined to both usher in and reflect a new moral way of being in the world. Rather than question their sincerity, however, our analytic focus should be on the conventionalization of self-reflexivity, the genres by which we appear and are recognized as ethical actors, moral subjects, valued interlocutors, authoritative scholars. Other anthropologists of global health have called on the discipline to be mindful of the capacity for our ethnographic representations to recapitulate the very images of suffering Africans we critique (McKay 2018), and to recognize that our research world is simply one among many and that we, like the global health professionals we observe, are constituted through our work (Biruk 2018). This book points toward the urgent need for a different mode of self-reflexivity, one that takes account of the stances we call on ourselves and our students to occupy by means of our own pedagogies. Its aspirations toward critique notwithstanding, critical global health has become a key site for the forging of a kind of moral insulation, a conjunction of subject-position and genre that requires an encounter with suffering in order to be redeemed by it insofar as the encounter gives rise to the type of story anthropologists have come to expect of themselves, the type of story we seek as consolation and reassurance. The stories that Molly and Michael told me and the roles to which they recruited me are as much products of American medical anthropology as they are of American biomedicine.

But what virtue is there in undoing global health at such an unsettled and unsettling time? Isn't saving the world exactly what we, anthropologists and physicians, need to learn—now more than ever? The danger lies in this: the more troubled the times, the more appealing uncritical salvific projects become, and the more tempting the deceptive appeal of an easy virtuousness. European missionaries arrived in southern Africa spurred by the abolition movement and thereby lay the ground, however inadvertently, for Africans' absorption into capitalist labor and colonial rule (J. Comaroff and J. L. Comaroff 1991; J. L. Comaroff and J. Comaroff 1997a). Despair and resentment born of thwarted righteousness, as Dr. James illustrated in chapter 4, do not necessarily lend themselves to the best medical practice, nor do they excuse the mistakes and even acts of violence that ensue. Moreover, the darkness of the past few years has only emphasized the enduring power of global health as a fantastical site of American redemption, as recent calls for America to "vaccinate the world" illustrate.[11] Even as I approached the completion of this book, a student in my class on global health told me that, upon visiting a medical school to which she had been accepted and asking about international rotations, a third-year medical student had assured her, "The best thing about it is that you know more than anyone there." That medical student might just as well have been the EUMS student who, a decade earlier, gushed at me that Botswana, as a zone of beneficent medical intervention, was "virgin territory"—a term that recalled nineteenth-century European images of an abject and bloodied Africa while also erasing nearly two centuries of the entanglement of Christianity, colonialism, capitalism, and medicine. Some things, not least among them an all-too-familiar rhetoric of dispossession, do not seem to have changed at all.

Notes

INTRODUCTION

1. Passed in 2003, PEPFAR originally pledged US$15 billion to fifteen focus countries, twelve of which are located in sub-Saharan Africa. Botswana is one of these focus countries. ARVs are most effective in combinations of drugs that interrupt the life cycle of the virus in different ways. This combination of medications, called highly active antiretroviral therapy (HAART), emerged as the standard of care in North America and Europe in the mid-1990s (Nguyen 2010, chap. 4).

2. Government of Botswana 2006; Joint United Nations Programme on HIV/AIDS (UNAIDS) 2004. Botswana's epidemic is typical of the region: In 2007 southern Africa accounted for nearly one-third of all new HIV infections and AIDS deaths worldwide (UNAIDS 2007).

3. *Batswana* (sing. *Motswana*) is a complex term, denoting citizens of Botswana but also indicating members of the Tswana *merafe* (kingdoms) that predated the arrival of European missionaries in the early nineteenth century, but whose constitution and recognition is also bound up in the colonial encounter (J. Comaroff and J. L. Comaroff 1991; Gulbrandsen 2012).

4. Throughout this book I follow the majority of my interlocutors by referring to individuals from and institutions based primarily in the United States as *American*. That said, *American*, like all identifications, is subject to fractal recursion (Gal 2002): not all the individuals I describe as *American* may recognize themselves as such in all instances. My use of the term gestures at a set of cultural, political, and institutional norms, but does not presume a bounded or fixed category.

5. Paul Farmer quoted in Kidder 2003, 293.

6. See also a special issue of *Medicine Anthropology Theory* 5 no. 2 (2018) edited by Nora Kenworthy, Lynn M. Thomas, Johanna Crane.

7. Some argue that anthropological research on global health only recapitulates global health's own logics and priorities, namely, a reduction of health and healing to biomedicine and a refusal to look beyond biomedicine's own spaces (Herrick 2017; Neely and Nading 2017; Scherz 2018).

8. I refer to these transformations as moral rather than ethical for two reasons. First, "ethics" in biomedicine and biomedical education tends to suggest a discursive domain that biomedicine already claims for itself but that partially overlaps at best with what scholars of self-cultivation, following Foucault, consider the ethical (e.g., Mahmood 2004; Zigon 2011; see Foucault 1978, 1998). In scholarship on biomedical education that does not take up this line of Foucauldian argument, "moral" suggests something cultivated yet implicit or embodied rather than a set of abstract, generalizable precepts (Taylor 2011). Second, ethnographers of Botswana tend to follow T. O. Beidelman (1993) when discussing, in contrast to abstract, generalizable precepts, the cultivation of sensibilities or dispositions Foucauldian scholars might consider the stuff of ethics, for example, the "moral imagination" (Livingston 2005); "moral passion" (Klaits 2010); and "moral intimacies of care" (Livingston 2012; cf. 2008).

9. I offer preliminary thoughts on why this is the case in Brada 2013. Certainly, there are scholars whose work bridges linguistic and medical anthropology (e.g., Arnold

2020; Black 2019; Briggs and Mantini-Briggs 2003; 2016; Buchbinder 2015; Carr 2010b; Faudree 2015; 2020), but *analytic* synergy between the two subdisciplines remains tenuous at best (Briggs and Faudree 2016). To the extent that medical anthropologists engage language, they often use the tools of science and technology studies (STS); see, for example, *Sociological Review* 68, no. 2 (2020). Anna Weichselbraun observes that, in contrast to STS approaches, scholarship informed by Peircean semiotics focuses on how social actors' assumptions about the world both prefigure meaningful social action and are produced by it (2019, 507), foregrounding how actors construe signs. Such an orientation is foundational to my analysis of how one learns to "do" global health.

10. Throughout the book the uppercase *Clinic* refers specifically to the Superlative Clinic. "Superlative Clinic" is a pseudonym.

11. Sometimes called simply the medical wards, the term *adult* differentiated them from the pediatric medical ward. EUMS's rotation was at this time limited to EUMS students, who were supervised and assessed by EUMS instructors. In this, it differed from the majority of international medical electives, which are facilitated by voluntary placement organizations; see Sullivan 2016; 2018; cf. Hanson, Harms, and Plamondon 2011.

12. In much of the British Commonwealth physicians begin their training directly after secondary school, completing two to three years of basic science education followed by two to three years of clinical training. In Botswana, holders of such degrees (e.g., MBBS) serve one-year internships, after which they qualify as medical officers. Plans for a medical school in Botswana began in the mid-1990s, but the University of Botswana School of Medicine began only in 2009, graduating its first class in 2015. A residency offers graduates of medical school training in specialized fields of medicine, such as internal medicine, pediatrics, and surgery.

13. Like the Superlative Clinic, Referral Hospital and EUMS are pseudonyms; all other institutions existed as named. With the exception of my research assistant, Patrick, the names of my interlocutors have been changed regardless of institutional affiliation. These pseudonyms are less an attempt at impeachable anonymity than a veneer of dissimulation that, in the ideal, helps the reader stay more invested in the book's narrative than in probing beneath its aliases.

14. Mark Nichter traces an early appearance of the term to a 1997 publication by the US Institute of Medicine, which defined global health as "health problems, issues, and concerns that transcend national boundaries, may be influenced by circumstances or experiences in other countries, and are best addressed by cooperative actions and solutions" (2018). Commentators tend to approach the term heuristically, focusing, for example, on "the transfer of knowledge and resources from Global North to Global South" and "efforts to act on and reduce the global burden of disease" (Herrick 2016, 674). Some scholars attempt to distinguish it from colonial-era tropical medicine and postwar international health (e.g., King 2002; Koplan et al. 2009); others emphasize continuities among these phenomena (Brown and Bell 2008).

15. Attempts to define global health, as many do, as a field, a discipline (Farmer et al. 2013), or "an area of research and practice" (Janes, and Corbett 2009, 169), subject to an "architecture" (Fidler 2007), or coalescing around a set of "compulsions" (Herrick 2016, 674) are generally overwhelmed in their efforts to catalogue its constituent parts.

16. Lakoff distinguishes between regimes of global health that organize themselves around global health security and those that organize themselves around humanitarian biomedicine, arguing that the latter "could be seen as offering a philanthropic palliative to nation-states lacking public health infrastructure in exchange for the right of international health organizations to monitor their populations for outbreaks that might threaten wealthy nations" (2010, 75). On global health's supposed anarchic qualities, see J. Biehl 2016; J. Biehl and Petryna 2014; Fidler 2008.

17. These include Kanye Seventh Day Adventist Hospital, which opened in 1922; Deborah Retief Memorial Hospital in Mochudi, which opened in 1932 and was supported by the Dutch Reformed Church mission among the BaKgatla baga Kgafela; Scottish Livingstone Hospital in Molepolole, which opened in 1933 and was financed by the United Free Church of Scotland; and Bamalete Lutheran Hospital (BLH) in Ramotswa, which opened in 1934. These hospitals now fall under the purview of Botswana's Ministry of Health, though BLH and Kanye SDA Hospital retain their commitments to their respective medical missions.

18. On the antecedents of the primary healthcare movement in the 1970s, its undoing, and its legacy, see Cueto 2004; Packard 2016.

19. On the relationship of Christian missionization in southern Africa to the slave trade (J. Comaroff and J. L. Comaroff 1991, chap. 3); on the productive tensions between healing bodies and saving souls (J. L. Comaroff and J. Comaroff 1997a, chap. 7; Vaughan 1991); on US postwar foreign policy vis-à-vis development (Escobar 1995; Ferguson 1990; Kelly and Kaplan 2001; Packard 1997). Sam Dubal persuasively argued that this abjectness, framed in terms of ethics rather than politics, preempted relations of political and social solidarity, diverting attention away from "enemies" and toward "structural violence" (Dubal 2012; cf. Birn and Brown 2013, 305–6; cf. Dubal 2018, 9–13). For an early attempt to grabble with this depoliticized abjectness, see Butt 2002b and responses (Butt 2002a; Irwin et al. 2002). I take up the disciplinary implications of these arguments for anthropology in the conclusion.

20. Bush made this comment in a press conference with then Prime Minister of Sweden Göran Persson in Göteborg, on June 14, 2001 (Bruni 2001).

21. President Donald Trump used this epithet in a meeting with members of Congress at the White House on January 11, 2018 (Davis, Stolberg, and Kaplan 2018).

22. This is not to suggest the eschatological and development frames cannot overlap or that they are no longer relevant; indeed, both were central, for example, to Bush's vision of PEPFAR. But they are not the primary frameworks on which global health's coherence depends.

23. The turn of the millennium saw the establishment of the Global Fund for AIDS, Tuberculosis and Malaria, the involvement of development institutions such as the World Bank and philanthropic foundations such as the Bill and Melinda Gates Foundation, and the World Health Organization's "3 by 5" program, as well as the US government's involvement in HIV/AIDS programming in sub-Saharan Africa via PEPFAR, and the explosion of global health activities in American universities (Crane 2010a; Kenworthy 2017; McGoey 2015; Rees 2014).

24. Elizabeth Harrison refers to it as "one of the most over-used and under-scrutinized words in the development lexicon" (2002, 589; Barnes, Brown, and Harman 2016; cf. Taylor 2018).

25. The two drugs were Crixivan and Stocrin. Their value is subject to debate: One physician who had treated HIV/AIDS in Botswana for more than a decade dismissed their utility, insisting that their benefits were outweighed by factors such as side effects and dosing difficulties. In fact, only Stocrin was part of Botswana's first-line regimen in 2006–2008. It was known to cause sleep disturbances, and many physicians preferred to prescribe other medications.

26. See, for example, Marseille, Hofmann, and Kahn 2002. The name, one American administrator told me in 2004, reflected the idea that if public treatment succeeded in Botswana, "it could be done anywhere." Elise Carpenter's doctoral thesis provides an important account of ACHAP and its early involvement with the treatment program (2008).

27. Fewer people than expected had voluntarily enrolled in the program, leading to a "bottleneck" wherein patients enrolled in the program at advanced stages the disease,

requiring a greater expenditure of resources and producing higher failure rates (CHGA 2004; Darkoh 2004). Program administrators expected routine testing, introduced in January 2006, to correct this problem, but human rights activists feared that patients were reluctant to question health professionals and would receive inadequate information (IRIN 2006; cf. Amon 2013).

28. An enrolled individual has not necessarily begun taking ARVs. Instead, they are expected to undergo regular clinical examinations and laboratory tests that should reveal when they qualify for (i.e., are sick enough to begin) treatment. They may also receive other services, such as counseling and nutritional support.

29. See Dreesch et al. 2007; AFA administers BPOMAS as well as Pula Medical Aid Fund, a private corporate scheme.

30. Botswana's Government has directly recruited health professionals, including pharmacists and pathologists as well as physicians, from countries such as Nigeria and India.

31. On South Africa (J. Comaroff 2007; Decoteau 2013); on Botswana's ARV program as a tool of state legitimation (Gulbrandsen 2012).

32. Gulbrandsen (2012) demonstrates the durability of redistribution as the performance of political legitimacy across Botswana's precolonial, colonial, and postcolonial eras; Livingston (2012) offers an account of this expectation of redistribution in healthcare settings.

33. The population of the Johannesburg metropolitan area neared 4 million in 2007; Harare, the capital of Zimbabwe, which borders Botswana to the east, was estimated at 2.8 million in 2006.

34. "Undeveloped" should not imply stasis: the discovery of mineral deposits in northern South Africa placed new value on the laboring bodies of African men. Taxation and other colonial interventions, a demand for firearms and other manufactured goods, and the effects of drought and rinderpest drove many Tswana in the Protectorate to join the underclass of industrial, menial, and domestic workers to the south (Morapedi 1999; Shillington 1985). They returned bearing broken and diseased bodies in addition to wages, thereby establishing an enduring regional circulation of bodies, capital, and pathogens (Livingston 2005; Packard 1989).

35. Botswana's status as a "miracle" has been a topic of scholarship since at least the mid-1980s. My objective is not to reinforce this narrative but to complicate Botswana's depiction as an uncomplicated success while also troubling the assumption that African public health services are necessarily weak and dependent on external support.

36. Staff grumbled that the hospital was never meant to do both and that Gaborone needed its own district hospital, freeing Referral Hospital to focus on the most complex and difficult cases.

37. Contradictions were everywhere: On one hand, patients or their families were responsible for their own laundry; drying clothing adorned the bushes along the hospital's breezeways. On the other, children were sent at the government's expense to South African hospitals for certain treatments unavailable in Botswana, such as the surgical repair of congenital heart defects. The admission fee increased in 2007 from to P5 for citizens; noncitizens paid higher fees. In 2007–2008 the exchange rate was roughly US$1/P6.5.

38. Setswana's polite forms of address for adults include *mma* and *rra* (and their many variations) for women and men, respectively. Setswana is Botswana's national language and is spoken by the majority of the population.

39. The history of the peoples who came to be known as "the Tswana" encompasses the colonial and national borders that eventually emerged in the region. To be sure, Botswana and South Africa have distinct national histories, but Tswana on both sides of

the border share experiences of missionization and colonization and recruitment into related pedagogical regimes. On the context and implications of the Soweto uprising, see J. Comaroff 1996; Reynolds 1995. On more recent movements to decolonize higher education in South Africa, see Booysen et al. 2016; Mbembe 2016; Nyamnjoh 2016.

40. Pedagogy has been an enduring site of anthropological attention across a broad range of approaches including: French sociology (Bourdieu 1977; Bourdieu and Passeron 1970; Mauss 1935); structural-functionalism (Richards 1956); culture and personality (Mead 1930); Marxism (Willis 2017; cf. Freire 1970; Giroux 1981); poststructuralist, postcolonial, and performative approaches (Butler 1990; Foucault 1977; Said 1979; Stoler 1995; cf. Rizvi, Lingard, and Lavia 2006), and linguistic anthropology (Levinson 1999; Mertz 2007; Pelissier 1991; Wortham 2008, 2012) and includes studies of language socialization (Garrett and Baquedano-López 2002; Ochs and Schieffelin 2017; Schieffelin and Ochs 1986). A more recent interest in experts and expertise (Boyer 2008; Carr 2010a; cf. Nader 1972) reflects the influence of science studies (cf. Collins and Evans 2002). For reviews, see Blum 2019; Pollock and Levinson 2016.

41. Accounts of patient subjectivization tend to leave practitioners in relative obscurity; conversely, ethnographic accounts of biomedical training, including those set in the Global South, focus predominantly on surgical training and treat patients as inert objects against which a trainee's technical and ethical formation takes place. I take up this point again in chapter 5. A growing literature examines the perspectives of African professionals in global health settings; see Crane 2013; Geissler 2013; Okwaro and Geissler 2015; Poleykett 2018; Prince and Marsland 2013; Prince and Otieno 2014; Redfield 2012b; Sullivan 2011, 2012, 2016, 2017; Wendland 2010, 2012b, 2012a, and a special issue of *Critical African Studies* 8, no. 3 (2016) edited by Rebecca Warne Peters and Claire Wendland.

42. Critical engagements with globalization across anthropology, geography and science studies have denaturalized scale as tool with which to perform comparisons and reconceptualized it as the outcome of a process and an expression of power. In these readings, scale is "neither ontologically given . . . nor a politically neutral discursive strategy in the construction of narratives" (Swyngedouw 1997, 140; cf. Herod and Wright 2008; Marston, Jones, and Woodward 2005), but a practice, something enacted in the world (Moore 2008; Smith 1996).

43. Anthropological scholarship on HIV has recently begun grappling with temporality as health policy discourses have begun to focus on "the end of AIDS"; see Benton, Sangaramoorthy, and Kalofonos 2017; Kenworthy, Thomann, and Parker 2018; Moyer 2015.

44. On the seeming self-evident urgency of global health, see Cohen 2012; Fassin 2012; cf. Carr and Fisher 2016; on how scales mutually reinforce one another, see Carr and Lempert 2016; Philips 2016.

45. As Englebretson and Jaffe both note, research on stance is heterogeneous and multidisciplinary, and has its roots in the turn in sociolinguistics and linguistic anthropology to language's performative and participatory aspects; see Austin 1962; Bauman 1977; Duranti and Goodwin 1992; Hall 1999; Hymes 1975.

46. On stance's intersubjective dimensions, see Du Bois and Kärkkäinen 2012; Kärkkäinen 2007; Scheibman 2007; on its indexical ones, see Du Bois 2007; Haviland 1989; Silverstein 1976.

47. See also Law 2004; Moore 2004. This point has a much deeper genealogy in anthropological analyses of development and globalization as well as a separate, if intertwined, genealogy in geography; see Appadurai 1996; J. Comaroff and J. L. Comaroff 2000; Escobar 1995; Harvey 1989, 2006; Malkki 1992; Massey 1994; Pigg 1992; Rodman 1992; Soja 1989.

48. On postwar development and international health: Escobar 1995; Ferguson 1990; Li 2007; Mitchell 2002; Packard 2016; Pigg 1997b; Scott 1998; on colonialism: J. L. Comaroff 1989; J. Comaroff and J. L. Comaroff 1991; J. L. Comaroff and J. Comaroff 1997a; F. Cooper 2005.

49. See, for example, Biehl 2016; Irwin et al. 2002.

1. SAVING MEDICATIONS VERSUS SAVING CHILDREN

1. A nurse was assigned to each consulting room to assist and translate. But the nurses had other duties, and a consultation would sometimes grind to a halt when a caregiver spoke little English and no nurse was available. Some nurses did not mind translating; others told me that they missed the work of caring for patients. That said, Elise Carpenter notes that the large number of expatriate physicians in Botswana's public sector means that translation is frequently part of nurses' day-to-day work (2008, chap. 4) On the position of nurses in Botswana and the moral and logistical challenges they face, see Barbee 1987; Brada 2016; Carpenter 2008; Fako and Forchen 2000; Kupe 1987; Livingston 2012.

2. Combination ARV therapy, or HAART, uses a combination of drugs to disrupt the virus's reproductive cycle at multiple points, with the goal of viral suppression, that is, a state wherein the virus, while still present, cannot reproduce in numbers sufficient to be detected by a standardized test. The Superlative Clinic's pediatricians held that intermittent exposure, or poor adherence, to these medications allows those strains of the virus least vulnerable to the medications to reproduce, giving rise to a virus resistant to a medication or perhaps even a whole class of medications. Crane's account complicates this narrative (2013, chap. 1), but in the Superlative Clinic, that poor adherence led to drug resistance was a key principle of treatment.

3. Pediatricians, nurses, and the Clinic's social worker conducted these training sessions, though the burden of explaining how ARVs worked vis-à-vis HIV infection in Setswana to a group of caregivers whose proficiency in English varied widely fell to the Clinic's Batswana staff.

4. Bianca Dahl observes that popular perceptions of the success of Botswana's prevention of mother-to-child transmission (PMTCT) program has led some Batswana to regard those children who are, in fact, living with the virus with ambivalence and suspicion (2012).

5. To "chase" children is not, for Tswana people, obviously inappropriate: Deborah Durham observes that, "Children are taught to fear adults physically . . . This fear is transformed into respect for the commands of adults; when told to do so, a child should bring water, run to the store, or carry a message for any adult" (2004, 595). Like Durham, I also heard *ke tlaa go betsa* [I'm going to beat you] both in jest and in earnest. That said, Batswana both within and outside the Clinic sometimes voiced concerns that men disciplined too vigorously the children a woman had borne in an earlier relationship.

6. CD4 cells (also called helper T cells) mobilize the body's response to infection. One of the aims of ARV treatment is to stabilize a patient's CD4 count (measured by the number of CD4 cells per cubic millimeter of blood) and maintain their production.

7. As a biomedical technology, pediatric antiretroviral adherence assessments have their roots in the establishment of a professionalized clinical biomedicine and its attendant doctor-patient relationships, as well as ideas about disease causation, understandings of the relation of the individual to the population, and the role of the state (Brodwin 2010; Greene 2004; Jones 2001; Lerner 1997; Mykhalovskiy, Mccoy, and Bresalier 2004; Trostle 1988). Compliance, in short, has emerged as the ground on which both patient autonomy and physician responsibility are conceptualized. In response to calls for patient

responsibility, Paul Farmer persuasively argued that accounts of noncompliance frequently exaggerate the agency of poor people and fail to recognize how structural violence places those with fewer resources at higher risk for disease and death (Farmer 2004; cf. Farmer 1999; Maskovsky 2005). The Clinic's pediatricians were aware of some of these criticisms and contradictions. They emphasized patient responsibility while trying to mitigate some of the factors that made adherence difficult for children and their caregivers to achieve. One could see responses to Farmer's critique, for example, in the funds available to help adolescent patients travel to and from the hospital, or in pediatricians' attempts to coordinate children's appointments with those of their HIV-positive caregivers, thereby reducing transportation costs. In some ways, however, these gestures simply highlighted the contradiction between a sympathetic attitude and the disciplinary aspects of the adherence assessment itself.

8. In 1990 the vast majority of reported cases of AIDS in Romania were in very young children, more than half of whom were living in public institutions when they were diagnosed; see Morrison 2004; Popovici et al. 1991.

9. The majority of HIV-positive African children are infected via perinatal transmission; without treatment more than half of such children will die before their second birthday (Newell et al. 2004). The landmark study demonstrating the efficacy of PMTCT was published in 1994, and through the late 1990s and early 2000s PMTCT programs were touted as the most cost-effective use of ARVs in poor countries, see, for example, Mansergh et al. 1998; Marseille, Kahn, and Saba 1998; Newell et al. 1998; Skordis and Nattrass 2002.

10. When the treatment program began, the guidelines recommended that any HIV-positive child under eighteen years of age begin taking ARVs unless there were clinical contraindications. Adults enrolled in treatment could begin taking ARVs if they had a CD4 count of less than 200 or an AIDS-defining illness (Darkoh 2004). The guidelines assumed that regular monitoring of a patient's clinical status and lab results would indicate when a patient should begin ARVs while rationing drug supply and avoiding patient burn-out and poor adherence. The threshold CD4 count for adults was later raised to 350, then to 500.

11. Offering a two-drug regimen when a three-drug one was freely available would have violated clinical research ethics guidelines, which state that trials must not test protocols that offer less than what has been established as the standard of care. I return to the topic of the Clinic's research program in chapter 6.

12. For critiques of evidence-based medicine, see Lambert 2006; Timmermans and Mauck 2005; Wendland 2007; with regard to HIV/AIDS specifically, see McDonnell 2016, chap. 3.

13. A row erupted in a continuing education session for nurses sponsored by the national blood transfusion service when it was discovered that the service had solicited donations from junior secondary school students. While national guidelines allow Batswana aged sixteen and above to donate blood, several nurses strenuously objected that those children could not consent to donation on their own behalf. In the case of an infant who required cranial surgery and whose mother was very young, consent to transfer the child to South Africa for treatment was sought from the mother's adult kin. Hospital staff did not consult the mother, nor did she offer input. These examples also reflect the efforts of adults to manage the simultaneous somatic and sentimental bonds between close kin, a topic I take up later in this chapter and in chapter 2.

14. Referral Hospital had a pediatric medical and a pediatric surgical ward; the Clinic and Squad generally had little to do with the latter. Some Squad pediatricians insisted they had never agreed to inpatient work; a few disagreed. But by early 2007 many were deeply dissatisfied with the arrangement, faulting Dr. Buyaga and Dr. Amy

for capitalizing their labor on the pediatric medical ward in order to smooth relations between ward and Clinic while dismissing Squad pediatricians' criticisms of what they saw as substandard medical practice on the ward.

15. The state of a child's body may also reflect care or its absence for Batswana, but they differ from Americans in how they assess this relationship and the stakes of bodily care (Durham 2005; Livingston 2008).

16. Analyzing pediatrics textbooks from the late nineteenth century, Jonathan Gilles observes the "striking continuity" (2005, 394) of this ambivalence toward parents, observing that the possibility of a duplicitous or inept parent, particularly a mother, has historically lent pediatricians the authority to monitor and intervene in intimate familial relations (Apple 1987; Gilles and Loughlan 2007; Trostle 1988; cf. Mattingly 2008; Rouse 2004). On anxieties over children's self-representation in clinical contexts, see Buchbinder 2009, 2015; Mattingly 2010; Tates and Meeuwesen 2001.

17. The idea that the epidemic in Africa is incommensurable with its manifestations elsewhere has long haunted debates over the nature of the disease, its origins, and the shape responses to it should take; see J. Comaroff 2007; Crane 2013, chap. 1; Farmer 1992; Hoad 2005; Patton 1999; Stillwaggon 2003; Treichler 1992; Watney 1989.

18. Fixed-dose combination tablets, such as Combivir (zidovudine plus lamivudine), are meant to improve adherence by reducing the number of pills a patient takes. These did not exist in pediatric formulations or as liquid suspensions at the time of my fieldwork.

19. Thanks to Julie Livingston for drawing my attention to this point.

20. See a special issue, "Kinship and Constellations of Care," *Social Dynamics* 42, no. 2 (2016) edited by Lenore Manderson and Ellen Block.

21. Child fosterage among close kin has a long history in Botswana (Ingstad 2004; Livingston 2005). Movement of children and adults amid households in towns, villages, farms, and cattle-posts is structured by the demands of schooling and employment and by patterns of reciprocation among extended kin (Lesetedi 2003; Townsend 1997; Upton 2003). These arrangements are understood to hold potential benefits for children as well as for the adults who foster them.

22. Formally, terms for agnatic and maternal kin are distinct among the Tswana as are their obligations, though in practice these distinctions are sometimes more flexible and subject to change over time than formal accounts suggest (Dahl 2009, 2016; Mookodi 2000; Townsend 1997; cf. J. L. Comaroff 1978; Schapera 1940, 1957). Indeed, some Setswana speakers used English terms such as "auntie" to sidestep the question of whether the adults caring for a child were agnatic or maternal kin, particularly if the arrangement was in any way contentious.

23. In the first case, the child as well as her family members might well refer to the woman in question as "mother" (Setswana: *mme/mmagwe*); moreover, the terms for parallel cousins (e.g., a mother's sister's children) are those used for siblings. In the second case, the Setswana term *batsadi* can refer to a child's mother and father or to a broader group of elder kin.

2. HOW TO DO THINGS TO CHILDREN WITH WORDS

1. My twist on John L. Austin's (1962) title highlights two points. First, while Austin attends to how subjects use language to transform social relationships, not all subjects have equal power to do so. Second, I foreground the role of language in a context wherein biomedical practitioners assume that language has no direct bearing on the condition requiring treatment.

2. *Go utlwa* can also mean to obey; its negation (e.g., *ga a utlwa*) can indicate disobedience or neglect of one's obligations in addition to a failure to hear or understand.

3. In their study of child-rearing in northeastern Botswana, Geiger and Alant note that "most of the verbal communication between caregivers and children was instructional, with very little verbal response encouraged or expected from the child" (2005, 186), adding that "children were taught not to initiate verbal communication or ask questions of adults" (2005, 187; cf. T. Maundeni 2002). Instead, children's speaking facilities are developed from infancy through multilevel play and in peer groups.

4. This is not to suggest that other clinicians never asked children personal questions. Squad pediatricians' insistence that children "speak for themselves," however, was distinct (cf. Guzmán 2014).

5. For a historical account of consumer preferences in Americans' perceptions of children's subjectivities, see Cook 2004; on children's popular culture as a *lingua franca* in clinical settings in the US, see Mattingly 2008.

6. This is not to presume that any person who declares herself to be HIV positive does so in these terms or that such declarations only ever work the way clinicians or activists assume they will. My goal is to draw attention to the ways that powerful institutions shape, if not utterly determine, the capacity of words such as *AIDS* to transform social relationships.

7. Even in the face of a terminal diagnosis, writes Julie Livingston, "to tell someone that they would die was the antithesis of care and resonated with forms of social pathos like witchcraft" (2012, 165; cf. Klaits 2010, 62–70).

8. Few scholars have examined the socialization of children to ARV treatment; exceptions include Bernays et al. 2017; Mattes 2014.

9. In 1999 the American Academy of Pediatrics published guidelines advocating disclosure, arguing that the benefits far outweigh any short-term negative effects. Although these guidelines were drawn largely from the experiences of US and European children, they have influenced expert practice globally. In the decades since their publication, the position that disclosure is psychosocially beneficial and necessary to ensure adherence has been echoed in clinical and psychological studies. The consensus that the benefits of disclosure outweigh the costs, however, seems to have been less clear prior to the guidelines publication (Funck-Brentano et al. 1997; Lipson 1994; Wiener et al. 2007). Additionally, one can view the position that children benefit from disclosure as a response by clinicians to studies showing that terminally ill American children were, in fact, aware of their diagnosis even when they received little direct information about it but maintained their social relations with adults, including clinicians, by acting as though they did not know (Bluebond-Langner 1974, 1978; cf. Gordon and Paci 1997).

10. I follow Irvine and Gal in conceiving of "language ideologies" as "conceptual schemes" subjects use to "frame their understandings" of language and "map those understandings onto people, events, and activities" (2000, 35). These schemes are ideological, they emphasize, because they are "suffused with the political and moral issues pervading the particular sociolinguistic field and are subject to the interests of their bearers' social positions" (2000, 35).

11. In her study of a pediatric pain clinic in the US, Mara Buchbinder suggests that the epistemological privilege in biomedicine of language's referential function—its capacity to refer to and make predications about things in the world—is overstated, pointing out that practitioners are aware of language's performative dimensions and that referring itself holds potential social consequences (2015, 181–82; see Wilce 2009). For Squad pediatricians, the catechism's social consequences lay precisely in its referential function, that is, biomedical explanations were innately persuasive and capable of shaping children's behavior *because they were true*. This may reflect the wider gap pediatricians perceived between the worlds they and their patients inhabited compared to clinical practice in the US.

12. "Ideological constructions of communication," Charles Briggs argues, "enable powerful actors to determine what will count as silences, lies, and surpluses, just as they create silences of their own" (2007, 328; cf. Gal 1991).

13. Thanks to Treasa Galvin for this point and for her insightful observations about this material.

3. THE METALANGUAGE OF HIV INTERVENTION

1. Secrecy is argued to undergird bureaucratic regimes (James 2012; Marcus and Powell 2003; West and Sanders 2003), research enterprises (Geissler 2013), social identities (Palmié 2007), and even anthropology itself (H. L. Moore 2010; Taussig 1999).

2. On expert patients in HIV treatment, see Kielmann and Cataldo 2010; Kyakuwa and Hardon 2012; Mattes 2011.

3. Anxieties over infection becoming the means of survival is a topic well covered in the anthropology of HIV/AIDS, see Biehl 2009a, 2009b; Kalofonos 2010; Nguyen 2010; Ticktin 2006.

4. These assumptions about stigma and normalization do not bear out empirically; see Maughan-Brown 2010; Wyrod 2011.

5. Link and Phelan observe that, "Even though Goffman initially advised that we needed 'a language of relationships, not attributes,' subsequent practice has often transformed stigmas or marks into attributes of persons" (2001, 366; cf. Fine and Asch 1988; R. Parker and Aggleton 2003).

6. *jwa* is a possessive marker; the missing term is presumably *bolwetsi*, illness (cf. Phorano, Nthomang, and Ngwenya 2005, 170). Setswana's grammatical noun classes limit the nouns that could be indexed by that marker (cf. Black 2013).

7. Also see Carr 2010b, chapter 6, on "flipping the script."

8. On enumeration and metrics in global health see Adams 2016b; Biruk 2018; Erikson 2015; Storeng and Béhague 2014, and a special issue, "Enumeration, Identity, and Health," *Medical Anthropology* 31, no. 4 (2012) edited by Thurka Sangaramoorthy and Adia Benton. On how numbers displace and transform other forms of evidence in global health, see Adams 2005, 2010, 2013, 2016a; Biehl and Adams 2016; Biehl and Petryna 2013, 2014.

9. These stamps could also be crucial to adult caregivers insofar as they constituted evidence for employers of the general reason for one's absence while not necessarily revealing details.

10. Dr. Chibesa may also have been responding to what many in the Clinic perceived as Dr. Amy's favoritism toward and patronage of Dr. Motlhabane. The Squad pediatricians were not all "white" in the sense that term tends to carry in the US, but during my fieldwork none would have been considered "Black" by the Clinic's Batswana staff.

11. On indexical impurities, see Carr 2010b; on downscaling, see Bauman 2016, 46.

12. Dr. Mendoza, by contrast, attributed the discrepancy in failure rates to the preponderance of the antiretroviral medication nevirapine in pediatric ARV regimens. Most children could not use the fixed-dose combinations that were preferred in adult treatment and were limited to the ARVs that were available in pediatric dosages and formulations.

13. These surveys of women attending antenatal clinics began in 1990. Estimates of Botswana's prevalence rate have shifted over time: In 2004 UNAIDS estimated the adult prevalence rate to be above 37 percent from 2001 to 2003 (2004). In 2014, however, UNAIDS retrospectively revised its estimate of Botswana's 2005 prevalence rate to have been closer to 25 percent (2014).

14. For this subheading, my use of this twist on James Scott's (1998) title is more in line with Hulsebosch 2017 than with Dinnen and Allen 2016.

15. I return to the topic of administrative and fiscal capacity building in chapter 6 (*Sunday Standard* 2007).

16. Critical perspectives on "good governance" in Africa include Anders 2009; Gruffydd Jones 2013; cf. Ferguson 2006b. Gruffydd Jones notes that good governance "has been an explicit component of World Bank policy in Africa since the late 1980s and remains a constant and commonplace referent underpinning virtually all other more specific international policy initiatives and agendas, from the promotion of democracy to sustainable cities" (2013, 50). On the issue of governance in global health specifically, see H. Brown 2015; Buse and Walt 2009; Fidler 2007; Gostin and Mok 2009.

17. H. Brown 2015; Biruk 2018; Sullivan 2017. The presumed horizontality of nation-states and their commensurability echoes Anderson's analysis of the emergence of "imagined communities," a horizontality that, as John Kelly and Martha Kaplan argue, has its roots in American postwar economic and political strategies (2001). "In so far as Africa was concerned," Putzel continues, "the Bank referred mainly to the experiences of Uganda and Senegal" (2004, 1132) Much more should be said about the ways Uganda has been "upscaled" as a reference point for HIV/AIDS management efforts across the African continent, see Allen and Heald 2004; Epstein 2007.

18. This should not imply no protests take place; see Burke 2000; Durham 2004; Werbner 2014.

19. This sentiment was not confined to Americans: one British development professional waxed nostalgic about his time in Kenya, where the NGO sector "really worked," that is, with what he considered a sufficient degree of independence from state agencies.

20. For a genealogy of the concept, see J. L. Comaroff and J. Comaroff 1999, who observe, first, that those "who impute to Africa a lack of anything qualified by the adjective 'civil' seldom ground their claims in empirical observation," and, second, that it is the very "slippery, equivocal quality" of this "polythetic clutch of signs" that makes it possible for it to serve so many purposes (1999, 2–3). Furthermore, they note that accounts of "civil society" in Africa often neglect "'uncool' forms of African association" (1999, 22). Burial societies, for example, or churches rarely figured in expatriate professionals' conversations about civil society in Botswana.

21. The age of consent for HIV testing was lowered to sixteen years in the 2013 Public Health Act.

4. THE GLOBAL HEALTH FRONTIER

1. Writing on the public/private distinction, Susan Gal notes that the establishment of this distinction does not depend on the use of the lexical items *public* and *private*. "The ideological distinction," she argues, "is a meta-commentary that regiments practices, sometimes implicitly, sometimes explicitly, mapping on them a grid of interpretation" (2002, 81).

2. This circular temporality also reflects the logic of the "war on terror" inasmuch as it emphasizes an infinite loop of unpreparedness (Lakoff 2008; cf. Masco 2014). Thanks to Joe Masco for this point.

3. As noted in the introduction, the rotation at this time was limited to EUMS students and is thus somewhat distinct among international medical experiences.

4. Merson observed that, "the number of 'comprehensive' global health . . . programs involving faculty and students from more than one school, engaged in both research and education, and partnered with at least one institution in the Global South . . . increased from 6 in 2001 to more than 78 in 2011" (2014, 1677). He noted that "approximately 250 North American universities now have global health education offerings . . . and one fifth

of U.S. medical specialty residency programs have global health activities" (1677). Kerry et al., looking at data from 2011, found "380 global health residency training programs . . . working in 141 countries" (2013).

5. Kerry et al. (2013) found "529 individual programmatic activities . . . at 1337 specific sites," and note that, "the majority of the activities consisted of elective–based rotations" analogous in structure and duration to the EUMS rotation at Referral Hospital.

6. Claire Wendland observes that "a substantial and high-quality body of research on the process of medical socialization seems to argue strongly for the existence—and persistence—of a durable moral order in medicine" (2010, 21) that emphasizes detachment, reductionism, cynicism, political conservatism, conformity, and "a defensive authoritarianism" (20). She also points out that social science accounts of the dehumanization entailed in biomedical education overlap considerably with physicians' own accounts of the process (18–21). Her excellent ethnography of Malawian medical students illustrates that this moral order is not inherent to biomedical training but is shaped by the circumstances under which training takes place.

7. Tine Hanrieder refers to this as the "outsourcing" of "doctors' moral education," thereby transforming global health sites in the Global South into "laboratories of compassion" (2019, 14).

8. Students sometimes asked nurses or me about these matters, and later groups took some advantage of Setswana lessons, but these topics were generally regarded as tangential to the task of learning and practicing medicine.

9. Since 1977 the WHO has prepared a list of essential medicines to meet the basic needs of a health system. National governments are encouraged to use this list as a basis from which to formulate one that meets the particular needs of their own populations (see Greene 2011).

10. A British Approved Name (BAN) is the official nonproprietary, or generic, name given to a pharmaceutical substance for use in the UK. These names are approved by the British Pharmacopoeia Commission. BANs also incorporate International Non-Proprietary Names, the selection of which is facilitated by the WHO.

11. Rather than suggesting that cardiac monitoring was entirely unavailable in the hospital, it is likely that Dr. Matheson was suggesting that, given the limited distribution of equipment at Referral Hospital, it would be difficult to arrange ongoing cardiac monitoring for a patient outside the confines of the intensive care unit.

12. Silverstein draws attention to the improvisational nature of this process: "Such a dynamic or processual figuration of participants' contextually created and transformed 'groupness' characteristics—in short a real social act—happens improvisationally each time there is discursive interaction" (1997, 282).

13. Attempts to authoritatively frame the space-time of heroic American medical action are evident across "global health," settings: Johanna Crane describes how one researcher visiting Uganda in 2005 found himself "almost nostalgic" for "the kind of doctor he had been able to be" in San Francisco's pretreatment era (Crane 2013, 89). This type of retrospective moral credentialization sparked desire and even envy among EUMS students at Referral Hospital (Brada 2017), who feared generational exclusion from moral stances such as these.

14. Indeed, when I visited, I found a young child who had been bitten by a venomous snake and transferred to the hospital in Ramotswa from the district hospital in Maun, a nine hundred-kilometer journey.

15. Bakalanga are an ethnic and linguistic minority within Botswana.

16. To be sure, there were gradations of "local" that tended to map, albeit unevenly, onto race and location of training: EUMS personnel sometimes expressed their approval of the few European doctors and some South Asian doctors for their "toughness"

in dealing with recalcitrant "local" (read: "Tswana") nursing staff, and the quality of their training went largely unquestioned.

17. In a conversation comparing hospitals within Botswana, the only Squad pediatrician who spent the vast majority of her time working in the northeast rather than at Referral Hospital insisted with exasperation, "Referral Hospital is *not* 'resource-poor'!"

18. Dr. Baum was "pimping" Mpho. This is a common phenomenon in American medical training in which a supervisor (e.g., attending or resident) fires a series of questions at a junior (e.g., student, intern), often in an aggressive manner, until the junior confesses her ignorance with regard to an aspect of the case at hand (see Bennett 1985; Brancati 1989). Many thanks to Dan Menchik for these references.

19. As John and Jean Comaroff have observed (1997a), frontiers as spaces suffused with demands, desires, and dialectical self-fashioning have a long and complex history in southern Africa. On the "tensions of empire" at colonial frontiers, see Cooper and Stoler 1997.

20. As noted in chapter 1, the Superlative Clinic also operated in accordance with these national guidelines, but the relative autonomy of the Clinic vis-à-vis Botswana's national healthcare system in general was an ongoing matter of contention. See Brada 2016.

21. Dr. James was likely prescribing three drugs in an attempt to cover as many possible bacterial organisms in the absence of laboratory tests identifying the pathogen. The other condition, a *Pseudomonas* infection, while less familiar than TB, also poses a serious threat as a nosocomial (i.e., hospital-acquired) infection in a setting where many patients are immunocompromised.

22. My thanks to China Scherz for this point.

5. EXPERIENCING AIDS IN AFRICA

1. As noted in the introduction: The idea that the epidemic in Africa is incommensurable with its manifestations elsewhere has long haunted debates over the nature of the disease, its origins, and the shape responses to it should take; see J. Comaroff 2007; Crane 2013, chap. 1; Farmer 1992; Hoad 2005; Patton 1999; Stillwaggon 2003; Treichler 1992; Watney 1989.

2. Patients who have developed resistance to first-line drugs are likely to have a higher viral load (i.e., number of copies of the virus in a unit of blood) and therefore an increased chance of infecting another person. Thanks to Kohar Jones, MD, for this point. The patient in question was something of a favorite of Molly's firm; she was not blamed for Molly's injury.

3. PEP is given in instances of exposure to the virus, such as needlesticks and rape, in an attempt to prevent a person from seroconverting, that is, developing an HIV infection. It is begun as soon as possible after the exposure; its efficacy decreases over time.

4. See Chelenyane and Endacott 2006; Newsom and Kiwanuka 2002.

5. On pragmatism and education, see Giles and Eyler 1994; Keane 2008; cf. Dewey 1938; on mediation and affect in the production of expertise, see Keller 1983; Knorr-Cetina 1999; Lakoff 2008; on how the body figures in claims to immediacy, see Allen 2009.

6. Studies of medical socialization have analyzed the embodied aspect of medical training in terms of homogenization and professionalization, that is, learning to "act like a doctor" (Beagan 2000; Becker et al. 1961; Bosk 2002; Cassell 1998; M.-J. D. Good 1995; Sinclair 1997); the cultivation of an expert sensorium (Fountain 2014; Hammer 2018; Rice 2008; cf. Wendland 2010, chap. 4); the reification of patients (Lock 1993, 2002; E. Martin 1987; Prentice 2013; Taussig 1980); and what Rachel Prentice calls "medical embodiment," that is, "the development of perceptions, affects, judgments, and ethics that occurs through bodily

practice in a clinical milieu" (2013, 6). As a number of scholars have noted, learning to see like a biomedical practitioner has been given far more scholarly attention than learning to touch, hear, or even smell like one, a fact emphasized by ethnographic studies of healing practices considered in contrast to biomedicine (see, e.g., Farquhar 1994, 2002). The classic study of the medical gaze is Foucault (1975), which emphasizes the violence of the engagement.

7. That this register is not generalizable to, for example, biomedicine in wealthy countries is highlighted by Yael Assor's analysis of a "moral sensibility for unemotionality" in Israeli healthcare (2021).

8. On these tensions, see R. Fox 1963; B. J. Good 1993a; M.-J. D. Good 1995; Kleinman 1995.

9. Arguably, this politicization has a much longer history (Starr 1982). For some physicians, these bureaucratic and political shifts of the latter decades of the twentieth century have undermined their professional legitimacy and political influence (Luft 1999; Schlesinger 2002); for a review see Light and Levine 1988; for a critique see Timmermans and Oh 2010.

10. See Gianakos 1996; Larson and Yao 2005; Spiro 1992; Spiro et al. 1996; Stepien and Baernstein 2006 and articles in *Academic Medicine* 84, no. 9 (2009). In pursuit of this transformation one US medical school invited students approaching the end of their preclinical training to be hospitalized themselves (Wilkes, Milgrom, and Hoffman 2002). This concern is not a new in medicine (Aring 1958), but its institutionalization as a learning objective is novel.

11. On shifts in training, see AAMC 2011, 2016; Hartocollis 2010; Rosenthal 2012; on bodily hexis in biomedical training, see Cassell 1996; Poirier 2006; Prentice 2007, 2013; expressions of anxiety that practitioners and trainees are too distant from patients' bodies include Grady 2010; Ofri 2010, 2014; Verghese 2009; Verghese and Horwitz 2009; on cultural insensitivity, see Jenks 2011; Shaw and Armin 2011; Taylor 2003.

12. Here Dr. Goldberg distinguishes between "managing," that is, keeping a patient stable and following orders placed by a superior, and actively participating in the processes of diagnosing a patient's condition, formulating a plan for treatment, and evaluating its effects.

13. Benton 2016; Crane 2013; Wendland 2012b; Wendland, Erikson, and Sullivan 2016. These racist logics exceed global health, of course, as illustrated by the number of physicians of color, particularly women, whose offers of assistance are ignored or whose credential are questioned or disbelieved in emergency situations in the US (Johnson 2016; Wible 2016).

14. This is not to suggest that the register of heroic American medicine is the provenance solely of US citizens. Following Berlant, however, it does seem very American, in light of weak commitments in the US to both social medicine and universal healthcare, to attempt to solve the problem of the politicization of medicine not by changing policy or infrastructure but by changing what medical trainees are made to feel and what they say about those feelings.

15. Quoted in EU's alumnae magazine, citation omitted to maintain anonymity; italics mine. On the temporal management of death in the US, see Kaufman 2010.

16. Why, Berlant asks, should shock be seen as productive of clarity when it "can as powerfully be said to produce panic, misrecognition, the shakiness of perception's ground?" (1999, 58).

17. Nurses in the US who lack specialized training in pediatrics also express anxiety with regard to providing care for children (Falgiani, Kennedy, and Jahnke 2014; McNeill 2016). A study at Mulago Hospital in Kampala found that 57 percent of the surveyed

nurses and midwives had experienced at least one needlestick injury in the previous year (Nsubuga and Jaakkola 2005).

18. The conflict escalated to the point that Dr. Mark brought to the ward a copy of the Nurses and Midwives Act, the law that laid out nurses' legal responsibilities. Its presence had little effect; the conflict was less a matter of legal interpretation than of what constituted moral medical practice. No Squad pediatrician ever framed this conflict for me in terms of their own risk of injury, but the fact remained that as attendings they effectively delegated the use of sharps and the risks those tools entailed to MOs, nurses, and other "local" staff. These tensions over authority and the division of biomedical labor in southern Africa should also be considered in terms of the colonial policies that inform them (Barbee 1987; Kupe 1987; Marks 1994).

19. Batswana MOs did complain about some of their patients and their patients' families, particularly if patients or families had delayed seeking care or had sought out *bongaka* (Tswana medicine). These complaints, however, did not tend to focus on holding patients responsible for their own illnesses, that is, as though patients had brought their illnesses on themselves.

20. This position was, of course, subject to fractal recursion (Gal 2002), as illustrated in chapter 4 by Dr. Chilube's discomfort on being asked to translate from Setswana. Conversely, foreigners could be incorporated into this community of health professionals by successfully performing a moral orientation toward the nation. Dr. Chibesa, a Zambian whose wife was Motswana, earned the approbation of some Clinic nurses for his wry commentary on the casual racism of some Squad pediatricians (see chapters 1 and 3). Given the circumspection with which individuals approached the topic of race across my field sites, Dr. Chibesa's frankness was unusual, and possibly afforded by his status as insider/outsider.

21. Indeed, Wendland speculates that Malawian medical students' nationalism was a product of their medical training and subsequent elite status, often facilitated by an urban upbringing (2010, 101–8; cf. Pigg 1992).

22. In my experience, Batswana health professionals' code-switching usage of *ga ke re* often indicated an effort to restrain anger and frustration. Together, Mpho's switch and the anonymized example following it reflect an indirectness that, many scholars have argued, is positively valued among Batswana as a marker of self-mastery in adulthood (Alverson 1978; J. L. Comaroff and J. Comaroff 2001; Durham and Klaits 2002; Klaits 2010; Livingston 2005, 2012). This indirectness is also evident in her oblique reference to the "subtle thing."

23. Tumelo also knew where to find and how to use the winged infusion (or "butterfly") needles that can make the placement of cannulas in very young children easier to carry out. These needles were largely unavailable on the hospital's pediatric medical ward.

24. See Kyakuwa and Hardon 2012 on the efforts of HIV-positive nurses in East Africa to conceal their serostatus.

25. It is unclear to me whether intermittent exposure to PEP would, in fact, render Tumelo more likely to develop resistance a particular antiretroviral drug or a class of drugs. Around 2004–2005, there was concern among health professionals in Botswana and elsewhere that the regimen of single-dose nevirapine used for prevention of mother-to-child transmission induced resistance to nevirapine in women who later began ARV treatment (see, e.g., Shapiro et al. 2006). At the time of our conversation, the "backbone" of ARV therapy in Botswana, including PEP, was AZT. Tumelo's speculation that intermittent exposure to AZT would render the drug less effective for her if she were to become infected with HIV was thus not unreasonable. Her wry commentary partially overlaps with the fatalism of the Malawian medical students in Wendland's study, conducted before treatment

became publicly available there, who saw exposure as an inevitable occupational hazard with a fatal outcome. Wendland notes that conversations about the inevitability of HIV exposure and its ramifications shifted as ARVs became more widely available in Malawi (2010, 126–29).

6. PEDAGOGY AS DISPOSSESSION

1. Concerns about the extractive aspects of clinical research reach back to the colonial era and, as many scholars have argued, point far beyond concerns with research itself to the broader social and political relationships upon which research projects depended and which they reshaped in the process (Geissler 2005, 2013; Geissler and Molyneux 2011; Graboyes 2015; Molyneux and Geissler 2008; Street 2014; Vaughan 1991; cf. White 2000).

2. The register was eventually made adaptable for use in South Africa, but its initial design was oriented toward the particularities of Botswana rather than as a "global public good" that circulated in search of an application (see Feierman 2011).

3. The grant included a training program for young scientists from southern Africa, though not specifically Batswana; see Harvard AIDS Institute 1999.

4. *Kitso* is Setswana for knowledge; cf. the verb *go itse*, to know. For BHP, KITSO stands for: Knowledge, Innovation & Training Shall Overcome AIDS.

5. Mokone et al. cite personal communication from Botswana's Ministry of Education indicating that only 10 percent of sponsored trainees returned to Botswana (2014). In 1975–1976, 90 percent of physicians in government hospitals were expatriates (Barbee 1986, 76); this ratio is unchanged in the 2005 WHO report alluded to by Parsons et al. 2012, though Parsons et al. do not indicate whether this is 90 percent of physicians in government service or 90 percent of all physicians in the country.

6. The phenomenon is not limited to doctors: a British company recruited away fifty nurses from one hospital in a single day (L. Garrett 2007; cf. Thupayagale-Tshweneagae 2007).

7. Studies from the late 1980s and 1990s indicate that pedagogical strategies in Botswana have historically been teacher-centric and that instructors have relied on closed-ended questions and collective recitation (Fuller and Snyder 1991), reflecting a confluence of colonial educational models, Tswana social hierarchies, and postcolonial polices (Tabulawa 1997). Seeming unresponsiveness could well have been a show of respect in line with pedagogic norms; see chapter 2 regarding language ideologies and social hierarchies in Botswana.

8. See chapter 1, note 1. The distinction Dr. Mark posits between the potential competence and mobility of MOs in contrast to the nurses' incompetence and immobility does not, in fact, bear out, as noted previously.

9. See note 7 in this chapter.

10. A computed tomography, or CAT scan, combines x-ray and computer technology to produce axial images, or "slices," of the body.

11. The question of who had been "poached" by whom was a constant source of gossip. Several health professionals in southeastern Botswana suggested I could map the institutional landscape of "the partners" by tracking the peripatetic careers of a few specific "local" doctors, both Batswana and expatriate Africans. Some African practitioners hinted, further, that doing so would reveal the "glass ceiling" of the partners, that is, the level of advancement beyond which brown-skinned health professionals could not rise, thus driving their circulation from one "partner" to the next.

12. In 2018 the AMA reported that almost 95 percent of US medical school graduates who applied to residencies were matched to a program, with more than 77 percent

offered their first choice of specialization. By contrast, the match rate for foreign graduates of medical schools outside the US and Canada was just over 50 percent (Murphy 2018; National Resident Matching Program 2018). "A doctor," explains Philip Sopher, "is only allowed to practice in the U.S. once he has obtained a license in the state in which he intends to work. The person must acquire a visa, pass the first two steps of the United States Medical-Licensing Exam (USMLE), then become certified by the Education Commission for Foreign Medical Graduates (ECFMG), get into an accredited U.S. or Canadian residency program, and finally, go back and pass step three of the USMLE. Each of these steps could take multiple years" (2014; Rios 2016).

13. In this inversion, Mma Modise jokingly emphasized some hierarchical distinctions between herself and Tshepo (doctor/nurse; male/female) while feigning unawareness of another (senior/junior). Tshepo had no formal supervisory role vis-à-vis Mma Modise. Variations of this inversion abounded, as when Dr. Chibesa greeted a fellow MO (or me!) as "chief" or when Mma Molefi, the Superlative Clinic's phlebotomist, consoled very young boys during blood draws using terms of address more appropriate to their grandfathers: *Sori, ntate . . . sori, papa.*

14. Before institutions can receive support from the US Department of Health and Human Services, including NIH funds, for research involving human subjects, they must have an FWA approved by the HHS Office for Human Research Protections (OHRP). Johanna Crane notes that, during the 2008 meetings of the Consortium of Universities for Global Health, an American researcher told her that "his university's program in Botswana had received 'one grant that was bigger than the whole local university budget,' which had, not surprisingly given its size, 'no idea how to manage it.' It's a real problem, he went on, because they 'desperately want to be treated like equals' but are not able to handle large NIH grants" (2013, 166). On the neglect of fiscal and administrative capacity in global health research partnerships, see Crane 2013, chap. 5; 2018; Crane et al. 2018; for a perspective from the University of Botswana's administration, see Holm and Malete 2010.

15. Citation withheld for anonymity. Structured interruptions in ARV therapy for HIV-infected adults was also a focus of HIV research around the same time; see, for example, the SMART trial.

16. Pediatric ETAT, as noted in an update to the guidelines, "is intended for use in low-resource settings where infants and children are likely to be managed by nonspecialists" (World Health Organization 2016, 2; see World Health Organization 2005).

17. See Thigpen et al. 2012, who note that animal studies demonstrated the superior efficacy of the drug used in the second trial (TDF2) compared to the first trial's study drug, but make no mention whatsoever of the controversy surrounding PrEP trials.

18. The views I heard are similar to those expressed in Toledo et al. 2015, whose data was collected from trial participants in 2010.

19. *Dikgosi* lack formal legislative power, but they have significant influence in Botswana. For them to object to the trial would not have been a trivial matter for BOTUSA's leadership.

20. This process of "replacing outsiders with insiders" mirrors earlier dynamics in the HIV treatment program (Carpenter 2008, chap. 2; cf. Nyamnjoh 2006), as well as a broader politics of capture with a much longer legacy in Botswana (Gulbrandsen 2012).

21. See https://aids.harvard.edu/the-mochudi-project/, dated November 7, 2009, accessed May 27, 2019.

22. I myself got caught up in this spiral as the HPRU expanded into transnational clinical research: Upon arriving in Gaborone in mid-2006, I stopped by BOTUSA at the invitation of an acquaintance, who introduced me around the office. The head of the HPRU, a physician, later contacted me to ask if I would join a study she was about to

begin. As noted, between 2004 and 2005, PrEP trials had been suspended and canceled due to activist protest (Singh and Mills 2005). The PrEP trial in Botswana, called TDF1, had begun enrolling participants had and formed both a Participant Advisory Group and a Community Advisory Group but had not yet begun to distribute the study drug. The Gates Foundation arranged a meeting in Seattle for researchers, activists, and other stakeholders in May 2005 to discuss the trials; one of the outcomes of that meeting was that Botswana's Participant and Community Advisory Groups should themselves be studied in order to determine why Botswana, unlike other sites, had not erupted in protest. This was explicitly framed as a search for generalizable principles: A draft of the study proposal in my possession suggests that, "By exploring community perceptions and describing the community participation in Botswana, information about involvement strategies and activities can be identified as 'best-practices'/lessons learned for the HIV prevention trials community." Before the study could begin, however, the head of the HPRU was transferred back to CDC headquarters in Atlanta for reasons that were never made clear to me. The study was put on indefinite hold and, to the best of my knowledge, never completed.

CONCLUSION

1. See Biehl 2009b; Kalofonos 2010; Kenworthy 2017; Marsland and Prince 2012; Parker 2000.

2. The timing of these shifts is important insofar as they occurred in conjunction with the broader geopolitical and ideological destabilizations of late Cold War (Trouillot 1991).

3. Critical global health (CGH) is not commensurate with, and is arguably generationally descendant from, critical medical anthropology. Those engaged in CGH are more influenced by Foucauldian ideas regarding knowledge, power, and subjectivity than critical medical anthropologists. Both groups, however, approach anthropology as a form of critique that can and should be directed toward the amelioration of human suffering. Thanks to Emily Yates-Doerr for this question.

4. See also Adams 2010, 2013, and 2016b.

5. See also Janes and Corbett 2009; Pfeiffer and Nichter 2008.

6. Michael is referring to photographs of Abu Ghraib prison published in the American media in 2004. Many of these photographs featured US personnel posing triumphantly with Iraqi detainees in positions of humiliation and torture.

7. On the primacy of suffering among human experiences, see Das et al. 2000; Kleinman 1988, 1992; Kleinman, Das, and Lock 1997; Scheper-Hughes 1993; cf. Boltanski 1999; Redfield 2006; Robbins 2013. Physician-anthropologists are not new, though their numbers have increased in recent years (Holmes et al. 2017). What is perhaps new is the position they claim at the juncture of the two disciplines with regard to a commitment to a "vision of health equity and social justice" (Hanna and Kleinman 2013, 16) irreducible to one discipline or the other, that is, a unique capacity to "socialize" suffering like anthropologists while insisting on the moral primacy of "bare life" as physicians. As a consequence, the anthropology of suffering tends to reflect biomedicine's commitments insofar as the primacy of a culturally and historically specific form of life is smuggled in through the back door.

8. Of course, the life story, or even an ethnographic account focused on a single individual, is not a recent invention nor the provenance of medical anthropology (see, e.g., Crapanzano 1980; Herzfeld 1997; Kroeber 1961; Shostak 1981), nor is such a text destined to index its author's moral subjectivity. That Biehl's text, in Robbins' words, "addresses its readers in their humanity" is not a feature inherent to either the method or the genre. We must look elsewhere for clues as to why it is successful in doing so.

9. See, for example, Biehl 2016; Wilkinson and Kleinman 2016.

10. Wary of depicting an "economy of good feeling" that "works only to conceal the despair on which it is built," Andrea Muehlebach reminds us that such an economy "is more than an ideological smoke screen or a psychological palliative. Rather, it is a profoundly indeterminate space of both love and loss, pleasure and pain, compassion and exclusion" (Muehlebach 2011, 75; cf. Stevenson 2009).

11. See, for example, Gayle, LaForge, and Slaughter 2021; Jha 2021.

Bibliography

AAMC (American Association of Medical Colleges). 1998. "Report I: Learning Objectives for Medical Student Education: Guidelines for Medical Schools. The Medical School Objectives Project." Washington, DC: AAMC.

——. 2011. "Behavioral and Social Science Foundations for Future Physicians: Report of the Behavioral and Social Science Expert Panel." Washington, DC: AAMC.

——. 2016. "Achieving Health Equity: How Academic Medicine Is Addressing the Social Determinants of Health." Washington, DC: AAMC.

Abadie, Roberto. 2010. *The Professional Guinea Pig: Big Pharma and the Risky World of Human Subjects*. Durham, NC: Duke University Press.

Adams, Vincanne. 2002. "Randomized Controlled Crime: Postcolonial Sciences in Alternative Medicine Research." *Social Studies of Science* 32 (5–6): 659–90.

——. 2005. "Saving Tibet? An Inquiry into Modernity, Lies, Truths, and Beliefs." *Medical Anthropology* 24 (1): 71–110.

——. 2010. "Against Global Health: Arbitrating Science, Non-Science, and Nonsense Through Health." In *Against Health: How Health Became the New Morality*, edited by Jonathan Metzl and Anna Kirkland, 40–60. New York: NYU Press.

——. 2013. "Evidence-Based Global Public Health: Subjects, Profits, Erasures." In *When People Come First: Critical Studies in Global Health*, edited by João Biehl and Adriana Petryna, 59–90. Princeton, NJ: Princeton University Press.

——. 2016a. "Metrics of the Global Sovereign: Numbers and Stories in Global Health." In *Metrics: What Counts in Global Health*, edited by Vincanne Adams, 19–56. Durham, NC: Duke University Press.

——, ed. 2016b. *Metrics: What Counts in Global Health*. Durham, NC: Duke University Press.

——. 2016c. "What Is Critical Global Health?" *Medicine Anthropology Theory* 3 (2): 186.

Agha, Asif. 2003. "The Social Life of Cultural Value." *Language & Communication* 23 (3–4): 231–73.

——. 2005. "Voice, Footing, Enregisterment." *Journal of Linguistic Anthropology* 15 (1): 38–59.

——. 2007. *Language and Social Relations*. Cambridge: Cambridge University Press.

Allen, Lori A. 2009. "Martyr Bodies in the Media: Human Rights, Aesthetics, and the Politics of Immediation in the Palestinian Intifada." *American Ethnologist* 36 (1): 161–80.

Allen, Tim, and Suzette Heald. 2004. "HIV/AIDS Policy in Africa: What Has Worked in Uganda and What Has Failed in Botswana?" *Journal of International Development* 16 (8): 1141–54.

Alverson, Hoyt. 1978. *Mind in the Heart of Darkness: Value and Self-Identity among the Tswana of Southern Africa*. New Haven, CT: Yale University Press.

Amon, Joseph J. 2013. "The 'Right to Know' or 'Know Your Rights'? Human Rights and a People-Centered Approach to Health Policy." In *When People Come First: Critical Studies in Global Health*, edited by João Biehl and Adriana Petryna, 91–108. Princeton, NJ: Princeton University Press.

Anders, Gerhard. 2009. *In the Shadow of Good Governance: An Ethnography of Civil Service Reform in Africa.* Leiden, Netherlands: Brill.

Anderson, Benedict. 1983. *Imagined Communities: Reflections on the Origin and Spread of Nationalism.* Rev. ed. London: Verso.

Anderson, Warwick. 2002. "Introduction: Postcolonial Technoscience." *Social Studies of Science* 32 (5/6): 643–58.

——. 2006. *Colonial Pathologies: American Tropical Medicine, Race, and Hygiene in the Philippines.* Durham, NC: Duke University Press.

——. 2008. *The Collectors of Lost Souls: Turning Kuru Scientists Into Whitemen.* Baltimore, MD: Johns Hopkins University Press.

Appadurai, Arjun. 1996. *Modernity at Large: Cultural Dimensions of Globalization.* Minneapolis: University of Minnesota Press.

Appel, Hannah. 2012. "Offshore Work: Oil, Modularity, and the How of Capitalism in Equatorial Guinea." *American Ethnologist* 39 (4): 692–709.

Apple, Rima D. 1987. *Mothers and Medicine: A Social History of Infant Feeding, 1890–1950.* Madison: University of Wisconsin Press.

Aring, Charles D. 1958. "Sympathy and Empathy." *Journal of the American Medical Association* 167 (4): 448–52.

Arnold, David. 1993. *Colonizing the Body: State Medicine and Epidemic Disease in Nineteenth-Century India.* Berkeley: University of California Press.

Arnold, Lynnette. 2020. "Cross-Border Communication and the Enregisterment of Collective Frameworks for Care." *Medical Anthropology* 39 (7): 624–37.

Assor, Yael. 2021. "'Objectivity' as a Bureaucratic Virtue." *American Ethnologist* 48 (1): 105–19.

Austin, John Langshaw. 1962. *How to Do Things with Words.* Cambridge, MA: Harvard University Press.

Baer, Hans A., Merrill Singer, and John H. Johnsen. 1986. "Toward a Critical Medical Anthropology." *Social Science & Medicine* 23 (2): 95–98.

Bagwasi, Mompoloki Mmangaka. 2012. "Perceptions, Contexts, Uses and Meanings of Silence in Setswana." *Journal of African Cultural Studies* 24 (2): 184–94.

Bakhtin, Mikhail Mikhaĭlovich. 1981. *The Dialogic Imagination: Four Essays.* Translated by Michael Holquist and Caryl Emerson. Austin: University of Texas Press.

——. 1984. *Problems of Dostoevsky's Poetics.* Translated by Caryl Emerson. Vol. 8 of *Theory and History of Literature.* Minneapolis: University of Minnesota Press.

Barbee, Evelyn L. 1986. "Biomedical Resistance to Ethnomedicine in Botswana." *Social Science & Medicine* 22 (1): 75–80.

——. 1987. "Tensions in the Brokerage Role: Nurses in Botswana." *Western Journal of Nursing Research* 9 (2): 244–56.

Barnes, Amy, Garrett W. Brown, and Sophie Harman. 2016. "Understanding Global Health and Development Partnerships: Perspectives from African and Global Health System Professionals." *Social Science & Medicine* 159 (June): 22–29.

Barr, Beth A. Tippet. 2006. "Pediatric Antiretroviral Adherence and Child Disclosure in Botswana." PhD diss., University of Texas School of Public Health.

Bataille, Georges. 1990. "Hegel, Death and Sacrifice." Translated by Jonathan Strauss. *Yale French Studies*, no. 78: 9–28.

Bauman, Richard. 1977. *Verbal Art as Performance.* Prospect Heights, IL: Waveland Press.

——. 2016. "Projecting Presence: Aura and Oratory in William Jennings Bryan's Presidential Races." In *Scale: Discourse and Dimensions of Social Life*, edited by E. Summerson Carr and Michael Lempert, 25–51. Berkeley: University of California Press.

Bauman, Richard, and Charles L. Briggs. 2003. *Voices of Modernity: Language Ideologies and the Politics of Inequality.* Cambridge: Cambridge University Press.

Beagan, Brenda L. 2000. "Neutralizing Differences: Producing Neutral Doctors for (Almost) Neutral Patients." *Social Science and Medicine* 51 (8): 1253–65.

Beaussier, Anne-Laure. 2014. "American Health Care Policy in a Time of Party Polarization." Translated by Sarah-Louise Raillard. *Revue Française de Science Politique* 64 (3): 383–405.

Becker, Howard Saul, Blanche Geer, Everett C. Hughes, and Anselm L. Strauss. 1961. *Boys in White: Student Culture in Medical School.* Chicago: University of Chicago Press.

Beidelman, T. O. 1993. *Moral Imagination in Kaguru Modes of Thought.* First Smithsonian ed. Smithsonian Institute Press.

Bennett, Bruce S. 1997. "'Suppose a Black Man Tells a Story': The Dialogues of John Mackenzie the Missionary and Sekgoma Kgari the King and Rainmaker." *Pula: Botswana Journal of African Studies* 11 (1): 43–53.

Bennett, Howard J. 1985. "How to Survive a Case Presentation." *Chest* 88 (2): 292–94.

Benton, Adia. 2012. "Exceptional Suffering? Enumeration and Vernacular Accounting in the HIV-Positive Experience." *Medical Anthropology* 31 (4): 310–28.

——. 2015. *HIV Exceptionalism: Development through Disease in Sierra Leone.* Minneapolis: University of Minnesota Press.

——. 2016. "African Expatriates and Race in the Anthropology of Humanitarianism." *Critical African Studies* 8 (3): 266–77.

Benton, Adia, Thurka Sangaramoorthy, and Ippolytos Kalofonos. 2017. "Temporality and Positive Living in the Age of HIV/AIDS: A Multisited Ethnography." *Current Anthropology* 58 (4): 454–76.

Benveniste, Emile. 1971. "The Nature of Pronouns." In *Problems in General Linguistics,* translated by Mary E. Meek, 217–22. Miami, FL: University of Miami Press.

Berg, Marc, and Annemarie Mol, eds. 1998. *Differences in Medicine: Unraveling Practices, Techniques, and Bodies.* Durham, NC: Duke University Press.

Berg, Marc, and Stefan Timmermans. 2000. "Orders and Their Others: On the Constitution of Universalities in Medical Work." *Configurations* 8 (1): 31–61.

Berlant, Lauren. 1999. "The Subject of True Feeling: Pain, Privacy, and Politics." In *Cultural Pluralism, Identity Politics, and the Law,* edited by Austin Sarat and Thomas R. Kearns, 49–84. Ann Arbor: University of Michigan Press.

——. 2008a. "Introduction: Intimacy, Publicity, Femininity." In *The Female Complaint: The Unfinished Business of Sentimentality in American Culture,* 1–31. Durham, NC: Duke University Press.

——. 2008b. "Poor Eliza." In *The Female Complaint: The Unfinished Business of Sentimentality in American Culture,* 33–67. Durham, NC: Duke University Press.

Berman, Ruth A. 2005. "Introduction: Developing Discourse Stance in Different Text Types and Languages." *Journal of Pragmatics* 37 (2): 105–24.

Bernays, Sarah, Sara Paparini, Janet Seeley, and Tim Rhodes. 2017. "'Not Taking It Will Just Be Like a Sin': Young People Living with HIV and the Stigmatization of Less-Than-Perfect Adherence to Antiretroviral Therapy." *Medical Anthropology* 36 (5): 485–99.

Berry, Nicole S. 2014. "Did We Do Good? NGOs, Conflicts of Interest and the Evaluation of Short-Term Medical Missions in Sololá, Guatemala." *Social Science & Medicine* 120 (November): 344–51.

Bialostok, Steven M., and Matt Aronson. 2016. "Making Emotional Connections in the Age of Neoliberalism." *Ethos* 44 (2): 96–117.

Bialostok, Steven M., and George Kamberelis. 2012. "The Play of Risk, Affect, and the Enterprising Self in a Fourth-Grade Classroom." *International Journal of Qualitative Studies in Education* 25 (4): 417–34.

Biehl, João. 2005. *Vita: Life in a Zone of Social Abandonment*. Berkeley: University of California Press.

——. 2009a. "Pharmaceuticalization: AIDS Treatment and Global Health Politics." *Anthropological Quarterly* 80 (4): 1083–1126.

——. 2009b. *Will to Live: AIDS Therapies and the Politics of Survival*. Princeton, NJ: Princeton University Press.

——. 2013. "Ethnography in the Way of Theory." *Cultural Anthropology* 28 (4): 573–97.

——. 2016. "Theorizing Global Health." *Medicine Anthropology Theory* 3 (2): 127–42.

Biehl, João, and Vincanne Adams. 2016. "The Work of Evidence in Critical Global Health." *Medicine Anthropology Theory* 3 (2): 123.

Biehl, João, and Ramah McKay. 2012. "Ethnography as Political Critique." *Anthropological Quarterly* 85 (4): 1209–28.

Biehl, João, and Adriana Petryna. 2013. *When People Come First: Critical Studies in Global Health*. Princeton, NJ: Princeton University Press.

——. 2014. "Peopling Global Health." *Saúde e Sociedade* 23 (June): 376–89.

Birn, Anne-Emanuelle, and Theodore M. Brown. 2013. "Across the Generations: Lessons from Health Internationalism." In *Comrades in Health: U.S. Health Internationalists, Abroad and at Home*, 303–18. New Brunswick, NJ: Rutgers University Press.

Biruk, C. 2012. "Seeing Like a Research Project: Producing 'High-Quality Data' in AIDS Research in Malawi." *Medical Anthropology* 31 (4): 347–66.

——. 2018. *Cooking Data: Culture and Politics in an African Research World*. Durham, NC: Duke University Press.

Biruk, C., and Ramah McKay. 2019. "Introduction: Objects of Critique in Critical Global Health Studies." *Medicine Anthropology Theory* 6 (2): 142–50.

Black, Steven P. 2013. "Stigma and Ideological Constructions of the Foreign: Facing HIV/AIDS in South Africa." *Language in Society* 42 (5): 481–502.

——. 2019. *Speech and Song at the Margins of Global Health: Zulu Tradition, HIV Stigma, and AIDS Activism in South Africa*. New Brunswick, NJ: Rutgers University Press.

Block, Ellen, and Will McGrath. 2019. *Infected Kin: Orphan Care and AIDS in Lesotho*. New Brunswick, NJ: Rutgers University Press.

Bluebond-Langner, Myra. 1974. "I Know, Do You? A Study of Awareness, Communication, and Coping in Terminally Ill Children." In *Anticipatory Grief*, edited by Bernard Schoenberg, Arthur C. Carr, Austin H. Kutscher, David Peretz, and Ivan K. Goldberg, 171–81. New York: Columbia University Press.

——. 1978. *The Private Worlds of Dying Children*. Princeton, NJ: Princeton University Press.

Blum, Susan D. 2019. "Why Don't Anthropologists Care about Learning (or Education or School)? An Immodest Proposal for an Integrative Anthropology of Learning Whose Time Has Finally Come." *American Anthropologist* 121 (3): 641–54.

Boellstorff, Tom. 2009. "Nuri's Testimony: HIV/AIDS in Indonesia and Bare Knowledge." *American Ethnologist* 36 (2): 351–63.

Boltanski, Luc. 1999. *Distant Suffering: Morality, Media and Politics*. Cambridge: Cambridge University Press.

Booysen, Susan, Gillian Godsell, Rekgotsofetse Chikane, and Sizwe Mpofu-Walsh, eds. 2016. *Fees Must Fall: Student Revolt, Decolonisation and Governance in South Africa*. Johannesburg: Wits University Press.

Bosk, Charles L. 2002. *Forgive and Remember: Managing Medical Failure*. 2nd ed. Chicago: University of Chicago Press.

Botlhomilwe, Mokganedi Zara, and David Sebududu. 2011. "Elections in Botswana: A Ritual Enterprise?" *The Open Area Studies Journal* 4 (1): 96–103.

Botlhomilwe, Mokganedi Zara, David Sebududu, and Bugalo Maripe. 2011. "Limited Freedom and Intolerance in Botswana." *Journal of Contemporary African Studies* 29 (3): 331–48.

Bourdieu, Pierre. 1977. *Outline of a Theory of Practice*. Translated by Richard Nice. Cambridge: Cambridge University Press.

——. 1990. "The Work of Time." In *The Logic of Practice*, translated by Richard Nice, 98–111. Cambridge, UK: Polity Press.

Bourdieu, Pierre, and Jean-Claude Passeron. 1970. *Reproduction in Education, Society and Culture*. Translated by Richard Nice. London: Sage.

Bourgois, Philippe. 2000. "Disciplining Addictions: The Bio-Politics of Methadone and Heroin in the United States." *Culture, Medicine and Psychiatry* 24 (2): 165–95.

Bowker, Geoffrey C., and Susan Leigh Star. 1999. *Sorting Things Out: Classification and Its Consequences*. Cambridge, MA: MIT Press.

Boyer, Dominic. 2008. "Thinking through the Anthropology of Experts." *Anthropology in Action* 15 (2): 38–46.

Brada, Betsey Behr. 2013. "How to Do Things to Children with Words: Language, Ritual, and Apocalypse in Pediatric HIV Treatment in Botswana." *American Ethnologist* 40 (3): 437–51.

——. 2016. "The Contingency of Humanitarianism: Moral Authority in an African HIV Clinic." *American Anthropologist* 118 (4): 755–71.

——. 2017. "Exemplary or Exceptional? The Production and Dismantling of Global Health in Botswana." In *Global Health Geographies*, edited by Clare Herrick and David Reubi, 40–53. New York: Routledge.

——. 2019. "Between Discipline and Empowerment: Temporal Ambivalence at a Sleepaway Camp for HIV-Positive Children in Botswana." *Anthropological Quarterly* 92 (1): 173–202.

Brancati, Frederick L. 1989. "The Art of Pimping." *Journal of the American Medical Association* 262 (1): 89–90.

Briggs, Charles L. 2004. "Theorizing Modernity Conspiratorially: Science, Scale, and the Political Economy of Public Discourse in Explanations of a Cholera Epidemic." *American Ethnologist* 31 (2): 164–187.

——. 2007. "Mediating Infanticide: Theorizing Relations between Narrative and Violence." *Cultural Anthropology* 22 (3): 315–56.

Briggs, Charles L., and Paja Faudree. 2016. "Communicating Bodies." *Anthropology News* 57 (5): e7–8.

Briggs, Charles L., and Clara Mantini-Briggs. 2003. *Stories in the Time of Cholera: Racial Profiling during a Medical Nightmare*. Berkeley: University of California Press.

——. 2016. *Tell Me Why My Children Died: Rabies, Indigenous Knowledge, and Communicative Justice*. Durham, NC: Duke University Press.

Briggs, Charles, and Mark Nichter. 2009. "Biocommunicability and the Biopolitics of Pandemic Threats: Medical Anthropology." *Medical Anthropology* 28 (3): 189–98.

Brodwin, Paul. 2010. "The Assemblage of Compliance in Psychiatric Case Management." *Anthropology & Medicine* 17 (2): 129–43.

——. 2011. "Futility in the Practice of Community Psychiatry." *Medical Anthropology Quarterly* 25 (2): 189–208.

Brown, Hannah. 2015. "Global Health Partnerships, Governance, and Sovereign Responsibility in Western Kenya." *American Ethnologist* 42 (2): 340–55.

Brown, Theodore M., Marcos Cueto, and Elizabeth Fee. 2006. "The World Health Organization and the Transition From 'International' to 'Global' Public Health." *American Journal of Public Health* 96 (1): 62–72.

Brown, Tim, and Morag Bell. 2008. "Imperial or Postcolonial Governance? Dissecting the Genealogy of a Global Public Health Strategy." *Social Science & Medicine* 67 (10): 1571–79.

Brown, Tim, Susan Craddock, and Alan Ingram. 2012. "Critical Interventions in Global Health: Governmentality, Risk, and Assemblage." *Annals of the Association of American Geographers* 102 (5): 1182–89.

Bruni, Frank. 2001. "Deep U.S.-Europe Split Casts Long Shadow on Bush Tour." *The New York Times*, June 15, 2001, A6. https://www.nytimes.com/2001/06/15/world/deep-us-europe-split-casts-long-shadow-on-bush-tour.html.

Bryant, Coralie, Betsy Stephens, and Sherry MacLiver. 1978. "Rural to Urban Migration: Some Data from Botswana." *African Studies Review* 21 (2): 85–99.

Buchbinder, Mara. 2009. "The Management of Autonomy in Adolescent Diabetes: A Case Study of Triadic Medical Interaction." *Health* 13 (2): 175–96.

——. 2015. *All in Your Head: Making Sense of Pediatric Pain*. Berkeley: University of California Press.

Bucholtz, Mary, and Kira Hall. 2005. "Identity and Interaction: A Sociocultural Linguistic Approach." *Discourse Studies* 7 (4–5): 585–614.

Burke, Charlanne. 2000. "They Cut Segametsi into Parts: Ritual Murder, Youth, and the Politics of Knowledge in Botswana." *Anthropological Quarterly* 73 (4): 204–14.

Buse, Kent, and Gill Walt. 2009. "The World Health Organization and Global Private-Public Health Partnerships: In Search of 'Good' Global Health Governance." In *The Global Social Policy Reader*, edited by Nicola Yeates and Chris Holden, 105–216. Bristol, UK: Policy Press.

Bussmann, Hermann, C. William Wester, Ndwapi Ndwapi, Chris Vanderwarker, Tendani Gaolathe, Geoffrey Tirelo, Ava Avalos, Howard Moffat, and Richard G. Marlink. 2006. "Hybrid Data Capture for Monitoring Patients on Highly Active Antiretroviral Therapy (HAART) in Urban Botswana." *Bulletin of the World Health Organization* 84 (2): 127–31.

Butler, Judith. 1990. *Gender Trouble: Feminism and the Subversion of Identity*. New York: Routledge.

Butt, Leslie. 2002a. "Reply to Alec Irwin, Joyce Millen, Jim Kim, John Gershman, Brooke G. Schoepf, and Paul Farmer." *Medical Anthropology* 21 (January): 31–33.

——. 2002b. "The Suffering Stranger: Medical Anthropology and International Morality." *Medical Anthropology* 21 (January): 1–24.

Byrd, W. Michael, and Linda A. Clayton. 2002. *An American Health Dilemma: Race, Medicine, and Health Care in the United States, 1900–2000*. Vol. 2. New York: Routledge.

Campbell, E. K. 2003. "Attitudes of Botswana Citizens toward Immigrants: Signs of Xenophobia?" *International Migration* 41 (4): 71–111.

Carpenter, Elise Audrey. 2008. "The Social Practice of HIV Drug Therapy in Botswana, 2002–2004: Experts, Bureaucrats, and Health Care Providers." PhD diss., Philadelphia: University of Pennsylvania.

Carr, E. Summerson. 2006. "'Secrets Keep You Sick': Metalinguistic Labor in a Drug Treatment Program for Homeless Women." *Language in Society* 35 (5): 631–53.

——. 2009. "Anticipating and Inhabiting Institutional Identities." *American Ethnologist* 36 (2): 317–36.

——. 2010a. "Enactments of Expertise." *Annual Review of Anthropology* 39 (October): 17–32.

——. 2010b. *Scripting Addiction: The Politics of Therapeutic Talk and American Sobriety.* Princeton, NJ: Princeton University Press.

Carr, E. Summerson, and Brooke Fisher. 2016. "Interscaling Awe, De-Escalating Disaster." In *Scale: Discourse and Dimensions of Social Life*, edited by E. Summerson Carr and Michael Lempert, 133–58. Berkeley: University of California Press.

Carr, E. Summerson, and Michael Lempert. 2016. "Introduction: Pragmatics of Scale." In *Scale: Discourse and Dimensions of Social Life*, edited by E. Summerson Carr, 1–24. Berkeley: University of California Press.

Cassell, Joan. 1996. "The Woman in the Surgeon's Body: Understanding Difference." *American Anthropologist* 98 (1): 41–53.

——. 1998. *The Woman in the Surgeon's Body.* Cambridge, MA: Harvard University Press.

Castro, Arachu, and Paul Farmer. 2005. "Understanding and Addressing AIDS-Related Stigma: From Anthropological Theory to Clinical Practice in Haiti." *American Journal of Public Health* 95 (1): 53–59.

Chelenyane, Mothusi, and Ruth Endacott. 2006. "Self-Reported Infection Control Practices and Perceptions of HIV/AIDS Risk amongst Emergency Department Nurses in Botswana." *Accident and Emergency Nursing* 14 (3): 148–54.

Chen, Peggy Guey-Chi, Leslie Ann Curry, Susannah May Bernheim, David Berg, Aysegul Gozu, and Marcella Nunez-Smith. 2011. "Professional Challenges of Non-U.S.-Born International Medical Graduates and Recommendations for Support during Residency Training." *Academic Medicine* 86 (11): 1383–88.

Chesney, Margaret A., and Ashley W. Smith. 1999. "Critical Delays in HIV Testing and Care: The Potential Role of Stigma." *American Behavioral Scientist* 42 (7): 1162–74.

CHGA (Commission on HIV/AIDS and Governance in Africa). 2004. "Scaling Up AIDS Treatment in Africa: Issues and Challenges. Background Paper for CHGA Interactive, Gaborone." Gaborone, Botswana.

Chumley, Lily Hope. 2013. "Evaluation Regimes and the Qualia of Quality." *Anthropological Theory* 13 (1/2): 169–83.

——. 2016. *Creativity Class: Art School and Culture Work in Postsocialist China.* Princeton, NJ: Princeton University Press.

Chumley, Lily Hope, and Nicholas Harkness. 2013. "Introduction: Qualia." *Anthropological Theory* 13 (1/2): 3–11.

Citrin, David. 2011. "'Paul Farmer Made Me Do It': A Qualitative Study of Short-Term Medical Volunteer Work in Northwest Nepal." Master's thesis, Department of Global Health, School of Public Health, Seattle, University of Washington.

Cohen, Lawrence. 2012. "Making Peasants Protestant and Other Projects: Medical Anthropology and Its Global Condition." In *Medical Anthropology at the Intersections: Histories, Activisms, and Futures*, edited by Marcia Inhorn and Emily Wentzell, 65–92. Durham, NC: Duke University Press.

Collins, H. M., and Robert Evans. 2002. "The Third Wave of Science Studies: Studies of Expertise and Experience." *Social Studies of Science* 32 (2): 235–96.

Comaroff, Jean. 1985. *Body of Power, Spirit of Resistance: The Culture and History of a South African People.* Chicago: University of Chicago Press.

——. 1993. "The Diseased Heart of Africa: Medicine, Colonialism, and the Black Body." In *Knowledge, Power and Practice: The Anthropology of Medicine and Everyday Life*, edited by Shirley Lindenbaum and Margaret Lock, 305–29. Berkeley: University of California Press.

——. 1996. "Reading, Rioting and Arithmetic: The Impact of Mission Education on Black Consciousness in South Africa." *Bulletin of the Institute of Ethnology, Academia Sinica* 82: 19–63.

——. 2007. "Beyond Bare Life: AIDS, (Bio)Politics, and the Neoliberal Order." *Public Culture* 19 (1): 197–219.

Comaroff, Jean, and John L. Comaroff. 1991. *Christianity, Colonialism, and Consciousness in South Africa*. Vol. 1 of *Of Revelation and Revolution*. Chicago: University of Chicago Press.

——. 2000. "Millennial Capitalism: First Thoughts on a Second Coming." *Public Culture* 12 (2): 291–343.

Comaroff, John L. 1978. "Rules and Rulers: Political Processes in a Tswana Chiefdom." *Man* 13 (1): 1.

——. 1989. "Images of Empire, Contests of Conscience: Models of Colonial Domination in South Africa." *American Ethnologist* 16 (4): 661–85.

Comaroff, John L., and Jean Comaroff. 1997a. *The Dialectics of Modernity on a South African Frontier*. Vol 2. of *Of Revelation and Revolution*. Chicago: University of Chicago Press.

——. 1997b. "Postcolonial Politics and Discourses of Democracy in Southern Africa: An Anthropological Reflection on African Political Modernities." *Journal of Anthropological Research* 53 (2): 123–46.

——. 1999. "Introduction." In *Civil Society and the Political Imagination in Africa: Critical Perspectives*, edited by John L. Comaroff and Jean Comaroff, 1–43. Chicago: University of Chicago Press.

——. 2001. "On Personhood: An Anthropological Perspective from Africa." *Social Identities* 7 (2): 267–83.

Cook, Daniel Thomas. 2004. *The Commodification of Childhood: The Children's Clothing Industry and the Rise of the Child Consumer*. Durham, NC: Duke University Press.

Cooper, Amy. 2015. "The Doctor's Political Body: Doctor–Patient Interactions and Sociopolitical Belonging in Venezuelan State Clinics." *American Ethnologist* 42 (3): 459–74.

Cooper, Frederick. 2005. *Colonialism in Question*. Berkeley: University of California Press.

Cooper, Frederick, and Randall Packard, eds. 1997. *International Development and the Social Sciences*. Berkeley: University of California Press.

Cooper, Frederick, and Ann Laura Stoler. 1997. *Tensions of Empire: Colonial Cultures in a Bourgeois World*. Berkeley: University of California Press.

Craig, Sienna R. 2011. "'Good' Manufacturing by Whose Standards? Remaking Concepts of Quality, Safety, and Value in the Production of Tibetan Medicines." *Anthropological Quarterly* 84 (2): 331–78.

Cramblit, M. Mackenzie. 2017. "Hopeful Engagement: The Sentimental Education of University-Sponsored Service Learning." In *Anthropological Perspectives on Student Futures: Youth and the Politics of Possibility*, edited by Amy Stambach and Kathleen D. Hall, 133–56. Anthropological Studies of Education. New York: Palgrave Macmillan US.

Crane, Johanna. 2010a. "Unequal 'Partners.' AIDS, Academia, and the Rise of Global Health." *Behemoth: A Journal on Civilisation* 3 (3): 78–97.

——. 2010b. "Adverse Events and Placebo Effects: African Scientists, HIV, and Ethics in the 'Global Health Sciences.'" *Social Studies of Science* 40 (6): 843–70.

——. 2013. *Scrambling for Africa: AIDS, Expertise, and the Rise of American Global Health Science*. Ithaca, NY: Cornell University Press.

——. 2018. "Global Health Enabling Systems: Accounting and Critique in the Era of 'America First.'" *Medicine Anthropology Theory: An Open-Access Journal in the Anthropology of Health, Illness, and Medicine* 5 (2): 167.

Crane, Johanna, Irene Andia Biraro, Tamer M. Fouad, Yap II Boum, and David R. Bangsberg. 2018. "The 'Indirect Costs' of Underfunding Foreign Partners in Global Health Research: A Case Study." *Global Public Health* 13 (10): 1422–29.

Crapanzano, Vincent. 1980. *Tuhami: A Portrait of a Morrocan*. Chicago: University of Chicago Press.

Csordas, Thomas J. 2007. "Review of Vita: Life in a Zone of Social Abandonment by João Biehl." *American Ethnologist* 34 (2): 12.

Cueto, Marcos. 2004. "The Origins of Primary Health Care and Selective Primary Health Care." *American Journal of Public Health* 94 (11): 1864–74.

Dahl, Bianca. 2009. "The 'Failures of Culture': Christianity, Kinship, and Moral Discourses about Orphans during Botswana's AIDS Crisis." *Africa Today* 56 (1): 22–43.

——. 2012. "Beyond the Blame Paradigm: Rethinking Witchcraft Gossip and Stigma around HIV-Positive Children in Southeastern Botswana." *African Historical Review* 44 (1): 53–79.

——. 2014. "'Too Fat to Be an Orphan': The Moral Semiotics of Food Aid in Botswana." *Cultural Anthropology* 29 (4): 626–47.

——. 2015. "Sexy Orphans and Sugar Daddies: The Sexual and Moral Politics of Aid for AIDS in Botswana." *Studies in Comparative International Development* 50 (4): 519–38.

——. 2016. "The Drama of De-Orphaning: Botswana's Old Orphans and the Rewriting of Kinship Relations." *Social Dynamics* 42 (2): 289–303.

Darkoh, Ernest. 2004. *Fighting HIV/AIDS in Africa: A Progress Report. Testimony before the Subcommittee on African Affairs of the Committee on Foreign Relations, United States Senate, April 7th*. Washington, DC.

Das, Veena, Arthur Kleinman, Mamphela Ramphele, and Pamela Reynolds, eds. 2000. *Violence and Subjectivity*. Berkeley: University of California Press.

Daston, Lorraine, and Peter Galison. 2010. *Objectivity*. Brooklyn, NY: Zone Books.

Davidson, Deanna. 2007. "East Spaces in West Times: Deictic Reference and Political Self-Positioning in a Post-Socialist East German Chronotope." *Language & Communication* 27 (3): 212–26.

Davis, Julie Hirschfeld, Sheryl Gay Stolberg, and Thomas Kaplan. 2018. "Trump Alarms Lawmakers with Disparaging Words for Haiti and Africa." *The New York Times*, January 11, 2018. https://www.nytimes.com/2018/01/11/us/politics/trump-shithole-countries.html.

de Beauvoir, Simone. 1989. *The Second Sex*. Edited and translated by H. M. Parshley. New York: Vintage Books.

Decoteau, Claire Laurier. 2013. *Ancestors and Antiretrovirals: The Biopolitics of HIV/AIDS in Post-Apartheid South Africa*. Chicago: University of Chicago Press.

Dewey, J. 1938. *Experience and Education*. New York: Collier Books.

Dilger, Hansjörg, and Dominik Mattes. 2018. "Im/Mobilities and Dis/Connectivities in Medical Globalisation: How Global Is Global Health?" *Global Public Health* 13 (3): 265–75.

Dinnen, Sinclair, and Matthew Allen. 2016. "State Absence and State Formation in Solomon Islands: Reflections on Agency, Scale and Hybridity." *Development and Change* 47 (1): 76–97.

Domek, Gretchen J. 2006. "Social Consequences of Antiretroviral Therapy: Preparing for the Unexpected Futures of HIV-Positive Children." *The Lancet* 367 (9519): 1367–69.

Douglas-Jones, Rachel, and Justin Shaffner. 2017. "Introduction: Capacity Building in Ethnographic Comparison." *Cambridge Journal of Anthropology* 35 (1): 1–16.

Drain, Paul K., Aron Primack, D. Dan Hunt, Wafaie W. Fawzi, King K. Holmes, and Pierce Gardner. 2007. "Global Health in Medical Education: A Call for More Training and Opportunities." *Academic Medicine* 82 (3): 226–30.

Dreesch, Norbert, Jennifer Nyoni, Ontlametse Mokopakgosi, Khumo Seipone, Jean Alfazema Kalilani, Owen Kaluwa, and Vincent Musowe. 2007. "Public-Private Options for Expanding Access to Human Resources for HIV/AIDS in Botswana." *Human Resources for Health* 5 (1): 25.

Du Bois, John W. 2007. "The Stance Triangle." In *Stancetaking in Discourse: Subjectivity, Evaluation, Interaction*, edited by Robert Englebretson, 139–82. Philadelphia: John Benjamins.

Du Bois, John W., and Elise Kärkkäinen. 2012. "Taking a Stance on Emotion: Affect, Sequence, and Intersubjectivity in Dialogic Interaction." *Text & Talk* 32 (4): 433–51.

Dubal, Sam. 2012. "Renouncing Paul Farmer: A Desperate Plea for Radical Political Medicine." *Being Ethical in an Unethical World* (blog). May 27, 2012. http://samdubal .blogspot.com/2012/05/renouncing-paul-farmer-desperate-plea.html.

——. 2018. *Against Humanity: Lessons from the Lord's Resistance Army*. Berkeley: University of California Press.

Duranti, Alessandro, and Charles Goodwin, eds. 1992. *Rethinking Context: Language as an Interactive Phenomenon*. Cambridge: Cambridge University Press.

Durham, Deborah. 1999. "Civil Lives: Leadership and Accomplishment in Botswana." In *Civil Society and the Political Imagination in Africa: Critical Perspectives*, edited by John L. Comaroff and Jean Comaroff, 192–218. Chicago: University of Chicago Press.

——. 2004. "Disappearing Youth: Youth as a Social Shifter in Botswana." *American Ethnologist* 31 (4): 589–605.

——. 2005. "Did You Bathe This Morning?: Baths and Morality in Botswana." In *Dirt, Undress, and Difference: Critical Perspectives on the Body's Surface*, edited by Adeline Masquelier, 190–212. Bloomington: Indiana University Press.

Durham, Deborah, and Frederick Klaits. 2002. "Funerals and the Public Space of Sentiment in Botswana." *Journal of Southern African Studies* 28 (4): 777–95.

Englebretson, Robert. 2007. "Stancetaking in Discourse: An Introduction." In *Stancetaking in Discourse: Subjectivity, Evaluation, Interaction*, edited by Robert Englebretson, 1–26. Philadelphia: John Benjamins.

Epstein, Helen. 2007. *The Invisible Cure: Africa, the West, and the Fight against AIDS*. New York: Farrar, Straus and Giroux.

Epstein, Steven. 2008. *Inclusion: The Politics of Difference in Medical Research*. Chicago: University of Chicago Press.

Erikson, Susan L. 2012. "Global Health Business: The Production and Performativity of Statistics in Sierra Leone and Germany." *Global Public Health* 31 (4): 367–84.

——. 2015. "Global Health Indicators and Maternal Health Futures: The Case of Intrauterine Growth Restriction." *Global Public Health* 10 (10): 1157–71.

Escobar, Arturo. 1995. *Encountering Development: The Making and Unmaking of the Third World*. Princeton, NJ: Princeton University Press.

Evert, Jessica, Andrew Bazemore, Allen Hixon, and Kelley Withy. 2007. "Going Global: Considerations for Introducing Global Health into Family Medicine Training Programs." *Family Medicine* 39 (9): 659–65.

Fabian, Johannes. 1983. *Time and the Other: How Anthropology Makes Its Object*. New York: Columbia University Press.

Fako, Thabo T., and Ntonghanwah Forchen. 2000. "Job Satisfaction among Nurses in Botswana." *Society in Transition* 31 (1): 10–21.

Falgiani, Tricia, Christopher Kennedy, and Sara Jahnke. 2014. "Exploration of the Barriers and Education Needs of Non-Pediatric Hospital Emergency Department Providers in Pediatric Trauma Care." *International Journal of Clinical Medicine* 5 (January): 56.

Farley, Maggie. 2001. "At AIDS Disaster's Epicenter, Botswana Is a Model of Action." *Los Angeles Times*, June 27, 2001. http://articles.latimes.com/2001/jun/27/news/mn -15017.

Farmer, Paul. 1992. "AIDS and an Anthropology of Suffering." In *AIDS and Accusation: Haiti and the Geography of Blame*, 211–20. Berkeley: University of California Press.

——. 1996. "On Suffering and Structural Violence: A View from Below." *Daedalus* 125 (1): 261–83.

——. 1999. *Infections and Inequalities: The Modern Plagues*. Berkeley: University of California Press.

——. 2004. "An Anthropology of Structural Violence." *Current Anthropology* 45 (3): 305–25.

Farmer, Paul, Jim Yong Kim, Arthur Kleinman, and Matthew Basilico. 2013. *Reimagining Global Health: An Introduction*. Berkeley: University of California Press.

Farquhar, Judith. 1994. "Eating Chinese Medicine." *Cultural Anthropology* 9 (4): 471–97.

——. 2002. *Appetites: Food and Sex in Post-Socialist China*. Durham, NC: Duke University Press.

Fassin, Didier. 2007. "Humanitarianism as a Politics of Life." *Public Culture* 19 (3): 499–520.

——. 2008. "The Humanitarian Politics of Testimony: Subjectification through Trauma in the Israeli–Palestinian Conflict." *Cultural Anthropology* 23 (3): 531–58.

——. 2012. "That Obscure Object of Global Health." In *Medical Anthropology at the Intersections: Histories, Activisms, and Futures*, edited by Marcia C. Inhorn and Emily A. Wentzell, 95–115. Durham, NC: Duke University Press.

——. 2013. "Children as Victims: The Moral Economy of Childhood in the Times of AIDS." In *When People Come First: Critical Studies in Global Health*, edited by João Guilherme Biehl and Adriana Petryna, 109–32. Princeton, NJ: Princeton University Press.

Faudree, Paja. 2015. "Tales from the Land of Magic Plants: Textual Ideologies and Fetishes of Indigeneity in Mexico's Sierra Mazateca." *Comparative Studies in Society and History* 57 (3): 838–69.

——. 2020. "'Making Medicine' with Salvia Divinorum: Competing Approaches and Their Implications." *Medical Anthropology* 39 (7): 582–96.

Feierman, Steven. 2011. "When Physicians Meet: Local Medical Knowledge and Global Public Goods." In *Evidence, Ethos and Ethnography: The Anthropology and History of Medical Research in Africa*, edited by P. Wenzel Geissler and Catherine Molyneux, 171–96. Oxford, UK: Berghahn.

Ferguson, James. 1990. *The Anti-Politics Machine: "Development," Depoliticization, and Bureaucratic Power in Lesotho*. Cambridge: Cambridge University Press.

——. 1997. "Anthropology and Its Evil Twin: 'Development' in the Constitution of a Discipline." In *International Development and the Social Sciences: Essays on the History and Politics of Knowledge*, edited by Frederick Cooper and Randall Packard, 150–75. Berkeley: University of California Press.

——. 1999. *Expectations of Modernity: Myths and Meanings of Urban Life on the Zambian Copperbelt*. Berkeley: University of California Press.

——. 2006a. "Decomposing Modernity: History and Hierarchy after Development." In *Global Shadows: Africa in the Neoliberal World Order*, 176–93. Durham, NC: Duke University Press.

——. 2006b. *Global Shadows: Africa in the Neoliberal World Order*. Durham, NC: Duke University Press.

Feudtner, Chris, Dimitri A. Christakis, and Nicholas A. Christakis. 1994. "Do Clinical Clerks Suffer Ethical Erosion? Students' Perceptions of Their Ethical Environment and Personal Development." *Academic Medicine* 69 (8): 670–79.

Fidler, David. 2007. "Architecture Amidst Anarchy: Global Health's Quest for Governance." *Articles by Maurer Faculty* 329: 18.

——. 2008. "A Theory of Open-Source Anarchy." *Indiana Journal of Global Legal Studies* 15 (1): 259–84.

Fine, Michelle, and Adrienne Asch. 1988. "Disability Beyond Stigma: Social Interaction, Discrimination, and Activism." *Journal of Social Issues* 44 (1): 3–21.

Foucault, Michel. 1975. *The Birth of the Clinic: An Archaeology of Medical Perception.* Translated by Alan M. Sheridan-Smith. New York: Vintage Books.

——. 1977. *Discipline and Punish: The Birth of the Prison.* Translated by Alan Sheridan. New York: Pantheon Books.

——. 1978. *The History of Sexuality: An Introduction.* Vol. 1. New York: Pantheon Books.

——. 1985. *The History of Sexuality: The Use of Pleasure.* Vol. 2. New York: Pantheon Books.

——. 1991. "Governmentality." In *The Foucault Effect*, edited by Graham Burchell, Colin Gordon, and Peter Miller, 87–104. Chicago: University of Chicago Press.

——. 1998. "Technologies of the Self." In *Technologies of the Self: A Seminar with Michel Foucault*, edited by Luther Martin, Huck Gutman, and Patrick H. Hutton, 16–49. Amherst: University of Massachusetts Press.

Fountain, T. Kenny. 2014. *Rhetoric in the Flesh: Trained Vision, Technical Expertise, and the Gross Anatomy Lab.* New York: Routledge.

Fox, Renée. 1963. "Training for 'Detached Concern' in Medical Students." In *The Psychological Basis of Medical Practice*, edited by Harold Lief, 12–35. New York: Harper and Row.

——. 1999. "Is Medical Education Asking Too Much of Bioethics?" *Daedalus* 128 (4): 1–25.

Fraser, Heather, and Nik Taylor. 2016. *Neoliberalization, Universities and the Public Intellectual: Species, Gender and Class and the Production of Knowledge.* New York: Springer.

Freire, Paulo. 1970. *Pedagogy of the Oppressed: 50th Anniversary Edition.* Translated by Myra Bergman Ramos. New York: Bloomsbury.

Friesen, Phoebe. 2018. "Educational Pelvic Exams on Anesthetized Women: Why Consent Matters." *Bioethics* 32 (5): 298–307.

Fuller, Bruce, and Conrad W. Snyder. 1991. "Vocal Teachers, Silent Pupils? Life in Botswana Classrooms." *Comparative Education Review* 35 (2): 274–94.

Fullwiley, Duana. 2011. *The Encultured Gene: Sickle Cell Health Politics and Biological Difference in West Africa.* Princeton, NJ: Princeton University Press.

Funck-Brentano, Isabelle, Dominique Costagliola, Nathalie Seibel, Elisabeth Straub, Marc Tardieu, and Stéphane Blanche. 1997. "Patterns of Disclosure and Perceptions of the Human Immunodeficiency Virus in Infected Elementary School-Age Children." *Archives of Pediatrics & Adolescent Medicine* 151 (10): 978–85.

Gal, Susan. 1991. "Between Speech and Silence: The Problematics of Research on Language and Gender." In *Gender at the Crossroads of Knowledge: Feminist Anthropology in the Postmodern Era*, edited by Micaela Di Leonardo, 175–203. Berkeley: University of California Press.

——. 2002. "A Semiotics of the Public/Private Distinction." *Differences: A Journal of Feminist Cultural Studies* 13 (1): 77–95.

——. 2005. "Language Ideologies Compared: Metaphors of Public/Private." *Journal of Linguistic Anthropology* 15 (1): 23–37.

———. 2016. "Scale-Making: Comparison and Perspective as Ideological Projects." In *Scale: Discourse and Dimensions of Social Life*, edited by E. Summerson Carr and Michael Lempert, 91–111. Berkeley: University of California Press.

Gamble, Vanessa Northington. 1997. "Under the Shadow of Tuskegee: African Americans and Health Care." *American Journal of Public Health* 87 (11): 1773–78.

Garrett, Laurie. 2007. "The Challenge of Global Health." *Foreign Affairs* 86 (1): 14–38.

Garrett, Paul B., and Patricia Baquedano-López. 2002. "Language Socialization: Reproduction and Continuity, Transformation and Change." *Annual Review of Anthropology* 31 (1): 339–61.

Gayle, Helene, Gordon LaForge, and Anne-Marie Slaughter. 2021. "America Can—and Should—Vaccinate the World." *Foreign Affairs*. https://www.foreignaffairs.com/articles/united-states/2021-03-19/america-can-and-should-vaccinate-the-world.

Geest, Sjaak van der, Susan Reynolds Whyte, and Anita Hardon. 1996. "The Anthropology of Pharmaceuticals: A Biographical Approach." *Annual Review of Anthropology* 25 (1): 153–78.

Geiger, Martha, and Erna Alant. 2005. "Child-Rearing Practices and Children's Communicative Interactions in a Village in Botswana." *Early Years* 25 (2): 183–91.

Geissler, P. Wenzel. 2005. "'Kachinja Are Coming!': Encounters around Medical Research Work in a Kenyan Village." *Africa* 75 (2): 173–202.

———. 2011. "Studying Trial Communities: Anthropological and Historical Inquiries into Ethos, Politics and Economy of Medical Research in Africa." In *Evidence, Ethos, and Experiment: The Anthropology and History of Medical Research in Africa*, edited by P. Wenzel Geissler and Catherine Molyneux, 1–28. New York: Berghahn.

———. 2013. "Public Secrets in Public Health: Knowing Not to Know While Making Scientific Knowledge." *American Ethnologist* 40 (1): 13–34.

———. 2015. *Para-States and Medical Science: Making African Global Health*. Durham, NC: Duke University Press.

Geissler, P. Wenzel, and Catherine Molyneux, eds. 2011. *Evidence, Ethos and Experiment: The Anthropology and History of Medical Research in Africa*. New York: Berghahn.

Geissler, P. Wenzel, and Noémi Tousignant. 2016. "Capacity as History and Horizon: Infrastructure, Autonomy and Future in African Health Science and Care." *Canadian Journal of African Studies/Revue Canadienne Des Études Africaines* 50 (3): 349–59.

Gerrets, Rene. 2015. "International Health and the Proliferation of 'Partnerships': (Un) Intended Boost for State Institutions in Tanzania?" In *Critical Global Health: Evidence, Efficacy, Ethnography*, edited by P. Wenzel Geissler, 176–206 Durham, NC: Duke University Press.

Gershon, Ilana. 2011. "'Neoliberal Agency.'" *Current Anthropology* 52 (4): 537–55.

Gianakos, Dean. 1996. "Empathy Revisited." *Archives of Internal Medicine* 156 (2): 135–36.

Giles, Dwight E., Jr., and Janet Eyler. 1994. "The Theoretical Roots of Service-Learning in John Dewey: Toward a Theory of Service-Learning." *Michigan Journal of Community Service Learning* 1 (1): 77–85.

Gilles, Jonathan. 2005. "Taking a Medical History in Childhood Illness: Representations of Parents in Pediatric Texts since 1850." *Bulletin of the History of Medicine* 79 (3): 393–429.

Gilles, Jonathan, and Patricia Loughlan. 2007. "Not Just Small Adults: The Metaphors of Pediatrics." *Archives of Disease in Childhood* 92 (11): 946–47.

Giroux, Henry A. 1981. *Ideology, Culture, and the Process of Schooling*. Philadelphia: Temple University Press.

Gluckman, Max. 1963. "Gossip and Scandal (Papers in Honor of Melville J. Herskovits)." *Current Anthropology* 4 (3): 307–16.

Goffman, Erving. 1956. "The Nature of Deference and Demeanor." *American Anthropologist* 58 (3): 473–502.

——. 1963. *Stigma: Notes on the Management of Spoiled Identity.* New York: Simon and Schuster.

——. 1967. *Interaction Ritual: Essays in Face to Face Behavior.* Chicago: Aldine Publishing Co.

Good, Byron J. 1993a. "How Medicine Constructs Its Objects." In *Medicine, Rationality, and Experience: An Anthropological Perspective*, 65–87. Cambridge: Cambridge University Press.

——. 1993b. *Medicine, Rationality and Experience: An Anthropological Perspective.* Cambridge University Press.

Good, Kenneth. 1992. "Interpreting the Exceptionality of Botswana." *Journal of Modern African Studies* 30 (1): 69–95.

——. 1993. "At the Ends of the Ladder: Radical Inequalities in Botswana." *Journal of Modern African Studies* 31 (2): 203–30.

——. 1996. "Authoritarian Liberalism: A Defining Characteristic of Botswana." *Journal of Contemporary African Studies* 14 (1): 29–51.

——. 1999. "The State and Extreme Poverty in Botswana: The San and Destitutes." *Journal of Modern African Studies* 37 (2): 185–205.

——. 2008. *Diamonds, Dispossession and Democracy in Botswana.* Oxford, UK: James Currey.

——. 2010. "The Presidency of General Ian Khama: The Militarization of the Botswana 'Miracle.'" *African Affairs* 109 (435): 315–24.

Good, Mary-Jo DelVecchio. 1995. *American Medicine: The Quest for Competence.* Berkeley: University of California Press.

Goodwin, Charles. 1994. "Professional Vision." *American Anthropologist* 96 (3): 606–33.

Gordon, Deborah R., and Eugenio Paci. 1997. "Disclosure Practices and Cultural Narratives: Understanding Concealment and Silence around Cancer in Tuscany, Italy." *Social Science & Medicine* 44 (10): 1433–52.

Gostin, Lawrence O., and Emily A. Mok. 2009. "Grand Challenges in Global Health Governance." *British Medical Bulletin* 90 (1): 7–18.

Government of Botswana. 2004. *Botswana HIV/AIDS Impact Survey II.* Gaborone: Government Press.

——. 2006. "Botswana Demographic Survey 2006." Gaborone, Botswana: Central Statistics Office.

Graboyes, Melissa. 2015. *The Experiment Must Continue: Medical Research and Ethics in East Africa, 1940–2014.* Athens: Ohio University Press.

Grady, Denise. 2010. "Restoring the Lost Art of the Physical Exam." *The New York Times*, October 11, 2010. https://www.nytimes.com/2010/10/12/health/12profile.html.

Gramsci, Antonio. 1971. *Selections from Prison Notebooks.* Edited by Q. Hoare and G. Nowell Smith. New York: International Publishers.

Grant, Jenna M. 2016. "From Subjects to Relations: Bioethics and the Articulation of Postcolonial Politics in the Cambodia Pre-Exposure Prophylaxis Trial." *Social Studies of Science* 46 (2): 236–58.

Gray, Glenda E. 2010. "Adolescent HIV—Cause for Concern in Southern Africa." *PLoS Medicine* 7 (2): 1–4.

Greene, Jeremy A. 2004. "Therapeutic Infidelities: 'Non-Compliance' Enters the Medical Literature, 1955–1975." *Social History of Medicine* 17 (3): 327–43.

——. 2011. "Making Medicines Essential: The Emergent Centrality of Pharmaceuticals in Global Health." *BioSocieties* 6 (1): 10–33.

Grudzen, Corita R., and Eric Legome. 2007. "Loss of International Medical Experiences: Knowledge, Attitudes and Skills at Risk." *BMC Medical Education* 7 (1): 1–5.

Gruffydd Jones, Branwen. 2013. "'Good Governance' and 'State Failure': Genealogies of Imperial Discourse." *Cambridge Review of International Affairs* 26 (1): 49–70.

Gulbrandsen, Ørnulf. 2012. *The State and the Social: State Formation in Botswana and Its Pre-Colonial and Colonial Genealogies.* New York: Berghahn.

Gupta, Akhil, and James Ferguson. 1992. "Beyond 'Culture': Space, Identity, and the Politics of Difference." *Cultural Anthropology* 7 (1): 6–23.

Guzmán, Jennifer R. 2014. "The Epistemics of Symptom Experience and Symptom Accounts in Mapuche Healing and Pediatric Primary Care in Southern Chile." *Journal of Linguistic Anthropology* 24 (3): 249–76.

Hacking, Ian. 1996. "The Disunity of the Sciences." In *The Disunity of Science: Boundaries, Contexts, and Power*, edited by Peter Louis Galison and David J. Stump, 37–74. Stanford, CA: Stanford University Press.

Hall, Kira. 1999. "Performativity." *Journal of Linguistic Anthropology* 9 (1–2): 184–87.

Hammer, Gili. 2018. "'You Can Learn Merely by Listening to the Way a Patient Walks through the Door': The Transmission of Sensory Medical Knowledge." *Medical Anthropology Quarterly* 32 (1): 138–54.

Hankins, Joseph D. 2014. *Working Skin: Making Leather, Making a Multicultural Japan.* Berkeley: University of California Press.

Hanna, Bridget, and Arthur Kleinman. 2013. "Unpacking Global Health: Theory and Critique." In *Reimagining Global Health: An Introduction*, edited by Paul Farmer, Jim Yong Kim, Arthur Kleinman, and Matthew Basilico, 15–32. Berkeley: University of California Press.

Hanrieder, Tine. 2019. "How Do Professions Globalize? Lessons from the Global South in US Medical Education." *International Political Sociology* 13 (3): 296–314.

Hanson, Lori, Sheila Harms, and Katrina Plamondon. 2011. "Undergraduate International Medical Electives: Some Ethical and Pedagogical Considerations." *Journal of Studies in International Education* 15 (2): 171–85.

Haq, Cynthia, Deborah Rothenberg, Craig Gjerde, James Bobula, Calvin Wilson, Lynn Bickley, Alberto Cardelle, and Abraham Joseph. 2000. "New World Views: Preparing Physicians in Training for Global Health Work." *Family Medicine* 32 (8): 566–72.

Haram, Liv. 1991. "Tswana Medicine in Interaction with Biomedicine." *Social Science & Medicine* 33 (2): 167–75.

Haraway, Donna. 1991. "Situated Knowledges: The Science Question in Feminism and the Privilege of Partial Perspective." In *Simians, Cyborgs, and Women: The Reinvention of Nature*, 183–201. New York: Routledge.

——. 1997. "The Virtual Speculum in the New World Order." *Feminist Review* 55: 22–72.

Harding, Sandra. 2008. "Postcolonial Science and Technologies Studies: Are There Multiple Sciences?" In *Sciences from Below*, 130–54. Durham, NC: Duke University Press.

Hardon, Anita, and Deborah Posel. 2012. "Secrecy as Embodied Practice: Beyond the Confessional Imperative." *Culture, Health & Sexuality* 14 (supp 1): S1–13.

Hardt, Michael. 1999. "Affective Labor." *Boundary* 2 (26): 89–100.

Harkness, Nicholas. 2013. "Softer Soju in South Korea." *Anthropological Theory* 13 (1–2): 12–30.

Harrison, Elizabeth. 2002. "'The Problem with the Locals': Partnership and Participation in Ethiopia." *Development and Change* 33 (4): 587–610.

Hartocollis, Anemona. 2010. "Getting Into Med School Without Hard Sciences." *The New York Times*, July 29, 2010. https://www.nytimes.com/2010/07/30/nyregion/30med schools.html.

Harvard AIDS Initiative. 2005. "Focus: The Mashi Study." Cambridge, MA: Harvard School of Public Health AIDS Initiative.

Harvard AIDS Institute. 1999. "Oak Foundation Gives Harvard AIDS Institute $2.5 Million for Southern African Research." March 24. http://archive.sph.harvard.edu /press-releases/archives/1999-releases/press03241999.html.

Harvey, David. 1989. *The Condition of Postmodernity: An Enquiry into the Origins of Cultural Change*. Cambridge, MA: Blackwell.

——. 2006. *Spaces of Global Capitalism*. London: Verso.

Haviland, John B. 1989. "'Sure, Sure': Evidence and Affect." *Text* 9 (1): 27–68.

Hayden, Cori. 2003. *When Nature Goes Public: The Making and Unmaking of Bioprospecting in Mexico*. Princeton, NJ: Princeton University Press.

He, Xiaopei, and Lisa Rofel. 2010. "'I Am AIDS': Living with HIV/AIDS in China." *Positions* 18 (2): 511–36.

Heald, Suzette. 2002. "It's Never as Easy as ABC: Understandings of AIDS in Botswana." *African Journal of AIDS Research* 1 (1): 1–11.

——. 2006. "Abstain or Die: The Development of HIV/AIDS Policy in Botswana." *Journal of Biosocial Science* 38 (1): 29–41.

Hecht, Gabrielle. 2018. "Interscalar Vehicles for an African Anthropocene: On Waste, Temporality, and Violence." *Cultural Anthropology* 33 (1): 109–41.

Helmreich, Stefan. 2009. *Alien Ocean: Anthropological Voyages in Microbial Seas*. Berkeley: University of California Press.

Herek, Gregory M. 1999. "AIDS and Stigma." *American Behavioral Scientist* 42 (7): 1106–16.

Herod, Andrew, and Melissa W. Wright. 2008. "Placing Scale: An Introduction." In *Geographies of Power*, 1–14. Hoboken, NJ: Wiley-Blackwell.

Herrick, Clare. 2016. "Global Health, Geographical Contingency, and Contingent Geographies." *Annals of the American Association of Geographers* 106 (3): 672–87.

——. 2017. "When Places Come First: Suffering, Archetypal Space and the Problematic Production of Global Health." *Transactions of the Institute of British Geographers* 42 (4): 530–43.

Herrick, Clare, and Andrew Brooks. 2018. "The Binds of Global Health Partnership: Working out Working Together in Sierra Leone: Global Health Partnership." *Medical Anthropology Quarterly* 32 (4): 520–38.

Herzfeld, Michael. 1997. *Portrait of a Greek Imagination: An Ethnographic Biography of Andreas Nenedakis*. Chicago: University Of Chicago Press.

Hindman, Heather. 2013. *Mediating the Global: Expatria's Forms and Consequences in Kathmandu*. Palo Alto, CA: Stanford University Press.

Ho, Karen. 2005. "Situating Global Capitalisms: A View from Wall Street Investment Banks." *Cultural Anthropology* 20 (1): 68–96.

——. 2009. *Liquidated: An Ethnography of Wall Street*. Durham, NC: Duke University Press.

Hoad, Neville. 2005. "Thabo Mbeki's AIDS Blues: The Intellectual, the Archive, and the Pandemic." *Public Culture* 17 (1): 101–28.

Hochschild, Arlie Russell. 1983. *The Managed Heart: Commercialization of Human Feeling*. Berkeley: University of California Press.

Hoffman, Beatrix. 2008. "Health Care Reform and Social Movements in the United States." *American Journal of Public Health* 98 (supp 1): S69–79.

Hoffman, Kelly M., Sophie Trawalter, Jordan R. Axt, and M. Norman Oliver. 2016. "Racial Bias in Pain Assessment and Treatment Recommendations, and False Beliefs about Biological Differences between Blacks and Whites." *Proceedings of the National Academy of Sciences* 113 (16): 4296–4301.

Høgh, Birthe, and Eskild Petersen. 1984. "The Basic Health Care System in Botswana: A Study of the Distribution and Cost in the Period 1973–1979." *Social Science & Medicine* 19 (8): 783–92.

Hojat, Mohammadreza, Michael J. Vergare, Kaye Maxwell, George Brainard, Steven K. Herrine, Gerald A. Isenberg, Jon Veloski, and Joseph S. Gonnella. 2009. "The Devil Is in the Third Year: A Longitudinal Study of Erosion of Empathy in Medical School." *Academic Medicine* 84 (9): 1182–91.

Holm, John D., and Leapetsewe Malete. 2010. "Nine Problems That Hinder Partnerships in Africa." *The Chronicle of Higher Education*, June 13. https://www.chronicle.com/article/Nine-Problems-That-Hinder/65892.

Holm, John D., and Patrick P. Molutsi. 1992. "State-Society Relations in Botswana: Beginning Liberalization." In *Governance and Politics in Africa*, edited by Goran Hyden and Michael Bratton, 75–96. Boulder, CO: Lynne Rienner.

Holmes, Seth M., Jeremy A. Greene, and Scott D. Stonington. 2014. "Locating Global Health in Social Medicine." *Global Public Health* 9 (5): 475–80.

Holmes, Seth M., Jennifer Karlin, Scott D. Stonington, and Diane L. Gottheil. 2017. "The First Nationwide Survey of MD-PhDs in the Social Sciences and Humanities: Training Patterns and Career Choices." *BMC Medical Education* 17 (1): 1–11.

Hope, Kempe Ronald. 2001. "Population Mobility and Multi-Partner Sex in Botswana: Implications for the Spread of HIV/AIDS." *African Journal of Reproductive Health* 5 (3): 73–83.

Horton, Richard. 2018. "Offline: Frantz Fanon and the Origins of Global Health." *The Lancet* 392 (10149): 720.

Hulsebosch, Daniel J. 2017. "Being Seen Like a State: How Americans (and Britons) Built the Constitutional Infrastructure of a Developing Nation." *William & Mary Law Review* 59 (March): 1239–1320.

Hunleth, Jean. 2017. *Children as Caregivers: The Global Fight against Tuberculosis and HIV in Zambia*. New Brunswick, NJ: Rutgers University Press.

Hyatt, Susan B., Boone W. Shear, and Susan Wright. 2015. *Learning Under Neoliberalism: Ethnographies of Governance in Higher Education*. New York: Berghahn Books.

Hymes, Dell. 1975. "Breakthrough into Performance." In *Folklore: Performance and Communication*, edited by Dan Ben-Amos and Kenneth S. Goldstein, 11–74. The Hague: Mouton.

Iliffe, John. 1998. *East African Doctors: A History of the Modern Profession*. Cambridge: Cambridge University Press.

Illouz, Eva. 2007. *Cold Intimacies: The Making of Emotional Capitalism*. Malden, MA: Polity.

Ingstad, Benedicte. 1990. "The Cultural Construction of AIDS and Its Consequences for Prevention in Botswana." *Medical Anthropology Quarterly* 4 (1): 28–40.

——. 2004. "The Value of Grandchildren: Changing Relations between Generations in Botswana." *Africa: Journal of the International African Institute* 74 (1): 62–75.

IRIN (Integrated Regional Information Networks of the United Nations Office for the Coordination of Humanitarian Affairs). 2006. "Botswana: Routine HIV Testing Not as Straightforward as It Sounds." *IRINNews*, February 1.

Irvine, Judith T. 1982. "Language and Affect: Some Cross-Cultural Issues." In *Contemporary Perceptions of Language: Interdisciplinary Dimensions*, edited by Heidi Byrnes, 31–48. Washington, DC: Georgetown University Press.

——. 2009. "Stance in a Colonial Encounter: How Mr. Taylor Lost His Footing." In *Stance: Sociolinguistic Perspectives*, edited by Alexandra Jaffe, 53–71. Oxford, UK: Oxford University Press.

——. 2016. "Going Upscale: Scales and Scale-Climbing as Ideological Projects." In *Scale: Discourse and Dimensions of Social Life*, edited by E. Summerson Carr and Michael Lempert, 213–32. Berkeley: University of California Press.

Irvine, Judith T., and Susan Gal. 2000. "Language Ideology and Linguistic Differentiation." In *Regimes of Language: Ideologies, Polities, and Identities*, edited by Paul V. Kroskrity, 35–83. Santa Fe, NM: School of American Research Press.

Irwin, Alec, Joyce Millen, Jim Kim, John Gershman, Brooke G. Schoepf, and Paul Farmer. 2002. "Suffering, Moral Claims, and Scholarly Responsibility: A Response to Leslie Butt." *Medical Anthropology* 21 (1): 25–30.

Jaffe, Alexandra M., ed. 2009a. "Introduction: The Sociolinguistics of Stance." In *Stance: Sociolinguistic Perspectives*, 3–29. Oxford Studies in Sociolinguistics. Oxford, UK: Oxford University Press.

——, ed. 2009b. *Stance: Sociolinguistic Perspectives*. Oxford Studies in Sociolinguistics. Oxford, UK: Oxford University Press.

Jakobson, Roman. 1960. "Closing Statement: Linguistics and Poetics." In *Style in Language*, edited by Thomas Albert Sebeok, 350–77. Cambridge, MA: MIT Press.

——. 1971. "Shifters, Verbal Categories, and the Russian Verb." *Word and Language*. Vol. 2 of *Selected Writings* 2:130–47. The Hague: Mouton.

James, Erica Caple. 2012. "Witchcraft, Bureaucraft, and the Social Life of (US)AID in Haiti." *Cultural Anthropology* 27 (1): 50–75.

Janes, Craig R., and Kitty K. Corbett. 2009. "Anthropology and Global Health." *Annual Review of Anthropology* 38: 167–83.

Jenks, Angela C. 2011. "From 'Lists of Traits' to 'Open-Mindedness': Emerging Issues in Cultural Competence Education." *Culture, Medicine, and Psychiatry* 35 (2): 209.

Jha, Ashish. 2021. "System Failure: America Needs a Global Health Policy for the Pandemic Age." *Foreign Affairs*.

Johnson, Carolyn Y. 2016. "The Disturbing Reason Why We Don't Believe Young, Black Women Are Really Doctors." *The Washington Post*, October 14. https://www.washingtonpost.com/news/wonk/wp/2016/10/14/a-black-doctor-wanted-to-save-a-mans-life-first-she-had-to-convince-the-flight-attendant-she-was-an-actual-physician/.

Johnstone, Barbara. 2013. *Speaking Pittsburghese: The Story of a Dialect*. Oxford, UK: Oxford University Press.

Joint United Nations Programme on HIV/AIDS (UNAIDS). 2004. "Epidemiological Fact Sheet on HIV/AIDS and Sexually Transmitted Diseases." Geneva: UNAIDS.

——. 2014. "The Gap Report." Geneva: UNAIDS.

Jones, David S. 2001. "Technologies of Compliance: Surveillance of Self-Administration of Tuberculosis Treatment, 1956–1966." *History and Technology* 17 (4): 279–318.

Jones, Graham M. 2014. "Secrecy." *Annual Review of Anthropology* 43 (1): 53–69.

Kalofonos, Ippolytos Andreas. 2008. "'All I Eat Is ARVs': Living with HIV/AIDS at the Dawn of the Treatment Era in Central Mozambique." PhD diss., Department of Anthropology, University of California, Berkeley with University of California, San Francisco.

——. 2010. "'All I Eat Is ARVs': The Paradox of AIDS Treatment Interventions in Central Mozambique." *Medical Anthropology Quarterly* 24 (3): 363–80.

Kärkkäinen, Elise. 2007. "Stance Taking in Conversation: From Subjectivity to Intersubjectivity." *Text & Talk* 26 (6): 699–731.

Kaufman, S. 2010. "Time, Clinic Technologies, and the Making of Reflexive Longevity: The Cultural Work of Time Left in an Ageing Society." *Sociology of Health and Illness* 32 (2): 225–37.

Keane, Webb. 2007. *Christian Moderns: Freedom and Fetish in the Mission Encounter.* Berkeley: University of California Press.

——. 2008. "Modes of Objectification in Educational Experience." *Linguistics and Education* 19 (3): 312–18.

Keller, Evelyn Fox. 1983. *A Feeling for the Organism: The Life and Work of Barbara McClintock.* New York: W. H. Freeman and Company.

Kelly, John D., and Martha Kaplan. 2001. "Nation and Decolonization: Toward a New Anthropology of Nationalism." *Anthropological Theory* 1 (4): 419–37.

Kenworthy, Nora J. 2017. *Mistreated: The Political Consequences of the Fight Against AIDS in Lesotho.* Nashville, TN: Vanderbilt University Press.

Kenworthy, Nora J., and Richard Parker. 2014. "HIV Scale-up and the Politics of Global Health." *Global Public Health* 9 (1–2): 1–6.

Kenworthy, Nora, Matthew Thomann, and Richard Parker. 2018. "Critical Perspectives on the 'End of AIDS.'" *Global Public Health* 13 (8): 957–59.

Kenworthy, Nora, Lynn M. Thomas, and Johanna Crane. 2018. "Introduction: Critical Perspectives on US Global Health Partnerships in Africa and Beyond." *Medicine Anthropology Theory* 5 (2): i.

Kerry, Vanessa B., Rochelle P. Walensky, Alexander C. Tsai, Regan W. Bergmark, Brian A. Bergmark, Chaturia Rouse, and David R. Bangsberg. 2013. "US Medical Specialty Global Health Training and the Global Burden of Disease." *Journal of Global Health* 3 (2): 020406. doi:10.7189/jogh.03.0202406.

Keshavjee, Salmaan. 2014. *Blind Spot: How Neoliberalism Infiltrated Global Health.* Berkeley: University of California Press.

Kidder, Tracy. 2003. *Mountains Beyond Mountains: The Quest of Dr. Paul Farmer, A Man Who Would Cure the World.* New York: Random House.

Kielmann, Karina, and Fabian Cataldo. 2010. "Tracking the Rise of the 'Expert Patient' in Evolving Paradigms of HIV Care." *AIDS Care: Psychological and Socio-Medical Aspects of AIDS/HIV* 22 (1): 21–28.

Kiley, Erin E., and Alice J. Hovorka. 2006. "Civil Society Organisations and the National HIV/AIDS Response in Botswana." *African Journal of AIDS Research* 5 (2): 167–78.

King, Nicholas B. 2002. "Security, Disease, Commerce: Ideologies of Postcolonial Global Health." *Social Studies of Science* 32 (5–6): 763–89.

Klaits, Frederick. 1998. "Making a Good Death: AIDS and Social Belonging in an Independent Church in Gaborone." *Botswana Notes and Records* 30: 101–19.

——. 2005. "The Widow in Blue: Blood and the Morality of Remembering during Botswana's Time of AIDS." *Africa* 75 (1): 46–62.

——. 2010. *Death in a Church of Life: Moral Passion during Botswana's Time of AIDS.* Berkeley: University of California Press.

Kleinman, Arthur. 1988. *The Illness Narratives: Suffering, Healing, and the Human Condition.* New York: Basic Books.

——. 1992. "Local Worlds of Suffering: An Interpersonal Focus for Ethnographies of Illness Experience." *Qualitative Health Research* 2 (2): 127–34.

——. 1995. "What Is Specific to Biomedicine?" In *Writing at the Margin: Discourse between Anthropology and Medicine*, 21–40. Berkeley: University of California Press.

——. 2006. *What Really Matters: Living a Moral Life Amidst Uncertainty and Danger.* Oxford, UK: Oxford University Press.

——. 2010. "Four Social Theories for Global Health." *The Lancet* 375 (9725): 1518–19.

Kleinman, Arthur, Veena Das, and Margaret Lock, eds. 1997. *Social Suffering.* Berkeley: University of California Press.

Kleinman, Arthur, and Joan Kleinman. 1996. "The Appeal of Experience; The Dismay of Images: Cultural Appropriations of Suffering in Our Times." *Daedalus* 125 (1): 1–23.

Klerk, Josien de. 2012. "The Compassion of Concealment: Silence Between Older Caregivers and Dying Patients in the AIDS Era, Northwest Tanzania." *Culture, Health & Sexuality* 14 (supp 1): S27–38.

Knorr-Cetina, Karin. 1999. *Epistemic Cultures: How the Sciences Make Knowledge.* Cambridge, MA: Harvard University Press.

Kohn, Abigail A. 2000. "'Imperfect Angels': Narrative 'Emplotment' in the Medical Management of Children with Craniofacial Anomalies." *Medical Anthropology Quarterly* 14 (2): 202–23.

Koplan, Jeffrey P., T. Christopher Bond, Michael H. Merson, K. Srinath Reddy, Mario Henry Rodriguez, Nelson K. Sewankambo, and Judith N. Wasserheit. 2009. "Towards a Common Definition of Global Health." *The Lancet* 373 (9679): 1993–95.

Kroeber, Theodora. 1961. *Ishi in Two Worlds: A Biography of the Last Wild Indian in North America.* Berkeley: University of California Press.

Kupe, Serera Segarona. 1987. "A History of the Evolution of Nursing Education in Botswana, 1922–1980." PhD diss., Teachers College, Columbia University.

Kyakuwa, Margaret, and Anita Hardon. 2012. "Concealment Tactics among HIV-Positive Nurses in Uganda." *Culture, Health & Sexuality* 14 (supp 1): S123–33.

LaHatte, Kristin. 2017. "Professionalizing Persons and Foretelling Futures: Capacity Building in Post-Earthquake Haiti." *Cambridge Journal of Anthropology* 35 (1): 17–30.

Lakoff, Andrew. 2008. "The Generic Biothreat, or, How We Became Unprepared." *Cultural Anthropology* 23 (3): 399–428.

——. 2010. "Two Regimes of Global Health." *Humanity* 1 (1): 59–79.

——. 2017. *Unprepared: Global Health in a Time of Emergency.* Berkeley: University of California Press.

Lambek, Michael, and Jacqueline S. Solway. 2001. "Just Anger: Scenarios of Indignation in Botswana and Madagascar." *Ethnos* 66 (1): 49–72.

Lambert, Helen. 2006. "Accounting for EBM: Notions of Evidence in Medicine." *Social Science & Medicine* 62 (11): 2633–45.

Lampland, Martha, and Susan Leigh Star. 2009. *Standards and Their Stories: How Quantifying, Classifying, and Formalizing Practices Shape Everyday Life.* Ithaca, NY: Cornell University Press.

Langwick, Stacey Ann. 2011. *Bodies, Politics, and African Healing: The Matter of Maladies in Tanzania.* Bloomington: Indiana University Press.

Larson, Eric B., and Xin Yao. 2005. "Clinical Empathy as Emotional Labor in the Patient-Physician Relationship." *Journal of the American Medical Association* 293 (9): 1100–1106.

Latour, Bruno. 2000. *We Have Never Been Modern.* Cambridge, MA: Harvard University Press.

——. 2005. *Reassembling the Social: An Introduction to Actor-Network-Theory.* Oxford, UK: Oxford University Press.

Law, John. 2004. "And If the Global Were Small and Noncoherent? Method, Complexity, and the Baroque." *Environment and Planning D: Society and Space* 22 (1): 13–26.

Le Marcis, Frédéric. 2004. "The Suffering Body of the City." Translated by Judith Inggs. *Public Culture* 16 (3): 453–77.

Lempert, Michael. 2016. "Interaction Rescaled: How Buddhist Debate Became a Diasporic Pedagogy." In *Scale: Discourse and Dimensions of Social Life*, edited by E. Summerson Carr and Michael Lempert, 52–69. Berkeley: University of California Press.

Lerner, Barron H. 1997. "From Careless Consumptives to Recalcitrant Patients: The Historical Construction of Noncompliance." *Social Science and Medicine* 45 (9): 1423–31.

Lesetedi, Gwen N. 2003. "Urban-Rural Linkages as an Urban Survival Strategy among Urban Dwellers in Botswana: The Case of Broadhurst Residents." *Journal of Political Ecology* 10 (1): 37.

Levinson, Bradley A. 1999. "Resituating the Place of Educational Discourse in Anthropology." *American Anthropologist* 101 (3): 594–604.

Li, Tania Murray. 2007. *The Will to Improve: Governmentality, Development, and the Practice of Politics*. Durham, NC: Duke University Press Books.

Light, Donald, and Sol Levine. 1988. "The Changing Character of the Medical Profession: A Theoretical Overview." *The Milbank Quarterly* 66 (supp 2): 10–32.

Link, Bruce G., and Jo C. Phelan. 2001. "Conceptualizing Stigma." *Annual Review of Sociology* 27: 363–85.

Lipson, Michael. 1994. "Disclosure of Diagnosis to Children with Human Immunodeficiency Virus or Acquired Immunodeficiency Syndrome." *Journal of Developmental and Behavioral Pediatrics* 15 (supp 3): S61–65.

Livingston, Julie. 2004. "AIDS as Chronic Illness: Epidemiological Transition and Health Care in South-Eastern Botswana." *African Journal of AIDS Research* 3 (1): 15–22.

——. 2005. *Debility and the Moral Imagination in Botswana*. Bloomington: Indiana University Press.

——. 2008. "Disgust, Bodily Aesthetics and the Ethic of Being Human in Botswana." *Africa* 78 (2): 288–307.

——. 2012. *Improvising Medicine: An African Oncology Ward in an Emerging Cancer Epidemic*. Durham, NC: Duke University Press.

——. 2019. *Self-Devouring Growth: A Planetary Parable as Told from Southern Africa*. Durham, NC: Duke University Press.

Lock, Margaret. 1993. "Cultivating the Body: Anthropology and Epistemologies of Bodily Practice and Knowledge." *Annual Review of Anthropology* 22: 133–55.

——. 2002. *Twice Dead: Organ Transplants and the Reinvention of Death*. Berkeley: University of California Press.

Luft, Harold S. 1999. "Why Are Physicians So Upset about Managed Care?" *Journal of Health Politics, Policy and Law* 24 (5): 957–66.

MacDonald, David S. 1996. "Notes on the Socio-Economic and Cultural Factors Influencing the Transmission of HIV in Botswana." *Social Science & Medicine* 42 (9): 1325–33.

Macfarlane, Sarah B., Marian Jacobs, and Ephata E. Kaaya. 2008. "In the Name of Global Health: Trends in Academic Institutions." *Journal of Public Health Policy* 29 (4): 383–401.

Maganu, Edward. 1997. "Access to Health Services and Its Impact on Quality of Life." In *Poverty and Plenty: The Botswana Experience*, edited by Doreen Nteta, Janet Hermans, and Pavla Jeskova, 291–301. Gaborone, Botswana: Botswana Society.

Mahajan, Anish P., Jennifer N. Sayles, Vishal A. Patel, Robert H. Remien, Daniel Ortiz, Greg Szekeres, and Thomas J. Coates. 2008. "Stigma in the HIV/AIDS Epidemic: A Review of the Literature and Recommendations for the Way Forward." *AIDS (London, England)* 22 (supp 2): S67–79.

Mahajan, Manjari. 2008. "Designing Epidemics: Models, Policy-Making, and Global Foreknowledge in India's AIDS Epidemic." *Science and Public Policy* 35 (8): 585–96.

Mahmood, Saba. 2004. *Politics of Piety: The Islamic Revival and the Feminist Subject*. Princeton, NJ: Princeton University Press.

Makgala, John, and Banyatsi Mmekwa. 2009. "Have Patronage and Paternalism Been Shaken in the BDP?" *Mmegi*, July 24.

Malkki, Liisa. 1992. "National Geographic: The Rooting of Peoples and the Territorialization of National Identity among Scholars and Refugees." *Cultural Anthropology* 7 (1): 24–44.

——. 2010. "Children, Humanity, and the Infantilization of Peace." In *In the Name of Humanity: The Government of Threat and Care*, edited by Ilana Feldman and Miriam Ticktin, 58–85. Durham, NC: Duke University Press.

Mangham, Lindsay J., and Kara Hanson. 2010. "Scaling up in International Health: What Are the Key Issues?" *Health Policy and Planning* 25 (2): 85–96.

Mansergh, Gordon, Anne C. Haddix, Richard W. Steketee, and R. J. Simonds. 1998. "Cost-Effectiveness of Zidovudine to Prevent Mother-to-Child Transmission of HIV in Sub-Saharan Africa." *Journal of the American Medical Association* 280 (1): 30–31.

Marcus, George E., and Michael G. Powell. 2003. "From Conspiracy Theories in the Incipient New World Order of the 1990s to Regimes of Transparency Now." *Anthropological Quarterly* 76 (2): 323–34.

Marks, Shula. 1994. *Divided Sisterhood: Race, Class, and Gender in the South African Nursing Profession*. New York: St. Martin's Press.

Marr, Stephen David. 2012. "'If You Are with Ten, Only Two Will Be Batswana': Nation-Making and the Public Discourse of Paranoia in Botswana." *Canadian Journal of African Studies/Revue Canadienne Des Études Africaines* 46 (1): 65–86.

Marseille, Elliot, Paul B. Hofmann, and James G. Kahn. 2002. "HIV Prevention before HAART in sub-Saharan Africa." *Lancet* 359 (9320): 1851–56.

Marseille, Elliot, James G. Kahn, and Joseph Saba. 1998. "Cost-Effectiveness of Antiviral Drug Therapy to Reduce Mother-to-Child HIV Transmission in Sub-Saharan Africa." *AIDS* 12 (8): 939–48.

Marsland, Rebecca, and Ruth J. Prince. 2012. "What Is Life Worth? Exploring Biomedical Interventions, Survival, and the Politics of Life." *Medical Anthropology Quarterly* 26 (4): 453–69.

Marston, Sallie A., John Paul Jones, and Keith Woodward. 2005. "Human Geography without Scale." *Transactions of the Institute of British Geographers* 30 (4): 416–32.

Martin, Emily. 1987. *The Woman in the Body: A Cultural Analysis of Reproduction*. Boston: Beacon Press.

——. 1990. "Toward an Anthropology of Immunology: The Body as Nation State." *Medical Anthropology Quarterly* 4 (4): 410–26.

Masco, Joseph. 2006. *The Nuclear Borderlands: The Manhattan Project in Post-Cold War New Mexico*. Princeton, NJ: Princeton University Press.

——. 2008. "'Survival Is Your Business': Engineering Ruins and Affect in Nuclear America." *Cultural Anthropology* 23 (2): 361–98.

——. 2014. *The Theater of Operations: National Security Affect from the Cold War to the War on Terror*. Durham, NC: Duke University Press.

Maskovsky, Jeff. 2005. "Do People Fail Drugs, or Do Drugs Fail People?: The Discourse of Adherence." *Transforming Anthropology* 13 (2): 136–42.

Massey, Doreen. 1994. *Space, Place and Gender*. Hoboken, NJ: John Wiley & Sons.

Matoesian, Gregory. 2005. "Struck by Speech Revisited: Embodied Stance in Jurisdictional Discourse." *Journal of Sociolinguistics* 9 (2): 167–93.

Mattes, Dominik. 2011. "'We Are Just Supposed to Be Quiet': The Production of Adherence to Antiretroviral Treatment in Urban Tanzania." *Medical Anthropology* 30 (2): 158–82.

——. 2014. "'Life Is Not a Rehearsal, It's a Performance': An Ethnographic Enquiry into the Subjectivities of Children and Adolescents Living with Antiretroviral Treatment in Northeastern Tanzania." *Children and Youth Services Review* 45 (October): 28–37.

Mattingly, Cheryl. 2008. "Pocahontas Goes to the Clinic: Popular Culture as Lingua Franca in a Cultural Borderland." *American Anthropologist* 108 (3): 494–501.

——. 2010. *The Paradox of Hope: Journeys through a Clinical Borderland*. Berkeley: University of California Press.

Maughan-Brown, Brendan. 2010. "Stigma Rises despite Antiretroviral Roll-out: A Longitudinal Analysis in South Africa." *Social Science & Medicine* 70 (3): 368–74.

Maundeni, Tapologo. 2002. "Seen But Not Heard?: Focusing on the Needs of Children of Divorced Parents in Gaborone and Surrounding Areas, Botswana." *Childhood* 9 (3): 277–302.

Maundeni, Zibani. 2004. "Mutual Criticism and State/Society Interaction in Botswana." *Journal of Modern African Studies* 42 (4): 619–36.

Mauss, Marcel. 1935. "Techniques of the Body." *Economy and Society* 2 (1): 70–88.

Mbembe, Achille. 2001. *On the Postcolony*. Berkeley: University of California Press.

——. 2016. "Decolonizing the University: New Directions." *Arts and Humanities in Higher Education* 15 (1): 29–45.

——. 2017. *Critique of Black Reason*. Durham, NC: Duke University Press.

McDonnell, Terence. 2016. *Best Laid Plans: Cultural Entropy and the Unraveling of AIDS Media Campaigns*. Chicago: University of Chicago Press.

McGoey, Linsey. 2015. *No Such Thing as a Free Gift: The Gates Foundation and the Price of Philanthropy*. London: Verso Books.

McKay, Ramah. 2018. *Medicine in the Meantime: The Work of Care in Mozambique*. Durham, NC: Duke University Press.

McNeill, Nancy. 2016. "Self-Efficacy and Select Characteristics in Nurses Who Respond to a Pediatric Emergency." PhD diss., Minneapolis, MN: Walden University.

McWilliam, Erica, and Caroline Hatcher. 2004. "Emotional Literacy as a Pedagogical Product." *Continuum: Journal of Media & Cultural Studies* 18 (2): 179–89.

Mead, Margaret. 1930. *Growing Up in New Guinea: A Comparative Study of Primitive Education*. New York: HarperCollins.

Merson, Michael H. 2014. "University Engagement in Global Health." *New England Journal of Medicine* 370 (18): 1676–78.

Merson, Michael H., and Chapman Page. 2009. "The Dramatic Expansion of University Engagement in Global Health: Implications for US Policy. A Report by the CSIS Global Health Policy Center." Washington, DC: Center for Strategic and International Studies.

Mertz, Elizabeth. 2007. *The Language of Law School: Learning to "Think Like a Lawyer."* Oxford, UK: Oxford University Press.

Metzl, Jonathan, and Anna Kirkland. 2010. *Against Health: How Health Became the New Morality*. New York: NYU Press.

Meyers, Todd, and Nancy Rose Hunt. 2014. "The Other Global South." *The Lancet* 384 (9958): 1921–22.

Mika, Marissa. 2016. "Fifty Years of Creativity, Crisis, and Cancer in Uganda." *Canadian Journal of African Studies/Revue Canadienne Des Études Africaines* 50 (3): 395–413.

——. 2021. *Africanizing Oncology: Creativity, Crisis, and Cancer in Uganda*. Athens, OH: Ohio University Press.

Minn, Pierre. 2015. "Troubling Objectivity: The Promises and Pitfalls of Training Haitian Clinicians in Qualitative Research Methods." *Medical Anthropology* 34 (1): 39–53.

Mitchell, Timothy. 2002. *Rule of Experts*. Berkeley: University of California Press.

Mmegi. 2007. "HIV/AIDS Organizations Speak Out on Global Fund Grant," February 1. https://allafrica.com/stories/200702011035.html.

Moffat, Robert. 1969. *Missionary Labours and Scenes in Southern Africa*. New York: Johnson Reprint Corporation.

Mokone, Gaonyadiwe G., Maikutlo Kebaetse, John Wright, Masego B. Kebaetse, Oarabile Makgabana-Dintwa, Poloko Kebaabetswe, Ludo Badlangana, Mpho Mogodi, Katie Bryant, and Oathokwa Nkomazana. 2014. "Establishing a New Medical School: Botswana's Experience." *Academic Medicine* 89 (supp 1): S83–87.

Mol, Annemarie. 2002. *The Body Multiple: Ontology in Medical Practice*. Durham, NC: Duke University Press.

Molefi, Rodgers Keteng Keokil. 1996. *A Medical History of Botswana, 1885–1966*. Gaborone: The Botswana Society.

Molutsi, Patrick P., and John D. Holm. 1990. "Developing Democracy When Civil Society Is Weak: The Case of Botswana." *African Affairs* 89 (July): 323–40.

Molyneux, Sassy, and P. Wenzel Geissler, eds. 2008. "Part Special Issue: Ethics and the Ethnography of Medical Research in Africa." *Social Science and Medicine* 67 (5): 685–799.

Montoya, Michael. 2011. *Making the Mexican Diabetic: Race, Science, and the Genetics of Inequality*. Berkeley: University of California Press.

Mookodi, Godisang B. 2000. "The Complexities of Female Household Headship in Botswana." *Pula: Botswana Journal of African Studies* 14 (2): 148–64.

Moore, Adam. 2008. "Rethinking Scale as a Geographical Category: From Analysis to Practice." *Progress in Human Geography* 32 (2): 203–25.

Moore, Henrietta L. 2004. "Global Anxieties: Concept-Metaphors and Pre-Theoretical Commitments in Anthropology." *Anthropological Theory* 4 (1): 71–88.

——. 2010. "Forms of Knowing and Un-Knowing: Secrets about Society, Sexuality and God in Northern Kenya." In *Secrecy and Silence in the Research Process*, edited by Roisin Ryan-Flood and Rosalind Gill, 49–60. London: Routledge.

Morapedi, Wazha G. 1999. "Migrant Labour and the Peasantry in the Bechuanaland Protectorate, 1930–1965." *Journal of Southern African Studies* 25 (2): 197–214.

Morgan, Kimberly J., and Andrea Louise Campbell. 2011. *The Delegated Welfare State: Medicare, Markets, and the Governance of Social Policy*. Oxford, UK: Oxford University Press.

Morrison, Lynn. 2004. "Ceausescu's Legacy: Family Struggles and Institutionalization of Children in Romania." *Journal of Family History* 29 (2): 168–82.

Moyer, Eileen. 2015. "The Anthropology of Life After AIDS: Epistemological Continuities in the Age of Antiretroviral Treatment." *Annual Review of Anthropology* 44 (1): 259–75.

Muehlebach, Andrea. 2011. "On Affective Labor in Post-Fordist Italy." *Cultural Anthropology* 26 (1): 59–82.

Munn, Nancy D. 1986. *The Fame of Gawa: A Symbolic Study of Value Transformation in a Massim Society (Papua New Guinea)*. Durham, NC: Duke University Press.

——. 1990. "Constructing Regional Worlds in Experience: Kula Exchange, Witchcraft and Gawan Local Events." *Man* 25 (1): 1–17.

Murphy, Brendan. 2018. "94% Match Rate in 2018 for U.S. Allopathic Med Students." *American Medical Association*, April 5, 2018. https://www.ama-assn.org/residents -students/match/94-match-rate-2018-us-allopathic-med-students.

Muzinda, Mark. 2007. "Monitoring and Evaluation Practices and Challenges of Gaborone Based Local NGOs Implementing HIV/AIDS Projects in Botswana." Master's thesis, Project Management, University of Botswana.

Mykhalovskiy, Eric, Liza Mccoy, and Michael Bresalier. 2004. "Compliance/Adherence, HIV, and the Critique of Medical Power." *Social Theory and Health* 2 (4): 315–40.

Nader, Laura. 1972. "Up the Anthropologist: Perspectives Gained From Studying Up." In *Reinventing Anthropology*, edited by Dell Hymes, 284–311. New York: Pantheon Books.

National Resident Matching Program. 2018. "Charting Outcomes in the Match: International Medical Graduates Characteristics of International Medical Graduates Who Matched to Their Preferred Specialty in the 2018 Main Residency Match." 2nd ed. National Resident Matching Program.

Nations, Marilyn K., and Linda-Anne Rebhun. 1988. "Mystification of a Simple Solution: Oral Rehydration Therapy in Northeast Brazil." *Social Science & Medicine* 27 (1): 25–38.

Neely, Abigail H., and Alex M. Nading. 2017. "Global Health from the Outside: The Promise of Place-Based Research." *Health & Place* 45 (May): 55–63.

Nelson, Brett D., Anne C. C. Lee, P. K. Newby, M. Robert Chamberlin, and Chi-Cheng Huang. 2008. "Global Health Training in Pediatric Residency Programs." *Pediatrics* 122 (1): 28–33.

Newell, Marie-Louise, Hoosen Coovadia, Marjo Cortina-Borja, Nigel Rollins, Philippe Gaillard, and Francois Dabis. 2004. "Mortality of Infected and Uninfected Infants Born to HIV-Infected Mothers in Africa: A Pooled Analysis." *The Lancet* 364 (9441): 1236–43.

Newell, Marie-Louise, Francois Dabis, Keith Tolley, and David Whynes. 1998. "Cost-Effectiveness and Cost-Benefit in the Prevention of Mother-to-Child Transmission of HIV in Developing Countries." *AIDS* 12 (13): 1571.

Newsom, D. H., and J. P. Kiwanuka. 2002. "Needle-Stick Injuries in an Ugandan Teaching Hospital." *Annals of Tropical Medicine and Parasitology* 96 (5): 517–22.

Nguyen, Vinh-Kim. 2005. "Antiretroviral Globalism, Biopolitics, and Therapeutic Citizenship." In *Global Assemblages: Technology, Politics, and Ethics*, edited by Aihwa Ong and Stephen J. Collier, 124–44. Malden, MA: Blackwell.

——. 2009. "Government-by-Exception: Enrolment and Experimentality in Mass HIV Treatment Programmes in Africa." *Social Theory and Health* 7 (3): 196–217.

——. 2010. *The Republic of Therapy: Triage and Sovereignty in West Africa's Time of AIDS*. Durham, NC: Duke University Press.

——. 2011. "Trial Communities: HIV and Therapeutic Citizenship in West Africa." In *Evidence, Ethos, and Experiment: The Anthropology and History of Medical Research in Africa*, edited by P. Wenzel Geissler, 429–44. New York: Berghahn Books.

Nguyen, Vinh-Kim, and Karine Peschard. 2003. "Anthropology, Inequality, and Disease: A Review." *Annual Review of Anthropology* 32 (1): 447–74.

Ngwane, Zolani. 2001a. "'Real Men Reawaken Their Fathers' Homesteads, the Educated Leave Them in Ruins': The Politics of Domestic Reproduction in Post-Apartheid Rural South Africa." *Journal of Religion in Africa* 31 (4): 402–26.

——. 2001b. "'The Long Conversation' The Enduring Salience of Nineteenth-Century Missionary/Colonial Encounters in Post-Apartheid South Africa." *Interventions* 3 (1): 65–75.

Nichter, Mark. 2018. "Global Health." In *The International Encyclopedia of Anthropology*, 1–14. John Wiley & Sons.

Nietzsche, Friedrich Wilhelm. 1969. *Thus Spoke Zarathustra*. Translated by R. J. Hollingdale. London: Penguin Books.

——. 1996. *Human, All Too Human: A Book for Free Spirits*. Translated by R. J. Hollingdale. Cambridge: Cambridge University Press.

Nsubuga, Fredrich M., and Maritta S. Jaakkola. 2005. "Needle Stick Injuries among Nurses in Sub-Saharan Africa." *Tropical Medicine & International Health* 10 (8): 773–81.

Nyamnjoh, Francis B. 2006. *Insiders and Outsiders: Citizenship and Xenophobia in Contemporary Southern Africa*. Dakar, Senegal: Codesria Books.

——. 2016. *#RhodesMustFall: Nibbling at Resilient Colonialism in South Africa*. Bamenda, Cameroon: Langaa RPCIG.

Ochs, Elinor. 1992. "Indexing Gender." In *Rethinking Context: Language as an Interactive Phenomenon*, edited by Alessandro Duranti and Charles Goodwin, 335–58. Cambridge: Cambridge University Press.

——. 1993. "Constructing Social Identity: A Language Socialization Perspective." *Research on Language and Social Interaction* 26 (3): 287–306.

——. 1996. "Resources for Socializing Humanity." In *Rethinking Linguistic Relativity*, edited by J. Gumperz and S. Levinson, 407–38. Cambridge: Cambridge University Press.

Ochs, Elinor, and Bambi Schieffelin. 2017. "Language Socialization: An Historical Overview." In *Language Socialization*, edited by Patricia A. Duff and Stephen May, 3rd ed., 3–17. New York: Springer International.

Ofri, Danielle. 2010. "No Longer on the Doctor's Checklist, but Physical Exam Still Matters." *The New York Times*, August 2. https://www.nytimes.com/2010/08/03/health/03case.html.

——. 2014. "The Physical Exam as Refuge." *The New York Times*, July 10. https://well.blogs.nytimes.com/2014/07/10/the-physical-exam-as-refuge/.

Okwaro, Ferdinand Moyi, and P. Wenzel Geissler. 2015. "In/Dependent Collaborations: Perceptions and Experiences of African Scientists in Transnational HIV Research." *Medical Anthropology Quarterly* 29 (4): 492–511.

Ong, Aihwa, and Stephen J. Collier. 2005. *Global Assemblages: Technology, Politics, and Ethics as Anthropological Problems*. Hoboken, NJ: Wiley.

Orr, Jackie. 2004. "The Militarization of Inner Space." *Critical Sociology* 30 (2): 451–81.

Ortner, Sherry B. 2016. "Dark Anthropology and Its Others: Theory Since the Eighties." *Hau: Journal of Ethnographic Theory* 6 (1): 47–73.

Owens, Deirdre Cooper. 2017. *Medical Bondage: Race, Gender, and the Origins of American Gynecology*. Athens: University of Georgia Press.

Packard, Randall M. 1989. *White Plague, Black Labor: Tuberculosis and the Political Economy of Health and Disease in South Africa*. Berkeley: University of California Press.

——. 1997. "Visions of Postwar Health and Development and Their Impact on Public Health Interventions in the Developing World." In *International Development and the Social Sciences: Essays on the History and Politics of Knowledge*, edited by Frederick Cooper and Randall M. Packard, 93–118. Berkeley: University of California Press.

———. 2016. *A History of Global Health: Interventions into the Lives of Other Peoples*. Baltimore, MD: Johns Hopkins University Press.

Palmié, Stephan. 2007. "Genomics, Divination, 'Racecraft.'" *American Ethnologist* 34 (2): 205–22.

Pandolfi, Mariella. 2003. "Contract of Mutual (In)Difference: Governance and the Humanitarian Apparatus in Contemporary Albania and Kosovo." *Indiana Journal of Global Legal Studies* 10 (1): 369–81.

Panosian, Claire, and Thomas J. Coates. 2006. "The New Medical 'Missionaries'— Grooming the Next Generation of Global Health Workers." *New England Journal of Medicine* 354 (17): 1771–73.

Panter-Brick, Catherine, Mark Eggerman, and Mark Tomlinson. 2014. "How Might Global Health Master Deadly Sins and Strive for Greater Virtues?" *Global Health Action* 7 (1). doi:10.3402/gha.v7.23411.

Parker, Richard. 2000. "Administering the Epidemic: HIV/AIDS Policy, Models of Development, and International Health." In *Global Health Policy, Local Realities: The Fallacy of the Level Playing Field*, edited by Linda M. Whiteford and Lenore Manderson, 39–58. Lynne Rienner Publishers.

Parker, Richard, and Peter Aggleton. 2003. "HIV and AIDS-Related Stigma and Discrimination: A Conceptual Framework and Implications for Action." *Social Science & Medicine* 57 (1): 13–24.

Parsons, Luise, Taatske Rijken, Deogratias O. Mbuka, and Oathokwa Nkomozana. 2012. "Potential for the Specialty of Family Medicine in Botswana: A Discussion Paper." *African Journal of Primary Health Care & Family Medicine* 4 (1): 1–6.

Patton, Cindy. 1999. "Inventing 'African AIDS.'" In *Culture, Society and Sexuality: A Reader*, edited by Richard Guy Parker and Peter Aggleton, 387–404. London: Psychology Press.

Peirce, Charles Sanders. 1932. *Collected Papers of Charles Sanders Peirce*. Vol. 2 of *Elements of Logic*, edited by Charles Hartshorne and Paul Weiss. Cambridge, MA: Harvard University Press.

Pelissier, Catherine. 1991. "The Anthropology of Teaching and Learning." *Annual Review of Anthropology* 20 (1): 75–95.

Pescosolido, Bernice A., Steven A. Tuch, and Jack K. Martin. 2001. "The Profession of Medicine and the Public: Examining Americans' Changing Confidence in Physician Authority from the Beginning of the 'Health Care Crisis' to the Era of Health Care Reform." *Journal of Health and Social Behavior* 42 (1): 1–16.

Peterson, Kristin. 2014. *Speculative Markets: Drug Circuits and Derivative Life in Nigeria*. Durham, NC: Duke University Press.

Peterson, Kristin, and Morenike O. Folayan. 2017. "A Research Alliance: Tracking the Politics of HIV-Prevention Trials in Africa." *Medicine Anthropology Theory* 4 (2): 18.

———. 2019. "Ethics and HIV Prevention Research: An Analysis of the Early Tenofovir PrEP Trial in Nigeria." *Bioethics* 33 (1): 35–42.

Peterson, Kristin, Morenike Oluwatoyin Folayan, Edward Chigwedere, and Evaristo Nthete. 2015. "Saying 'No' to PrEP Research in Malawi: What Constitutes 'Failure' in Offshored HIV Prevention Research?" *Anthropology & Medicine* 22 (3): 278–94.

Petryna, Adriana. 2002. *Life Exposed: Biological Citizens After Chernobyl*. Princeton, NJ: Princeton University Press.

——. 2005. "Ethical Variability: Drug Development and Globalizing Clinical Trials." *American Ethnologist* 32 (2): 183–97.

——. 2009. *When Experiments Travel: Clinical Trials and the Global Search for Human Subjects*. Princeton, NJ: Princeton University Press.

Pfeiffer, James, and Rachel Chapman. 2010. "Anthropological Perspectives on Structural Adjustment and Public Health." *Annual Review of Anthropology* 39 (1): 149–65.

Pfeiffer, James, and Mark Nichter. 2008. "What Can Critical Medical Anthropology Contribute to Global Health?" *Medical Anthropology Quarterly* 22 (4): 410–15.

Philips, Susan U. 2016. "Balancing the Scales of Justice in Tonga." In *Scale: Discourse and Dimensions of Social Life*, edited by E. Summerson Carr and Michael Lempert, 112–32. Berkeley: University of California Press.

Phorano, O. M., K. Nthomang, and B. N. Ngwenya. 2005. "HIV/AIDS, Home Care and Human Waste Disposal in Botswana." *Botswana Notes and Records* 37: 161–78.

Pigg, Stacy Leigh. 1992. "Inventing Social Categories through Place: Social Representations and Development in Nepal." *Comparative Studies in Society and History* 34 (3): 491–513.

——. 1997. "'Found in Most Traditional Societies': Traditional Medical Practioners between Culture and Development." In *International Development and the Social Sciences: Essays on the History and Politics of Knowledge*, edited by Frederick Cooper and Randall Packard, 259–90. Berkeley: University of California Press.

——. 2001. "Languages of Sex and AIDS in Nepal: Notes on the Social Production of Commensurability." *Cultural Anthropology* 16 (4): 481–541.

——. 2013. "On Sitting and Doing: Ethnography as Action in Global Health." *Social Science & Medicine* 99 (December): 127–34.

Piot, Charles D. 1993. "Secrecy, Ambiguity, and the Everyday in Kabre Culture." *American Anthropologist* 95 (2): 353–70.

Pitse, Reuben. 2008. "Botswana Prepares for War?" *Sunday Standard*, July 2.

Poirier, Suzanne. 2006. "Medical Education and the Embodied Physician." *Literature and Medicine* 25 (2): 522–52.

Poku, Nana K. 2006. *AIDS in Africa: How the Poor Are Dying*. Cambridge, UK: Polity.

Poleykett, Branwyn. 2018. "Made in Denmark: Scientific Mobilities and the Place of Pedagogy in Global Health." *Global Public Health* 13 (3): 276–87.

Pollock, Mica, and Bradley A. Levinson. 2016. "Introduction." In *A Companion to the Anthropology of Education*, edited by Bradley A. Levinson and Mica Pollock, 1–8. Malden, MA: Wiley-Blackwell Publishers.

Popovici, F., R. C. Apetrei, L. Zolotusca, N. Beldescu, A. Calomfirescu, Z. Jezek, D. L. Heymann, A. Gromyko, B. S. Hersh, and M. J. Oxtoby. 1991. "Acquired Immunodeficiency Syndrome in Romania." *The Lancet* 338 (8768): 645–49.

Povinelli, Elizabeth A. 2006. *The Empire of Love: Toward a Theory of Intimacy, Genealogy, and Carnality*. Durham, NC: Duke University Press.

Prentice, Rachel. 2007. "Drilling Surgeons: The Social Lessons of Embodied Surgical Learning." *Science, Technology, & Human Values* 32 (5): 534–53.

——. 2013. *Bodies in Formation: An Ethnography of Anatomy and Surgery Education*. Experimental Futures. Durham, NC: Duke University Press.

Preston-Whyte, Eleanor M. 2003. "Contexts of Vulnerability: Sex, Secrecy and HIV/AIDS." *African Journal of AIDS Research* 2 (2): 89–94.

Prince, Ruth J. 2014. "Situating Health and the Public in Africa." In *Making and Unmaking Public Health in Africa: Ethnographic and Historical Perspectives*, edited by Ruth J. Prince and Rebecca Marsland, 1–54. Athens: Ohio University Press.

Prince, Ruth J., and Hannah Brown, eds. 2016. *Volunteer Economies: The Politics and Ethics of Voluntary Labour in Africa*. Woodbridge, Suffolk, UK: Boydell & Brewer.

Prince, Ruth J., and Rebecca Marsland, eds. 2013. *Making and Unmaking Public Health in Africa: Ethnographic and Historical Perspectives*. Athens: Ohio University Press.

Prince, Ruth J., and Phelgona Otieno. 2014. "In the Shadowlands of Global Health: Observations from Health Workers in Kenya." *Global Public Health* 9 (8): 927–45.

Putzel, James. 2004. "The Global Fight against AIDS: How Adequate Are the National Commissions?" *Journal of International Development* 16 (8): 1129–40.

Rabinow, Paul. 1992. "Artificiality and Enlightenment: From Sociobiology to Biosociality." In *Incorporations*, edited by Jonathan Crary and Sanford Kwinter, 234–52. New York: Bradbury Tamblyn and Boorne.

——. 2003. *Anthropos Today: Reflections on Modern Equipment*. Princeton, NJ: Princeton University Press.

Rajan, Kaushik Sunder. 2006. *Biocapital: The Constitution of Postgenomic Life*. Durham, NC: Duke University Press.

Ramiah, Ilavenil, and Michael R. Reich. 2005. "Public-Private Partnerships And Antiretroviral Drugs For HIV/AIDS: Lessons From Botswana." *Health Affairs* 24 (2): 545–51.

Ramsey, Alan H., Cynthia Haq, Craig L. Gjerde, and Deborah Rothenberg. 2004. "Career Influence of an International Health Experience during Medical School." *Family Medicine* 36 (June): 412–16.

Redfield, Peter. 2006. "A Less Modest Witness." *American Ethnologist* 33 (1): 3–26.

——. 2012a. *Life in Crisis: The Ethical Journey of Doctors Without Borders*. Berkeley: University of California Press.

——. 2012b. "The Unbearable Lightness of Expats: Double Binds of Humanitarian Mobility." *Cultural Anthropology* 27 (2): 358–82.

Rees, Tobias. 2014. "Humanity/Plan; or, On the 'Stateless' Today (Also Being an Anthropology of Global Health)." *Cultural Anthropology* 29 (3): 457–78.

Reich, Michael. 2002. *Public-Private Partnerships for Public Health*. Cambridge, MA: Harvard Center for Population and Development Studies.

Reynolds, Lindsey. 2014a. "'Low-Hanging Fruit': Counting and Accounting for Children in PEPFAR-Funded HIV/AIDS Programmes in South Africa." *Global Public Health* 9 (1–2): 124–43.

——. 2014b. "'Making Known' or 'Counting Our Children'? Constructing and Caring for Children in Epidemic South Africa." *Medicine Anthropology Theory* 1 (1): 114.

Reynolds, Pamela. 1995. "Youth and the Politics of Culture in South Africa." In *Children and the Politics of Culture*, edited by Sharon Stephens, 218–40. Princeton, NJ: Princeton University Press.

Rhine, Kathryn A. 2009. "Support Groups, Marriage, and the Management of Ambiguity among HIV-Positive Women in Northern Nigeria." *Anthropological Quarterly* 82 (2): 369–400.

——. 2016. *The Unseen Things: Women, Secrecy, and HIV in Northern Nigeria*. Bloomington: Indiana University Press.

Rice, Tom. 2008. "'Beautiful Murmurs': Stethoscopic Listening and Acoustic Objectification." *Senses and Society* 3 (3): 293–306.

Richards, Audrey. 1956. *Chisungu: A Girl's Initiation Ceremony Among the Bemba of Zambia*. New York: Routledge.

Riles, Annelise. 2001. *The Network Inside Out*. Ann Arbor: University of Michigan Press.

Rios, Simón. 2016. "For Doctors Trained Abroad, Challenges To Practicing Medicine Often Insurmountable." *WBUR*, September 30, 2016. https://www.wbur.org/common health/2016/09/30/foreign-trained-doctors-challenges.

Rizvi, Fazal, Bob Lingard, and Jennifer Lavia. 2006. "Postcolonialism and Education: Negotiating a Contested Terrain." *Pedagogy, Culture & Society* 14 (3): 249–62.

Robbins, Joel. 2013. "Beyond the Suffering Subject: Toward an Anthropology of the Good." *Journal of the Royal Anthropological Institute* 19 (3): 447–62.

Robins, Steven. 2006. "From 'Rights' to 'Ritual': AIDS Activism in South Africa." *American Anthropologist* 108 (2): 312–23.

Rodman, Margaret C. 1992. "Empowering Place: Multilocality and Multivocality." *American Anthropologist* 94 (3): 640–56.

Rose, Nikolas. 1999. *Governing the Soul: The Shaping of the Private Self.* 2nd ed. London: Free Association Books.

Rose, Nikolas, and Carlos Novas. 2005. "Biological Citizenship." In *Global Assemblages: Technology, Politics, and Ethics as Anthropological Problems*, edited by Aihwa Ong and Stephen Collier, 439–63. Malden, MA: Blackwell.

Rosen, David M. 2007. "Child Soldiers, International Humanitarian Law, and the Globalization of Childhood." *American Anthropologist* 109 (2): 296–306.

Rosenthal, Elisabeth. 2012. "Pre-Med's New Priorities: Heart and Soul and Social Science." *The New York Times*, April 13, 2012. https://www.nytimes.com/2012/04/15/education/edlife/pre-meds-new-priorities-heart-and-soul-and-social-science.html.

Rothman, David J. 1991. *Strangers at the Bedside: A History of How Law and Bioethics Transformed Medical Decision Making.* New York: Basic Books.

Roura, Maria, M. Urassa, J. Busza, D. Mbata, A. Wringe, and B. Zaba. 2009. "Scaling Up Stigma? The Effects of Antiretroviral Roll-Out on Stigma and HIV Testing. Early Evidence from Rural Tanzania." *Sexually Transmitted Infections* 85 (4): 308–12.

Rouse, C. 2004. "'If She's a Vegetable, We'll Be Her Garden': Embodiment, Transcendence, and Citations of Competing Cultural Metaphors in the Case of a Dying Child." *American Ethnologist* 31 (4): 514–29.

Said, Edward W. 1979. *Orientalism.* New York: Vintage Books.

Sanders, Todd, and Harry G. West. 2003. "Power Revealed and Concealed in the New World Order." In *Transparency and Conspiracy: Ethnographies of Suspicion in the New World Order*, edited by Harry G. West and Todd Sanders, 1–37. Durham, NC: Duke University Press.

Sangaramoorthy, Thurka. 2012. "Treating the Numbers: HIV/AIDS Surveillance, Subjectivity, and Risk." *Medical Anthropology* 31 (4): 292–309.

Sangaramoorthy, Thurka, and Adia Benton. 2012. "Enumeration, Identity, and Health." *Medical Anthropology* 31 (4): 287–91.

Schapera, Isaac. 1933. "Premarital Pregnancy and Native Opinion: A Note on Social Change." *Africa* 6 (1): 59–89.

——. 1940. *Married Life in an African Tribe.* London: Faber and Faber.

——. 1947. *Migrant Labour and Tribal Life: A Study of Conditions in the Bechuanaland Protectorate.* London: Oxford University Press.

——. 1957. "Marriage of Near Kin among the Tswana." *Africa: Journal of the International African Institute* 27 (2): 139–59.

——. 1971. *Rainmaking Rites of Tswana Tribes.* Leiden, Netherlands: Afrika-Studiecentrum.

Schegloff, Emanuel A. 1972. "Notes on a Conversational Practice: Formulating Place." In *Studies in Social Interaction*, edited by Pier P. Giglioli, 95–135. Harmondsworth, UK: Penguin Books.

Scheibman, Joanne. 2007. "Subjective and Intersubjective Uses of Generalizations in English Conversations." In *Stancetaking in Discourse: Subjectivity, Evaluation, Interaction*, edited by Robert Englebretson, 111–38. Philadelphia: John Benjamins.

Scheper-Hughes, Nancy. 1990. "Three Propositions for a Critically Applied Medical Anthropology." *Social Science & Medicine* 30 (2): 189–97.

——. 1993. *Death without Weeping: The Violence of Everyday Life in Brazil*. Berkeley: University of California Press.

——. 1995. "The Primacy of the Ethical: Propositions for a Militant Anthropology." *Current Anthropology* 36 (3): 409–40.

Scherz, China. 2013. "Let Us Make God Our Banker: Ethics, Temporality, and Agency in a Ugandan Charity Home." *American Ethnologist* 40 (4): 624–36.

——. 2014. *Having People, Having Heart: Charity, Sustainable Development, and Problems of Dependence in Central Uganda*. Chicago: University of Chicago Press.

——. 2018. "Stuck in the Clinic: Vernacular Healing and Medical Anthropology in Contemporary Sub-Saharan Africa." *Medical Anthropology Quarterly* 32 (4): 539–55.

Schieffelin, Bambi B., and Elinor Ochs, eds. 1986. *Language Socialization across Cultures*. Cambridge: Cambridge University Press.

Schieffelin, Bambi B., Kathryn A. Woolard, and Paul V. Kroskrity, eds. 1998. *Language Ideologies: Practice and Theory*. New York: Oxford University Press.

Schlesinger, Mark. 2002. "On Values and Democratic Policy Making: The Deceptively Fragile Consensus around Market-Oriented Medical Care." *Journal of Health Politics, Policy and Law* 27 (6): 889–92.

Schoepf, Brooke Grundfest. 2001. "International AIDS Research in Anthropology: Taking a Critical Perspective on the Crisis." *Annual Review of Anthropology* 30: 335–61.

Scott, James C. 1985. *Weapons of the Weak: Everyday Forms of Peasant Resistance*. New Haven, CT: Yale University Press.

——. 1998. *Seeing Like a State: How Certain Schemes to Improve the Human Condition Have Failed*. New Haven, CT: Yale University Press.

Seboni, Naomi M. 2012. "Botswana." In *The State of Nursing and Nursing Education in Africa: A Country-by-Country Review*, edited by Hester Klopper and Leana Uys, 25–41. Indianapolis, IN: Sigma Theta Tau International.

Seitio, Onalenna S., and Jamesetta A. Newland. 2008. "Improving the Quality of Nurse Practitioner Education: The Case of Botswana." *The Nurse Practitioner* 33 (3): 40–45.

Serite, S. 2006. "Accountability Is Primary." *Botswana Guardian*, August 31.

Shapiro, Roger L, Ibou Thior, Peter B Gilbert, Shahin Lockman, Carolyn Wester, Laura M Smeaton, Lisa Stevens, et al. 2006. "Maternal Single-Dose Nevirapine versus Placebo as Part of an Antiretroviral Strategy to Prevent Mother-to-Child HIV Transmission in Botswana." *AIDS* 20 (9): 1281–88.

Sharma, Kevshav C., and Thabo Lucas Seleke. 2008. "HIV/AIDS in Africa: Botswana's Response to the Pandemic." In *Disaster Management Handbook*, edited by Jack Pinkowski, 321–35. Boca Raton, FL: CRC Press.

Shaw, Susan J., and Julie Armin. 2011. "The Ethical Self-Fashioning of Physicians and Health Care Systems in Culturally Appropriate Health Care." *Culture, Medicine, and Psychiatry* 35 (2): 236–61.

Sheon, Nicolas, and G. Michael Crosby. 2004. "Ambivalent Tales of HIV Disclosure in San Francisco." *Social Science & Medicine* 58 (11): 2105–18.

Sheon, Nicolas, and Seung-Hee Lee. 2009. "Sero-Skeptics: Discussions between Test Counselors and Their Clients about Sexual Partner HIV Status Disclosure." *AIDS Care* 21 (2): 133–39.

Shillington, Kevin. 1985. *The Colonisation of the Southern Tswana, 1879–1900*. Braamfontein, South Africa: Ravan Press.

Shore, Cris, and Susan Wright. 2000. "Coercive Accountability: The Rise of Audit Culture in Higher Education." In *Audit Cultures: Anthropological Studies in Accountability, Ethics and the Academy*, edited by Marilyn Strathern, 57–89. London: Routledge.

Shostak, Marjorie. 1981. *Nisa: The Life and Words of a !Kung Woman*. Cambridge, MA: Harvard University Press.

Silverstein, Michael. 1976. "Shifters, Linguistic Categories, and Cultural Description." In *Meaning in Anthropology*, edited by Keith Basso and Henry Selby, 11–55. Albuquerque: University of New Mexico Press.

——. 1979. "Language Structure and Linguistic Ideology." In *The Elements, a Parasession on Linguistic Units and Levels*, edited by Paul R. Clyne, William F. Hanks, and Carol L. Hofbauer, 193–247. Chicago: Chicago Linguistic Society.

——. 1993. "Metapragmatic Discourse and Metapragmatic Function." In *Reflexive Language: Reported Speech and Metapragmatics*, edited by John A. Lucy, 33–58. Cambridge: Cambridge University Press.

——. 1995. "Shifters, Linguistic Categories, and Cultural Description." In *Language, Culture, and Society: A Book of Readings*, edited by Ben G. Blount, 187–221. Prospect Heights, IL: Waveland Press.

——. 1997. "The Improvisational Performance of Culture in Realtime Discursive Practice." In *Creativity in Performance*, edited by Robert Keith Sawyer, 265–312. Greenwich, CT: Ablex Publishing Corp.

——. 1998. "The Uses and Utility of Ideology." In *Language Ideologies: Practice and Theory*, edited by Bambi B. Schieffelin, Kathryn A. Woolard, and Paul V. Kroskrity, 123–45. New York: Oxford University Press.

——. 2003. "Indexical Order and the Dialectics of Sociolinguistic Life." *Language & Communication* 23 (3–4): 193–229.

——. 2004. "'Cultural' Concepts and the Language-Culture Nexus." *Current Anthropology* 45 (5): 621–52.

——. 2005. "Axes of Evals: Token versus Type Interdiscursivity." *Journal of Linguistic Anthropology* 15 (1): 6–22.

——. 2009. "Private Ritual Encounters, Public Ritual Indexes." In *Ritual Communication*, edited by Gunter Senft and Ellen B. Basso, 271–92. New York: Berg Books.

Simmel, Georg. 1906. "The Sociology of Secrecy and of Secret Societies." *American Journal of Sociology* 11 (4): 441–98.

Sinclair, Simon. 1997. *Making Doctors: An Institutional Apprenticeship*. Oxford, UK: Berg Books.

Singer, Merrill. 1989. "The Coming of Age of Critical Medical Anthropology." *Social Science & Medicine* 28 (11): 1193–1203.

Singer, Merrill, and Hans Baer. 1995. *Critical Medical Anthropology*. Amityville, NY: Baywood Publishing Company.

Singh, Jerome A., and Edward J. Mills. 2005. "The Abandoned Trials of Pre-Exposure Prophylaxis for HIV: What Went Wrong?" *PLoS Medicine* 2 (9): 234.

Skordis, Jolene, and Nicoli Nattrass. 2002. "Paying to Waste Lives: The Affordability of Reducing Mother-to-Child Transmission of HIV in South Africa." *Journal of Health Economics* 21 (3): 405–21.

Smith, Daniel Jordan. 2003. "Patronage, Per Diems and the 'Workshop Mentality': The Practice of Family Planning Programs in Southeastern Nigeria." *World Development* 31 (4): 703–15.

Smith, Neil. 1979. "Toward a Theory of Gentrification A Back to the City Movement by Capital, Not People." *Journal of the American Planning Association* 45 (4): 538–48.

——. 1996. "Spaces of Vulnerability: The Space of Flows and the Politics of Scale." *Critique of Anthropology* 16 (1): 63–77.

Smith-Oka, Vania. 2012. "Bodies of Risk: Constructing Motherhood in a Mexican Public Hospital." *Social Science & Medicine* 75 (12): 2275–82.

Snyman, Charles S., Philippe Boucher, Suzanne Cloutier, John A. Puvimanasinghea, and Ndwapi Ndwapi. 2007. "Establishing a Data Warehouse for Patients on ART in Botswana." https://citeseerx.ist.psu.edu/viewdoc/download?doi=10.1.1.93.7595&rep=rep1&type=pdf.

Soja, Edward W. 1989. *Postmodern Geographies: The Reassertion of Space in Critical Social Theory*. London: Verso.

Sopher, Philip. 2014. "Doctors With Borders: How the U.S. Shuts Out Foreign Physicians." *The Atlantic*, November 18, 2014. https://www.theatlantic.com/health/archive/2014/11/doctors-with-borders-how-the-us-shuts-out-foreign-physicians/382723/.

Spiro, Howard M. 1992. "What Is Empathy and Can It Be Taught?" *Annals of Internal Medicine* 116 (10): 843–46.

Spiro, Howard M., Mary G. McCrea Curnen, Enid Peschel, and Deborah St. James, eds. 1996. *Empathy and the Practice of Medicine: Beyond Pills and the Scalpel*. Rev. ed. New Haven, CT: Yale University Press.

Stambach, Amy. 2010. "Education, Religion, and Anthropology in Africa." *Annual Review of Anthropology* 39: 361–79.

Starr, Paul. 1982. *The Social Transformation of American Medicine: The Rise of a Sovereign Profession and the Making of a Vast Industry*. New York: Basic Books.

Stasch, Rupert. 2011. "Ritual and Oratory Revisited: The Semiotics of Effective Action." *Annual Review of Anthropology* 40 (October): 159–74.

Stein, Jo. 2003. "HIV/AIDS Stigma: The Latest Dirty Secret." *African Journal of AIDS Research* 2 (2): 95–101.

Stepien, Kathy A., and Amy Baernstein. 2006. "Educating for Empathy: A Review." *Journal of General Internal Medicine* 21 (5): 524–30.

Stevenson, Lisa. 2009. "The Suicidal Wound and Fieldwork among Canadian Inuit." In *Being There: The Fieldwork Encounter and the Making of Truth*, edited by John Borneman and Abdellah Hammoundi, 55–76. Berkeley: University of California Press.

Stewart, Kearsley A. 2013. "The Undergraduate Field-Research Experience in Global Health: Study Abroad, Service Learning, Professional Training or 'None of the Above'?" *Learning and Teaching* 6 (2): 53–71.

Stillwaggon, Eileen. 2003. "Racial Metaphors: Interpreting Sex and AIDS in Africa." *Development and Change* 34 (5): 809–32.

Stoler, Ann Laura. 1995. *Race and the Education of Desire: Foucault's History of Sexuality and the Colonial Order of Things*. Durham, NC: Duke University Press.

Storeng, Katerini T., and Dominique P. Béhague. 2014. "'Playing the Numbers Game': Evidence-Based Advocacy and the Technocratic Narrowing of the Safe Motherhood Initiative." *Medical Anthropology Quarterly* 28 (2): 260–79.

Strain, Robert M. 2008. "Battle from the Bottom: The Role of Indigenous AIDS NGOs in Botswana." *College Undergraduate Research Electronic Journal* 81 (April): 1–66.

Strathern, Marilyn. 1999. *Property, Substance, and Effect: Anthropological Essays on Persons and Things*. London: Athlone Press.

Street, Alice. 2014. *Biomedicine in an Unstable Place: Infrastructure and Personhood in a Papua New Guinean Hospita*. Durham, NC: Duke University Press.

Suggs, David N. 1987. "Female Status and Role Transition in the Tswana Life Cycle." *Ethnology* 26 (2): 107–20.

——. 2002. *A Bagful of Locusts and the Baboon Woman: Constructions of Gender, Change, and Continuity in Botswana*. San Diego, CA: Northam: Cengage Learning.

Sullivan, Noelle. 2011. "Mediating Abundance and Scarcity: Implementing an HIV/AIDS-Targeted Project Within a Government Hospital in Tanzania." *Medical Anthropology* 30 (2): 202–21.

——. 2012. "Enacting Spaces of Inequality: Placing Global/State Governance Within a Tanzanian Hospital." *Space and Culture* 15 (1): 57–67.

——. 2016. "Hosting Gazes: Clinical Volunteer Tourism and Hospital Hospitality in Tanzania." In *Volunteer Economies: The Politics and Ethics of Voluntary Labour in Africa*, edited by Ruth J. Prince and Hannah Brown, 140–63. Rochester, NY: James Currey.

——. 2017. "Multiple Accountabilities: Development Cooperation, Transparency, and the Politics of Unknowing in Tanzania's Health Sector." *Critical Public Health* 27 (2): 193–204.

——. 2018. "International Clinical Volunteering in Tanzania: A Postcolonial Analysis of a Global Health Business." *Global Public Health* 13 (3): 310–24.

Sunday Standard. 2007. "NACA Applies for Fresh Money from Global Fund," March 26.

Swidler, Ann. 2006. "Syncretism and Subversion in AIDS Governance: How Locals Cope with Global Demands." *International Affairs* 82 (2): 269–84.

Swyngedouw, Erik. 1997. "Neither Global nor Local: 'Glocalization' and the Politics of Scale." In *Spaces of Globalization: Reasserting the Power of the Local*, edited by Cox, Kevin R., 137–66. New York: Guilford Press.

Tabulawa, Richard. 1997. "Pedagogical Classroom Practice and the Social Context: The Case of Botswana." *International Journal of Educational Development* 17 (2): 189–204.

Taha, Maisa C. 2017. "Shadow Subjects: A Category of Analysis for Empathic Stance-taking." *Journal of Linguistic Anthropology* 27 (2): 190–209.

Tambiah, Stanley J. 1985. "A Performative Approach to Ritual." In *Culture, Thought and Social Action: An Anthropological Perspective*, 123–66. Cambridge, MA: Harvard University Press.

Tappan, Jennifer. 2014. "Blood Work and 'Rumors' of Blood: Nutritional Research and Insurrection in Buganda, 1935–1970." *International Journal of African Historical Studies* 47 (3): 473–94.

Tates, Kiek, and Ludwien Meeuwesen. 2001. "Doctor–Parent–Child Communication. A (Re)View of the Literature." *Social Science & Medicine* 52 (6): 839–51.

Taussig, Michael T. 1980. "Reification and the Consciousness of the Patient." *Social Science & Medicine, Medical Anthropology* 14B (February): 3–13.

——. 1999. "Pity Those Weak in Lying." In *Defacement: Public Secrecy and the Labor of the Negative*, 59–77. Stanford, CA: Stanford University Press.

——. 2003. "The Adult's Imagination of the Child's Imagination." In *Aesthetic Subjects*, edited by Pamela R. Matthews and David McWhirter, 449–67. Minneapolis: University of Minnesota Press.

Taylor, Janelle S. 2003. "Confronting 'Culture' in Medicine's 'Culture of No Culture.'" *Academic Medicine* 78 (6): 5.

——. 2011. "The Moral Aesthetics of Simulated Suffering in Standardized Patient Performances." *Culture, Medicine & Psychiatry* 35 (2): 134–62.

——. 2014. "The Demise of the Bumbler and the Crock: From Experience to Accountability in Medical Education and Ethnography." *American Anthropologist* 116 (3): 523–34.

——. 2018. "What the Word 'Partnership' Conjoins, and What It Does." *Medicine Anthropology Theory* 5 (2): 6.

Thigpen, Michael C., Poloko M. Kebaabetswe, Lynn A. Paxton, Dawn K. Smith, Charles E. Rose, Tebogo M. Segolodi, Faith L. Henderson, et al. 2012. "Antiretroviral Preexposure Prophylaxis for Heterosexual HIV Transmission in Botswana." *New England Journal of Medicine* 367 (5): 423–34.

Thomas, S. B., and S. C. Quinn. 1991. "The Tuskegee Syphilis Study, 1932 to 1972: Implications for HIV Education and AIDS Risk Education Programs in the Black Community." *American Journal of Public Health* 81 (11): 1498–1505.

Thupayagale-Tshweneagae, Gloria. 2007. "Migration of Nurses: Is There Any Other Option?" *International Nursing Review* 54 (1): 107–9.

———. 2010. "Behaviors Used by HIV-Positive Adolescents to Prevent Stigmatization in Botswana." *International Nursing Review* 57 (2): 260–64.

Tichenor, Marlee. 2017. "Data Performativity, Performing Health Work: Malaria and Labor in Senegal." *Medical Anthropology* 36 (5): 436–48.

Ticktin, Miriam. 2006. "Where Ethics and Politics Meet: The Violence of Humanitarianism in France." *American Ethnologist* 33 (1): 33–49.

———. 2014. "Transnational Humanitarianism." *Annual Review of Anthropology* 43: 273–89.

———. 2017. "A World without Innocence." *American Ethnologist* 44 (4): 577–90.

Tilley, Helen. 2011. *Africa as a Living Laboratory: Empire, Development, and the Problem of Scientific Knowledge, 1870–1950.* Chicago: University of Chicago Press.

Timberg, Craig. 2005. "Botswana's Gains Against AIDS Put U.S. Claims to Test." *Washington Post*, July 1, 2005. http://www.washingtonpost.com/wp-dyn/content/article/2005/06/30/AR2005063002158.html.

Timmermans, Stefan, and Marc Berg. 1997. "Standardization in Action: Achieving Local Universality through Medical Protocols." *Social Studies of Science* 27 (2): 273–305.

Timmermans, Stefan, and Steven Epstein. 2010. "A World of Standards but Not a Standard World: Toward a Sociology of Standards and Standardization." *Annual Review of Sociology* 36 (1): 69–89.

Timmermans, Stefan, and Aaron Mauck. 2005. "The Promises and Pitfalls of Evidence-Based Medicine." *Health Affairs* 24 (1): 18–28.

Timmermans, Stefan, and Hyeyoung Oh. 2010. "The Continued Social Transformation of the Medical Profession." *Journal of Health and Social Behavior* 51 (1): S94–106.

Tlou, S. D., and R. L. Tobias. 2005. "A Successful Partnership to Fight AIDS." *Washington Post*, July 24.

Toledo, Lauren, Eleanor McLellan-Lemal, Faith L. Henderson, and Poloko M. Kebaabetswe. 2015. "Knowledge, Attitudes, and Experiences of HIV Pre-Exposure Prophylaxis (PrEP) Trial Participants in Botswana." *World Journal of AIDS* 5: 10–20.

Townsend, Nicholas W. 1997. "Men, Migration, and Households in Botswana: An Exploration of Connections over Time and Space." *Journal of Southern African Studies* 23 (3): 405–20.

Treichler, Paula. 1992. "AIDS and HIV Infection in the Third World: A First World Chronicle." In *AIDS: The Making of a Chronic Disease*, edited by Elizabeth Fee and Daniel M. Fox, 377–412. Berkeley: University of California Press.

Trilling, Lionel. 1972. *Sincerity and Authenticity.* Cambridge, MA: Harvard University Press.

Trostle, James A. 1988. "Medical Compliance as an Ideology." *Social Science & Medicine* 27 (12): 1299–1308.

Trouillot, Michel-Rolph. 1991. "Anthropology and the Savage Slot: The Poetics and Politics of Otherness." In *Recapturing Anthropology: Working in the Present*, edited by Richard Gabriel Fox, 17–44. Santa Fe, NM: School of American Research Press.

———. 1995. "An Unthinkable History: The Haitian Revolution as a Non-Event." In *Silencing the Past: Power and the Production of History*, 70–107. Boston: Beacon Press.

Tsie, Balefi. 1996. "The Political Context of Botswana's Development Performance." *Journal of Southern African Studies* 22 (4): 599–616.

Tsing, Anna Lowenhaupt. 2000. "The Global Situation." *Cultural Anthropology* 15 (3): 327–60.

——. 2005. *Friction: An Ethnography of Global Connection.* Princeton, NJ: Princeton University Press.

——. 2015. *The Mushroom at the End of the World: On the Possibility of Life in Capitalist Ruins.* Princeton, NJ: Princeton University Press.

UNAIDS, Joint United Nations Programme on HIV/AIDS. 2004. "Epidemiological Fact Sheet on HIV/AIDS and Sexually Transmitted Diseases." Geneva: UNAIDS.

——. 2007. "AIDS Epidemic Update." Geneva: UNAIDS.

——. 2014. "The Gap Report." Geneva: UNAIDS.

UNICEF. 1993. *The State of the World's Children, 1992.* Edited by James P. Grant. Oxford, UK: Oxford University Press.

Upton, Rebecca L. 2003. "'Women Have No Tribe': Connecting Carework, Gender, and Migration in an Era of HIV/AIDS in Botswana." *Gender and Society* 17 (2): 314–22.

Urciuoli, Bonnie. 2003. "Excellence, Leadership, Skills, Diversity: Marketing Liberal Arts Education." *Language & Communication* 33 (3): 385–408.

——. 2008. "Skills and Selves in the New Workplace." *American Ethnologist* 35 (2): 211–28.

——. 2010. "Neoliberal Education: Preparing the Student for the New Workplace." In *Ethnographies of Neoliberalism,* edited by Carol Greenhouse, 162–76. Philadelphia: University of Pennsylvania Press.

——. 2013. "Introduction: The Promise and Practice of Service Learning and Engaged Scholarship." *Learning and Teaching* 6 (2): 1–10.

——, ed. 2018. *The Experience of Neoliberal Education.* Berghahn Books.

Vaughan, Megan. 1991. *Curing Their Ills: Colonial Power and African Illness.* Cambridge, UK: Polity Press.

Verghese, Abraham. 2009. "A Touch Of Sense." *Health Affairs* 28 (4): 1177–82.

Verghese, Abraham, and Ralph I. Horwitz. 2009. "In Praise of the Physical Exam." *BMJ (Online)* 339 (December): b5448.

Vinson, Alexandra H., and Kelly Underman. 2020. "Clinical Empathy as Emotional Labor in Medical Work." *Social Science & Medicine* 251 (April): 112904.

Wainaina, Binyavanga. 2005. "How to Write About Africa." *Granta,* 2005.

Wardlow, Holly. 2012. "The Task of the HIV Translator: Transforming Global AIDS Knowledge in an Awareness Workshop." *Medical Anthropology* 31 (5): 404–19.

Wark, McKenzie. 1995. "Fresh Maimed Babies: The Uses of Innocence." *Transition,* no. 65: 36–47.

Washington, Harriet. 2006. *Medical Apartheid: The Dark History of Medical Experimentation on Black Americans from Colonial Times to the Present.* New York: Harlem Moon.

Watkins, Susan Cotts, and Ann Swidler. 2013. "Working Misunderstandings: Donors, Brokers, and Villagers in Africa's AIDS Industry." *Population and Development Review* 38 (supp 1): 197–218.

Watney, Simon. 1989. "Missionary Positions: AIDS, 'Africa', and Race." *Critical Quarterly* 31 (3): 45–62.

Wear, Delese, Julie M. Aultman, Joseph D. Varley, and Joseph Zarconi. 2006. "Making Fun of Patients: Medical Students' Perceptions and Use of Derogatory and Cynical Humor in Clinical Settings." *Academic Medicine* 81 (5): 454–62.

Weichselbraun, Anna. 2019. "Of Broken Seals and Broken Promises: Attributing Intention at the IAEA." *Cultural Anthropology* 34 (4): 503–28.

Wendland, Claire L. 2007. "The Vanishing Mother: Cesarean Section and 'Evidence-Based Obstetrics.'" *Medical Anthropology Quarterly* 21 (2): 218–33.

——. 2010. *A Heart for the Work: Journeys through an African Medical School.* Chicago: University of Chicago Press.

——. 2012a. "Animating Biomedicine's Moral Order: The Crisis of Practice in Malawian Medical Training." *Current Anthropology* 53 (6): 755–88.

——. 2012b. "Moral Maps and Medical Imaginaries: Clinical Tourism at Malawi's College of Medicine." *American Anthropologist* 114 (1): 108–22.

——. 2016. "Opening up the Black Box: Looking for a More Capacious Version of Capacity in Global Health Partnerships." *Canadian Journal of African Studies/Revue Canadienne Des Études Africaines* 50 (3): 415–35.

Wendland, Claire L., Susan L Erikson, and Noelle Sullivan. 2016. "Beneath the Spin: Moral Complexity & Rhetorical Simplicity in 'Global Health' Volunteering." In *Volunteer Economies: The Politics and Ethics of Voluntary Labour in Africa*, edited by Ruth J. Prince and Hannah Brown, 164–82. Melton, UK: James Currey.

Werbner, Pnina. 2014. *The Making of an African Working Class: Politics, Law, and Cultural Protest in the Manual Workers' Union of Botswana*. London: Pluto Press.

West, Anna. 2016. "Body Politics in the Postcolony: Global Health and Local Governance in Malawi." PhD diss., Stanford University.

West, Harry G., and Todd Sanders, eds. 2003. *Transparency and Conspiracy: Ethnographies of Suspicion in the New World Order*. Durham, NC: Duke University Press.

West, Paige. 2016. *Dispossession and the Environment: Rhetoric and Inequality in Papua New Guinea*. New York: Columbia University Press.

White, Luise. 2000. *Speaking with Vampires: Rumor and History in Colonial Africa*. Berkeley: University of California Press.

WHO (World Health Organization). 2005. "Emergency Triage Assessment and Treatment (ETAT): Manual for Participants." Geneva: Department of Child and Adolescent Health and Development, World Health Organization. https://www.who .int/publications/i/item/9241546875

——. 2008. "XDR-TB: Extensively Drug-Resistant Tuberculosis, February 2008." Geneva: Stop TB Department, World Health Organization. https://www.who.int/tb /challenges/xdr/news_feb08.pdf.

——. 2016. *Guideline: Updates on Pediatric Emergency Triage, Assessment and Treatment: Care of Critically-Ill Children*. Geneva: World Health Organization. https://apps .who.int/iris/bitstream/handle/10665/204463/9789241510219_eng.pdf

WHO, UNAIDS. 2003. *Treating 3 Million by 2005: Making It Happen. The WHO Strategy*. Geneva: WHO, UNAIDS.

Whyte, Susan Reynolds, ed. 2014. *Second Chances: Surviving AIDS in Uganda*. Durham, NC: Duke University Press.

Whyte, Susan Reynolds, Sjaak van der Geest, and Anita Hardon. 2002. *Social Lives of Medicines*. Cambridge: Cambridge University Press.

Whyte, Susan Reynolds, Michael A. Whyte, Lotte Meinert, and Jenipher Twebaze. 2013. "Therapeutic Clientship: Belonging in Uganda's Projectified Landscape of AIDS Care." In *When People Come First: Critical Studies in Global Health*, edited by João Guilherme Biehl and Adriana Petryna, 140–65. Princeton, NJ: Princeton University Press.

Wible, Pamela. 2016. "Her Story Went Viral. But She Is Not the Only Black Doctor Ignored in an Airplane Emergency." *The Washington Post*, October 20, 2016. https:// www.washingtonpost.com/national/health-science/tamika-cross-is-not-the -only-black-doctor-ignored-in-an-airplane-emergency/2016/10/20/3f59ac08 -9544-11e6-bc79-af1cd3d2984b_story.html.

Wiener, Lori, Claude Ann Mellins, Stephanie Marhefka, and Haven B. Battles. 2007. "Disclosure of an HIV Diagnosis to Children: History, Current Research, and Future Directions." *Journal of Developmental and Behavioral Pediatrics* 28 (2): 155–66.

Wilce, James M. 2009. "Medical Discourse." *Annual Review of Anthropology* 38: 199–215.

Wilce, James M., and Janina Fenigsen. 2016. "Emotion Pedagogies: What Are They, and Why Do They Matter?" *Ethos* 44 (2): 81–95.

Wilf, Eitan. 2014. *School for Cool: The Academic Jazz Program and the Paradox of Institutionalized Creativity.* Chicago: University Of Chicago Press.

Wilkes, Michael, Etan Milgrom, and Jerome R. Hoffman. 2002. "Towards More Empathic Medical Students: A Medical Student Hospitalization Experience." *Medical Education* 36 (6): 528–33.

Wilkinson, Iain, and Arthur Kleinman. 2016. *A Passion for Society: How We Think about Human Suffering.* Berkeley: University of California Press.

Williams, Raymond. 1975. *The Country and the City.* Oxford, UK: Oxford University Press.

Willis, Paul. 2017. *Learning to Labour: How Working Class Kids Get Working Class Jobs.* New York: Routledge.

Wood, Kate, and Helen Lambert. 2008. "Coded Talk, Scripted Omissions: The Micro-Politics of AIDS Talk in an Affected Community in South Africa." *Medical Anthropology Quarterly* 22 (3): 213–33.

Woolard, Katherine, and Bambi Schieffelin. 1994. "Language Ideology." *Annual Review of Anthropology* 23: 55–82.

Wortham, Stanton. 2008. "Linguistic Anthropology of Education." *Annual Review of Anthropology* 37 (1): 37–51.

——. 2012. "Beyond Macro and Micro in the Linguistic Anthropology of Education." *Anthropology & Education Quarterly* 43 (2): 128–37.

Wyrod, Robert. 2011. "Masculinity and the Persistence of AIDS Stigma." *Culture, Health & Sexuality* 13 (4): 443–56.

Yates-Doerr, Emily. 2012. "The Weight of the Self: Care and Compassion in Guatemalan Dietary Choices." *Medical Anthropology Quarterly* 26 (1): 136–58.

——. 2015. "Intervals of Confidence: Uncertain Accounts of Global Hunger." *BioSocieties* 10 (2): 229–46.

——. 2019. "Whose Global, Which Health? Unsettling Collaboration with Careful Equivocation." *American Anthropologist* 121 (2): 297–310.

Zigon, Jarrett. 2011. *"HIV Is God's Blessing": Rehabilitating Morality in Neoliberal Russia.* Berkeley: University of California Press.

Index

Note: Page numbers in *italics* indicate figures.

Ingram Content Group UK Ltd.
Milton Keynes UK
UKHW010152310523
422595UK00003B/93

9 781501 762413